The Magic of Pointe Shoes

Everything a Dancer Needs to Know About Pointe Shoes
All the Secrets Revealed by the Experts

by
Patricia Storelli, RADRTS
A Registered Teacher of the Royal Academy of Dance
RAD Teaching Diploma

With a Foreword by Michele Attfield MBE – Pointe Shoe Expert with Freed of London

© 2011 Patricia Storelli

Cover photos © 2011 by Celeste Mannerud, www.flipflopproductions.com

All rights reserved. No part of this publication may be reproduced or transmitted in any form or by any means electronic or mechanical, including photocopy, recording, or any information storage and retrieval system, without permission in writing from both the copyright owner and the publisher.

Requests for permission to make copies of any part of this work should be mailed to Permissions Department, Llumina Press, 7101 W. Commercial Blvd., Ste. 4E, Tamarac, FL 33319.

ISBN: 978-1-60594-691-7

Printed in the United States of America by Llumina Press

Library of Congress Control Number: 2011904203

*This book is dedicated to my mother, Angela, who took
me to my first ballet class and guided me throughout the way.*

To my students: Before, now, and always.

When you are able to make a graceful bow, you unconsciously acquire a taste for dancing.
—Pierre Rameau (1674-1748)

Contents

Foreword by Michele Attfield	i
Acknowledgments	iii
Preface	v
PART I: The History of Pointe Shoes	
Chapter 1: A Short History of Pointe Shoes and Their Evolution	1
Chapter 2: Marie Taglioni: Her Influence on Classical Ballet and Pointe Work	5
Chapter 3: Anna Pavlova: Her Shoes, Her Art and Her Feet	9
PART II: The Process of Making Pointe Shoes	11
Chapter 1: Technology Works Side by Side with Art: The New Pointe Shoes Compared to the Old Ones	13
Chapter 2: The Making of Pointe Shoes and Their Life Span	15
Chapter 3: Visit to a Pointe Shoe Factory: Freed of London	17
Chapter 4: Meeting a Pointe Shoe Maker: Ushi Nagar	26
Chapter 5: The Anatomy of a Pointe Shoe	30
Chapter 6: Demi Pointe Shoes and Soft Slippers	35
PART III: Everything a Dancer Needs to Know About Feet	39
Chapter 1: The Anatomy of the Foot	41
Chapter 2: Types of Legs	42
Chapter 3: Types of Feet	44
Chapter 4: Taking Care of Your Feet	47
Chapter 5: Arches	50
Chapter 6: Different Ways of Rising Up to Pointe	52
PART IV: Pointe Work	53
Chapter 1: Beginning Pointe Work	55
Chapter 2: The Right Age to Start Pointe	57
Chapter 3: Buying the Right Shoes	61

Chapter 4: Toe Pads: Which Are the Best Toe Pads to Buy? Are they Really Necessary? 67
Chapter 5: Fitting Help from Grishko Pointe Shoe Fitter Judy Weiss 69
Chapter 6: Teachers' Guidelines: Step-by-Step on How to Check the Fit of a Pointe Shoe 70
Chapter 7: Bringing the Shoes Home and How to Prepare Them 72
Chapter 8: Ribbons and Elastics 80
Chapter 9: Padding 84
Chapter 10: Softening Pointe Shoes and Break-in Techniques 86
Chapter 11: How to Take Care of Pointe Shoes 90
Chapter 12: Some Sample Exercises for the First Week on Pointe 92

PART V: How to Solve Problems with Pointe Shoes and How to Modify Them 93
Chapter 1: What to Do If the Shoe Is Slipping Off the Heel 95

PART VI: Brands and Types of Pointe Shoes 103
Chapter 1: The Pointe Shoe Market 105
Chapter 2: Finding the Right Shoe for Every Foot 123
Chapter 3: Pointe Shoes and Ballet Companies 126
Chapter 4: 32 Famous Ballerinas and Their Pointe Shoes 127
Chapter 5: Pointe Shoe Master an Unusual but Fascinating Job! 129
Chapter 6: Interviews 131
    Michael Clifford: Pointe Shoe Master, Birmingham Royal Ballet 131
    Julie Heggie: Pointe Shoe Mistress, English National Ballet 134
    Jane Latimer: Pointe Shoe Mistress, London's Royal Ballet 137

PART VII: Interviews with Pointe Shoe Makers 141

PART VIII: Interviews with Pointe Shoe Fitters and Specialists 161

PART IX: Ballet and Pointe-Related Injuries: How to Prevent and Treat Them 181
Chapter 1: Common Problems 183
Chapter 2: Different Types of Injuries 184
Chapter 3: Treating Minor Injuries 194
Chapter 4: Little Accessories to Make Life Easier 198
Chapter 5: Interviews with Health Specialists 202

PART X: Prestigious Schools Around the World and Interviews with Professional Students   213

PART XI: All the Secrets Revealed by the Experts!   249
Chapter 1: Interviews with Thirteen Ballet Masters   251
Chapter 2: Interviews with Thirty-One Famous Ballerinas   283
Chapter 3: Sample Pointe Classes   334

Famous Dancers' Statements About Shoes   336
Glossary   337
Bibliography   338
Resources   340
Index   341

Foreword

For anyone involved or interested in Dance, the Pointe Shoe is iconic, at once beautiful and mysterious.

In this book Ms Storelli explores every aspect pertaining to both the shoe and the discipline it is designed for.

Within its pages you will find an answer to any query you have, and also many you may not yet have thought of!

A wonderful read for dancers, would be dancers, teachers and enthusiasts.

Self evidently written with wisdom and love.

Michele Attfield MBE, Pointe Shoe Expert at Freed of London

Acknowledgments

I would like to thank all the people and friends who helped me in the preparation of this book, the ones who believed in me and encouraged me up to this point. Without them this book would have never been published.

Special thanks to Michele Attfield MBE, who shared some of her extensive experience and knowledge on pointe shoes and accepted to write a foreword to this book.

I am extremely grateful to Freed of London, in particular to Gary Brooks, manager at the pointe shoe factory, for explaining with so much patience how pointe shoes are made. Special thanks to all the staff at Freed's in St. Martins Lane, especially to Michele and Beth Chivers, for their kind help throughout.

I am indebted to Kyla Owens of English National Ballet School for letting me visit the school and watch classes and rehearsals, and to Anya Evans, ballet teacher, also of ENBS.

My warmest thanks to Ushi Nagar, my pointe shoe maker, for the time he spent with me, the wonderful shoes he makes, for his friendship, and much more.

I gratefully acknowledge the Philip Richardson Library at the Royal Academy of Dance London Headquarters, in particular Miss Helen, the librarian, for allowing me to use the Academy's journals, magazines, and books as reference resource for my book.

Thanks to Dawn Terlizzi, manager of the Special Makeup Wholesale Division at Capezio Pointe Shoe Factory, for her interest in my book and for helping me with the history of Salvatore Capezio.

I am deeply grateful to Zoe Cleland, Mary Carpenter, and Judy Weiss, professional pointe fitters in New York, for unveiling some of the secrets of their fantastic job.

Once again I am indebted to Cecilia Kerche, for her friendship and for endorsing this book. I love you, Cecilia.

Special thanks to Michael Clifford, pointe shoe master at Birmingham Royal Ballet; Jane Latimer, pointe shoe mistress at London's Royal Ballet; and Julie Heggie, pointe shoe mistress at English National Ballet, for allowing me to interview them.

Thanks to Melissa Sand for providing interviews with some of the dancers.

I am grateful to Linda Villella and Alexander Carter of Miami City Ballet for inviting me to their school and letting me observe classes and interview the teachers.

Special thanks to Sports for Girls and Dance Gear in Tampa, Florida, for allowing me to take pictures of pointe shoes and accessories, and to Troy Jansen of Jansen Dance Project for letting me use the studio and the students, and for supporting me throughout this project.

I am grateful to Dr. Frank Sinkoe, DPM, at Atlanta ballet, for imparting medical advice and sharing precious information. My warmest appreciation of the help given by Dr. Simon Costain, DPM, of the Gait Posture Centre Ltd. in London and by Dr. Margaret Papoutsis, DO, of the Margaret Papoutsis Practice in London.

My deepest thanks to all the dancers, ballet teachers, pointe shoe fitters, and doctors who contributed to this book by letting me interview them.

I would like to express my gratitude to Llumina Press, for the hard and highly professional work and for turning my manuscript into a beautiful book. My deepest thanks to my Publishing Consultant Gary Roen, for his precious advice and for guiding me step by step through the writing, publishing and marketing process. I would like to acknowledge my photographer Celeste Mannerud of Flip Flop Productions for the exceptional artistic quality of the front and back cover pictures of this book.

To my best friend, Brandon Nguyen, for his support, for always believing in me, and following me in my "pilgrimages" to ballet schools and pointe shoe makers. He will always be my very best friend.

To all of my students, for patiently waiting for this book to be published. This book is for you all.

And last, but not least, to Paul, for encouraging me, giving me the right advice always, and believing this book will one day be published.

Preface

Pointe shoes are beautiful: they are pink, shiny, and they create the magic! In my long dancing career, pointe classes have always been my favorite. I loved pointe work, and pointe shoes! There was something magical about those beautiful pink satin slippers and ballerinas balancing on their toes. Like every little girl, I waited for the day I would have my own pointe shoes and finally get to dance in them, like a real ballerina!

When that special day finally came, it was a truly wonderful experience to try and balance "on pointe" for the very first time! It was like defying the laws of physics, a unique feeling never experienced before. I have to admit that it was a little more painful than it looked, but I immediately thought that my reward for enduring some discomfort would be worth it, tried to forget about my sore toes, and just dance!

I still remember the smell of my first pair of pointe shoes, the day we bought them at Porselli, the official pointe shoe maker of the Teatro alla Scala in Milan. Porselli, located in Piazza Paolo Ferrari, right by the theater, is the smallest store I can remember. Beautiful tutus were always artistically displayed in the window, with pink pointe shoes arranged on top of them or hanging nearby. The interior of the shop looked like a sacred temple to me: golden chairs with brocade fabric to sit and try shoes on, ancient mirrors, and everywhere, that particular smell of new pointe shoes! So many memories are related to that smell, and so many years have gone by.

When I finally got my first pair of pointe shoes, after the initial joy and excitement, I also experienced pain and frustration, the first blisters, tears, disappointment if I could not perform a step as my teacher wanted, and the eternal struggle to find the right pair of shoes had eventually started!

Today, as a ballet teacher, I would like young dancers to have the most enjoyable and positive experience possible with their pointe shoes. Every day I face students struggling to make the right choice, looking for a suitable brand and type, and I know that this search can be long and frustrating. Too often I see dancers wearing the wrong type of shoes and struggling with them without success. This is why I decided to write this book, hoping it will assist dancers and students in finding the correct fit, and also help them gain some understanding of their shoes and their feet. Hopefully it will also guide teachers in their hard task of monitoring students in transition from soft shoes to pointe.

Ballet lovers reading this book will get to know more about these "magic shoes" and their history. Parents will find this book a thorough guide, enlightening them on many hidden aspects of pointe shoe practice, and possibly help them save money. In my long career—first as a dancer and later on as a teacher—I have come across thousands of students who really needed help with their pointe shoes, especially beginners buying their first pair.

In vocational schools, the transition from soft shoes to pointe is generally carefully planned and teachers spend plenty of time answering questions and giving feedback. In private schools, though, where time is always short, students generally have no time to ask specific questions about their feet and their shoes. Guidelines on how to sew ribbons and elastics are not always specifically given.

Students are often embarrassed to ask questions, or they feel that the rest of the class would make fun of them; and many teachers still lack the proper training and knowledge to provide safe training, particularly to young students. Inevitably, this leads to serious damage to feet, backs, and knees, as well as to future injuries.

This book is the result of a long period of research; study; traveling; and interviews with famous ballerinas, ballet masters, pointe shoe fitters, and doctors—in addition to the experience brought by a life dedicated to ballet. It was created to give dancers, teachers, parents, and especially pointe beginners, a better understanding about pointe work and pointe shoes. It is my hope that by reading this book they will find answers to their questions, and even more.

While looking through the pages, the reader will find useful advice on how to sew ribbons and elastics and take care of pointe shoes, as well as how to prevent or deal with blisters, bunions, and other problems related to the use of pointe shoes.

I also tried to give as many tips as possible on how to modify the shoes and adapt them to a dancer's foot, and a few notions about anatomy and history.

Professional dancers from major ballet companies and advanced students from world-famous ballet schools contributed to this book, revealed their secrets, and shared their own experiences, while master ballet teachers gave their precious advice.

A visit to Freed's pointe shoe factory in London is documented in this book, revealing how a pointe shoe is made, what materials go into it, as well as how much care, effort, and . . . sweat! A long and extremely useful interview with Michele Attfield, Freed's official fitter and world-acclaimed pointe shoe expert, acquaints the reader with the principles of proper fitting.

Ushi Nagar, a cobbler who has been crafting custom-made pointe shoes for fifty-five years for major ballet companies and principal dancers, tells the story of his life and his unconditional love for ballet shoes. Birmingham Royal Ballet's pointe shoe master, Royal Ballet's and English National Ballet's pointe shoe mistresses give an insight on how a major ballet company deals with pointe shoes—from ordering, measuring, altering, and dying.

Capezio Pointe Shoe Factory's official fitter and Capezio's manager provide an insight into their daily job at the factory and during fittings.

Samples of barre and center exercises are provided, as well as a peek into the best schools around the globe.

Buying a new pair of pointe shoes is such a special event in a young dancer's life; it opens a secret door into a magic world, and maybe marks the beginning of a bright and fulfilling career. But regardless of whether you will become a famous dancer or not, choosing the right shoes is extremely important, and this book wants to be your silent but faithful guide throughout the whole process. Finding your dream shoes and adapting them to your feet can be a long process, but a rewarding one in the end; and it is my hope this book will make your search easier.

Good luck and enjoy every single minute of your dancing!

Part I

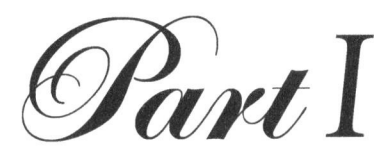

THE HISTORY OF POINTE SHOES

Chapter 1

A Short History of Pointe Shoes and Their Evolution

Contrary to what most people believe, Marie Taglioni, (1804–1884) was not the first to dance on pointe. It is reported that other ballerinas had been seen "standing on the tips of their toes."

In 1778, an Italian dancer, Cecilia Castellini from Milan, performed in a ballet by Jean-Georges Noverre (1727-1809) and obtained the first written critique praising her "flexible points." More ballerinas were seen dancing on pointe: Maria del Caro around 1804; Maria Danilova (1793-1810) in 1808 in St. Petersburg, in the ballet Flore et Zéphire choreographed by Charles Louis Didelot; Geneviève Gosselin (1791-1818) in France around 1813; Avdotia Istomina (1799-1848) in 1820; and Amalia Brugnoli (1802-1892) around 1823. Here is how the Countess of Blessington, in her book The Idler in Italy, described Brugnoli seen in 1823:

She advances rapidly across the stage on the extreme point of her toes, without for a moment losing her aplomb, cuts into the air, and alights again on the point of her feet as if she were no heavier than gossamer. (Judith Chazin-Bennahum, The Lure of Perfection: Fashion and Ballet, 1780-1830 [New York and London: Routledge, 2005])

Brugnoli's pointe work was described as something amazing, striking the audience's imagination. In the same book, Chazin-Bennahum also mentions that the 1833 London Morning Herald wrote,

Mme. Brugnoli's toe is quite unequalled by anything within our recollection, except Paganini's bow or single string. She performs evolutions on it such as no other dancer could accomplish with their ten, with unerring precision and nonchalance.

A dancer of the Paris Opera named Geneviève Gosselin seems to have been the first who really "balanced" on her toes "for a full minute" back in 1813, something considered extraordinary and almost impossible at the time. On August 3, 1827, the newspaper Journal des Débats (Journal of Debates) reported that "the power of Miss Gosselin's muscles kept her suspended for one minute on the tips of her toes." Geneviève had been a pupil of Jean-François Coulon. Her sister Constance (also known as Madame Anatole) was also acclaimed for her capacity to dance "on pointe." Earlier statements acknowledge two German sisters as the first to dance on pointe. These ballerinas must have had steel muscles, if we take into account that pointe shoes at the time were nothing but soft slippers with some darning to provide support! In the book The Lure of Perfection: Fashion and Ballet, 1780-1830 by Judith Chazin-Bennahum, Camille Roqueplan, French painter and lithographer, described the dancer's pain this way:

The public thinks that the dancer's foot is so beautifully arched, so supple, so graceful when it is encased in a silk stocking and a piqué shoe. However when examining the nude foot of a dancer, one discovers a monstrous appendage with a fat lot of red and tumified skin as a result of the violent and continuous exercises of ossified articulation, twisted toes, ingrown nails, corns, irritated skin and protrusions.

In 1830 and 1831, a French dancer of the Paris Opera, Léon Michel, wrote about dancing "sur les orteils" (on pointe), and so did E. A. Théleur, the ballet master at the Paris Opera, in his 1830 treatise, Letters on Dancing.

Pauline Montessu (1805-187) was another French dancer who first created the role of Lise in La Fille Mal Gardée. In 1833, she was seen in Covent Garden executing "a gracefully slow tip-toe circumvolution." Taglioni's rival, Fanny Elssler (1810-1884), wrote that she could use up to three pairs of shoes every time she performed. Around 1845, an Italian dancer named Sofia Fuoco was nicknamed "La pointue" by the Parisian audience, who was amazed by the brilliance of her pointe work.

The Romantic ballet found the ideal tool in pointe shoes, which created the illusion of weightlessness. Pointe shoes perfectly expressed the image of the ethereal ballerina almost "floating" on the stage, and the most famous ballets of the times were filled with sylphs, ghost-like creatures, Willis, and other creatures from the underworld. But how did pointe shoes look at the time?

Old lithographs show dancers of the Paris Opera wearing some kind of unpadded slippers with cross-stitching as reinforcement, and Marie Taglioni's unblocked pointe shoes (such shoes also had no shanks), made by Janssen of Paris, can still be seen at the library of the Paris Opera. Lucile Grahn's shoes are kept at the German Dance Archive in Cologne and still bear her signature. "The manufacturers of ballet shoes became a specialized industry in the nineteenth century," relates Ivor Guest in his article "Pioneers of the Pointes." The first real pointe shoe manufacturers were Italian, followed by the French and Russian makers. One of the most famous was Janssen of Paris, where both Taglioni and Elssler used to order shoes.

Another famous manufacturer from Paris was Crait (this brand still exists today), who became the official shoe supplier for the Paris Opera Ballet. Ebermann of Berlin used to make shoes for Adeline Genée, while Romeo Nicolini in Milan was Anna Pavlova's shoe supplier. By that time, however, shoes were already made with a block, although not totally hard like modern pointe shoes. Italy was considered the center of the pointe shoe manufacturing, in particular Milan, home of the La Scala Theater and its prestigious ballet school.

In 1866, Théophile Gautier wrote that "the sole, which is very hollowed out in the centre, does not reach the tip of the foot but ends squarely, leaving about two fingers-breadths of material projecting." Marius Petipa (1818-1910), in his days at the Imperial Ballet, kept refining pointe work, claiming that, "pointes are the finishing touch to the women's side of classical dance" (Petipa, ed. Moore, 1958). Pierina Legnani (1868-1930) performed the famous 32 fouettés en tournant during Act III of Swan Lake, thanks to the harder toe box, which had replaced Taglioni's soft slippers.

The Magic of Pointe Shoes

The famous prima ballerina assoluta of the Maryinsky, Mathilde Kschessinska (1879-1971), was also well known for her ability on pointe. In 1891, the St. Petersburg Gazette reported her success in The Tulip of Harlem. "M.lle Kschessinska astonished the connoisseurs with the audacity of her tours and her steel pointes." Kschessinska, who was barely five feet tall and wore a size 3, used to wear pointe shoes manufactured in Italy.

The construction of modern pointe shoes is widely attributed to the famous twentieth-century Russian ballerina Anna Pavlova (1881-1931). Anna had beautifully arched feet, with a very high instep, but she always had a lot of trouble in finding the right shoe to fit her perfectly. Her companion, Victor Dandré, wrote in Anna Pavlova in Art and Life, "Her thin and nervous foot with a very high instep, slender and beautifully shaped gave, at the same time, great difficulty in the matter of choice and fitting of shoes" (London: Benjamin Bloom, 1932).

Dandré, recalls that "Pavlova had a lot of shoemakers—one in London, several in Paris, in Italy and everywhere where we stayed more than three weeks—in Berlin, Sydney, Buenos Aires, Calcutta, and Johannesburg." All these shoe manufacturers were doing their best—and even more—to satisfy Pavlova's difficult taste and feet requirements. But Pavlova was very hard to please, especially when it came to shoes.

As we have already discussed, ancient ballet shoes were more similar to soft ballroom slippers, but the evolution of the technique in dance began to mark a change in the shape of the shoes and also in the way they were made. Shoemakers, particularly the Italian ones, were the first to feel the impact of this change.

In Italy, ballerinas were starting to show a stronger technique that required sturdier shoes. One of the best known of these shoemakers was the Italian Romeo Nicolini, who supplied Pavlova with pointe shoes for years. She used to give him very precise directions about how she wanted her shoes and would get very angry with him when he could not understand her. Nicolini spoke only Italian, and they had to use his son who spoke a little French as an interpreter. Pavlova ended up modifying her shoes by herself, by inserting leather soles inside them for extra support and would flatten and harden the toe area to form a box. Wherever she traveled and performed, the audiences were mesmerized when she danced for three minutes on pointe during her famous solo The Dying Swan.

Pavlova was said to use pointe shoes with a very wide platform for more balance; she then carefully retouched every single picture to make the tips of her shoes look narrower. Modern pointe shoes are a perfected tool, able to suit every dancer's requirement. Thousands of types of stock shoes are on the market, offering different widths, strength of blocks, shanks and a variety of vamps, from round to V shaped. Professional dancers can order custom-made shoes, crafted according to their own specifications and fitting their foot perfectly. Special materials have been introduced to maximize the dancer's comfort when on pointe, and while some makers still craft their shoes as in the nineteenth century, other manufacturers have introduced high technology to create "the perfect shoe."

Accessories of all types are available to minimize the pain and to help with minor problems affecting the foot, and more and more specialized doctors work side by side with ballet companies to provide dancers with medical advice and advanced therapies for injuries. As a conclusion, we can surely assert that today's ballerinas are very lucky compared to the ones of the last two centuries.

The choice of a pointe shoe is still hard, as it is dancing on them; but hundreds of types of shoes are now available to the delight of today's dancers, as well as a huge range of "accessories" to reduce pain and discomfort and to adapt the shoe to each type of foot. George Balanchine used to stress the importance for all the classes to be taken on pointe and not on demi-pointe. He wanted his dancers to become used to dancing on pointe at any speed.

During my visit to Miami City Ballet School, I observed that all intermediate and advanced classes were taught on pointe, starting from barre work and finishing with the grand allegro. It is crucial for the future professional dancer to start wearing pointe shoes for barre and center work in order to get accustomed to the feeling of the harder insole.

Of all the choreographers, the one who was the most fascinated with pointe shoes was George Balanchine, Mr. B. to his students. He loved pointe work, and his dancers had to dance all the time in pointe shoes. Balanchine wanted them to be able to jump, run, turn, and execute adagios and grand pliés in pointe shoes. He also liked the look of new shiny pointe shoes and was against the use of Pan-Cake to make shoes matte and match the tights. He wanted his dancers to control the shoes, rather than the other way around.

Based on Balanchine's suggestions, ballet shoemakers developed new types of shoes. Mr. B. also wanted pointe shoes to be silent; he didn't like noisy or squeaky shoes. Since rosin would at times make pointe shoes squeak, he sometimes removed the rosin box from backstage, saying that he would rather see a dancer slip than hear the squeaking of the shoes. Dancers in his company would roughen the soles of their shoes using knives or razors.

Today pointe shoe manufacturers continue their research, aiming to produce the perfect shoes, improving balance and turning, minimizing pain, and reducing the risk for injury.

Chapter 2

Marie Taglioni (1804-1884)
Her Influence on Classical Ballet and Pointe Work

She floats like a spirit in a transparent mist of white muslin with which she loves to surround herself, and she resembles a contented soul scarcely bending the petals of celestial flowers with the tips of her rosy feet.
—Théophile Gautier, on Marie Taglioni, 1837

Marie Taglioni, with her ethereal grace and romantic style, influenced not only the dancers of her time but many other generations of dancers who came after her death. This delicate image of the ballerina almost completely erased from the stage the figure of the male dancer. Théophile Gautier himself wrote:

For nothing is more abominable than a man who displays his red neck, his great muscular arms . . . the dancers at the Opera are of a nature to encourage the opinion which will only allow women in ballet." (Priddin, 1952)

Nobody can think about the ballet La Sylphide without recalling the image of Marie in her long white tutu sitting next to James, or standing at the window in the beginning of the first act. In 1844, the poet Théophile Gautier wrote of Marie, "What lightness, what rhythm of movement, what mobility of gesture, what poetry of attitude, and above all, what sweet melancholy, what chaste abandon."

Admired by kings, artists, and poets (Victor Hugo dedicated a book "to her feet, to her wings"), Marie Taglioni has even left her trace on the French language: the verb taglionniser became part of the French vocabulary, to suggest how original her style was. And so did the noun sylphide. All women wanted to imitate her looks, be as thin and ethereal as she was, and dress like her. The best compliment for the ladies of the time was to be compared to a sylph, and they also started wearing white gowns with a long veil for their wedding day. A hat baptized sylph was created, and a fashion newspaper of the time called La Sylphide!

Marie Taglioni, however, was not the first ballerina to dance on pointe. A common misnomer is to credit her for being the first to dance on the tips of her toes. Other ballerinas (like Fanny Bias or Amanda Brugnoli) had already danced on pointe before her, but none of them could make pointe dancing look as ethereal and delicate as she did. Of all the ballerinas who attempted pointe work before her, Marie Taglioni was the first to make it seem effortless, thus creating that illusion of etherealness and grace that all dancers would like to achieve. Thanks to her, pointe dancing became famous and made all dancers want to imitate her and be as light and graceful as she was. Taglioni did not perform in the hard-blocked pointe shoes of today but in fragile, narrow tubelike slippers made of silk ribbon with paper-thin soles. As only reinforcement, she would darn the sides and stiff the block with cotton. Janssen of Paris, who in 1879 became the official shoemaker of the Paris Opera, used to supply Taglioni with her ballet slippers.

Marie was certainly not a pretty girl. Very thin, with rounded shoulders and very long arms, it seems unbelievable that she might have been worshipped everywhere she danced. Her ballet teacher, Jean-François Coulon (1764-1836), used to say, "Will that little hunchback ever learn to dance?" What created the magic of her dancing?

Most of the credits go to her father, Filippo Taglioni (1777-1871).

Marie was born in Stockholm, Sweden, on April 23, 1804. Her mother was a Swedish painter and dancer named Sophie Karsten. Her father, Filippo Taglioni, was an acclaimed maître de ballet and former dancer of his time. Her childhood was spent traveling from one European city to the other, following her father's engagements as ballet master. In Paris, and more precisely in Montmartre, Marie started to work on her technique. She was about eleven years old, and her teacher was Maître Jean-François Coulon, who had been her father's teacher. Coulon, however, didn't think Marie's technique was strong enough to make her debut yet. Her father then took charge of her training and started a five-month period of exhausting work, determined to improve her technique and her natural grace, lightness, and elevation.

Ivor Guest, in his book The Romantic Ballet in Paris (London: Pitman, 1966), reports that "for five months he made her work at a ferocious pitch which few others could have endured." He also reports that the training Marie underwent with her father prepared her to represent a new romantic style of ballet. He created a style that minimized his daughter's excessively long arms and neck, her facial features, and her rounded shoulders.

As we see in lithographs of Marie, Filippo Taglioni created for his daughter special positions in which the arms were bent in front of her chest or in a lower fifth position to disguise their length. It is said that Taglioni made his daughter work for hours and hours without a break and at night she was so exhausted that she had to have someone undressing her and putting her in bed! Her daily training basically consisted of two hours spent in slowly developed positions and sustained balances, two hours dedicated to stretching exercises and two hours to the improvement of her technique, particularly with exercises on pointe.

Nathaniel Willis, an American visiting Paris (quoted by Ivor Guest) wrote the following words:

She swims in your eye like a curl of smoke, or a flake of down. Her difficulty seems to be to keep to the floor. You have the feeling while you gaze upon her that, if she were to rise and float away like Ariel, you would scarce be surprised. (Guest, p.104)

On June 20, 1822, shortly after her eighteenth birthday, Marie was ready for her debut, which proved to be a triumph. In Vienna, she appeared in a ballet choreographed by her father to music by Rossini: La Reception d'une Jeune Nymphe à la Cour de Terpsichore. But it was not until five years later that Marie danced at the Paris Opera, with her brother Paul as partner.

In 1831 she appeared in the Pas de Fascination in Meyerbeer's opera Robert le Diable, but it was only in 1832 that Marie became the one and only queen of romantic ballet. On March 12, 1832—a historical date—Marie appeared as the sylph in the ballet La Sylphide, choreographed especially for her by her father, and whose libretto was written by Adolphe Nourrit.

On July 14, 1835, at St. Pancras Church in London, Marie married Count Gilbert de Voisins, who was a close friend of Louis-Désiré Véron, director of the Paris Opera. Their marriage was meant to last only three years, ending in divorce. Count de Voisins did not appreciate his wife's career and therefore asked her to abandon dancing. Marie refused, and this became a reason for constant disagreement, which eventually led to the split.

Taglioni was left alone with two young children: a son, Georges-Philippe Marie (called Youry), and a daughter, Eugénie-Marie Edwige. Marie had been good managing her finances throughout her career, but after her divorce, she became very concerned about money. She bargained over contracts and demanded higher fees for her performances, although she was being paid more money than any other dancer. If she could not get what she asked for, she would refuse to appear on stage, even if the audience was waiting.

For seven years after her success in La Sylphide, Marie reigned at the Opera, until the arrival of other brilliant and virtuoso dancers like Fanny Elssler, whose technique was the opposite of Taglioni's. The presence of these dancers and the strong competition obliged Marie Taglioni to tour extensively for more than ten years. Gautier, who had been such a great admirer of Marie's, started to be fascinated by her rival Fanny Elssler and began writing that Taglioni's technique was not the same anymore. "Marie Taglioni, worn out after her interminable travels, is no longer what she was," he wrote.

When she makes her entrance, she is still the same white mist bathed in transparent muslin, the same ethereal, chaste vision, the same divine delight we know so well, but after a few bars signs of fatigue appear, she grows short of breath perspiration dabbles her brow, her muscles tense up with strain and her arms and bosom become flushed. She who a few moments before was a real Sylphide is now a mere dancer – the greatest dancer in the world, if you wish, but no more than that.

Taglioni toured in England and, most of all, in Russia, especially in St. Petersburg, where she was worshipped. In Russia, a pair of her pointe shoes was sold for two hundred rubles, cooked with a special sauce, and eaten at a memorial dinner of fanatical admirers.

Although past the age of forty, Marie still practiced daily under the strict supervision of her father. In 1847, while her niece Marie was ready for her debut, the elder Marie and her father retired to Switzerland with enough money to take care of their needs for the rest of their lives. In 1859, Taglioni became Inspectrice de la Danse at the Paris Opera and is credited for creating the school's examination system.

Marie started to teach and found a young protégé whom she took under her protection. Her name was Emma Livry, and she had all the qualities to continue the Taglioni dancing tradition. Marie created a ballet for her called The Butterfly, which was performed in 1860 at the Paris

Opera. Unfortunately, Emma's skirt caught fire by one of the open gas jets lighting the stage, and she was burned to death. Marie was devastated. She sank into even deeper depression when her niece retired three years later, thus ending the Taglioni dancing tradition.

Marie lost her money and investments during the Franco-Prussian War, and she and her father were left without anything. Marie moved to London and opened a school for ballet and deportment, but in spite of her reputation, knowledge of several languages, and her education, she had very few pupils. She spent the last years of her life in Marseille, close to her son, Georges. She died in 1884, one day before her 80th birthday, almost in misery. She is buried at Pere Lachaise Cemetery (rue Pacthod, région 94) in Paris, France, under the name of her ex-husband.

The success of La Sylphide and of Taglioni, who had been a symbol of the Romantic era, was absolute. La Sylphide changed the nature of ballet throughout Europe. The costume she wore, the famous tutu designed by Eugène Lamy, is still considered the model for a Ballet Blanc. The tight-fitting bodice left the neck and shoulders bare, the midcalf bell-shaped skirt was made of white tulle, which gave it a cloudlike appearance. The little garland of flowers in her hair, the wings behind her back, and a thin string of pearls around her neck, created the immortal image of Marie as the sylph. Even Queen Victoria, when she was a child, dressed her dolls as Marie Taglioni, who would later give Princess Mary ballet lessons at White Lodge in the 1870s.

Taglioni invented a new vision of dancing. The dancers who came after her could never match her etherealness or the modest grace she brought to her roles. Taglioni remained the first ballerina of her era; even today her image is for us the essential picture of the Romantic dancer. Taglioni will never die. Her technical strength and the incredible lightness associated with her name are immortal and serve as an example for all ballerinas today.

Ivor Guest said, "Taglioni's dancing was supremely lyrical and modest, and her supremacy, which was never seriously challenged throughout her career, was all the more remarkable in that the age was so exceptionally rich in ballerinas."

Although many extremely talented dancers followed Taglioni after her death, no other ballerina has been described as light and ethereal as she was. But the illusion that she could create didn't die with her. It keeps inspiring dancers and choreographers and will always be an example of beauty.

The elegiac chooses the symbolic and abstract language of dance steps.... With her body she traces hieroglyphics, legible signs made indelible through her emotion.
—Andre Levinson on Marie Taglioni

Chapter 3

Anna Pavlova (1881–1931)
Her Shoes, Her Art, and Her Feet

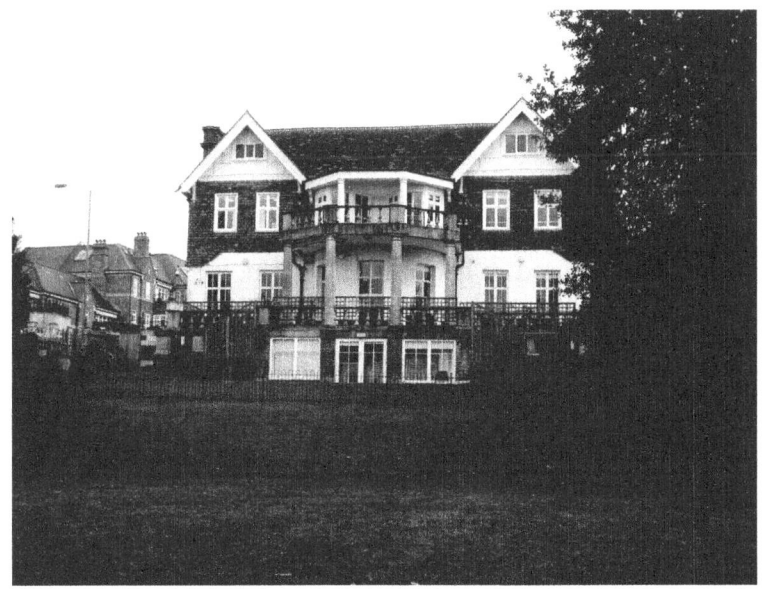

Anna Pavlova's Ivy House in Golders Green

Anna Pavlova is undoubtedly the greatest dancer of all times. Endless pages have been written about her life, her art, and also about her feet! From pictures we can easily see that they were extremely arched, and this was for her a blessing and a curse at the same time.

Pavlova was really picky about her pointe shoes. None of the shoes especially made for her really seemed to please her. She had different makers, but the one she used almost throughout her career was the Italian Romeo Nicolini. His workshop, located in Milan, was a family business, run only by him and by members of his family. Pavlova used to place large orders of shoes, but for some reason and in spite of the detailed explanations she gave of what she wanted, the shoes would never totally fit her.

We have to point out that Nicolini spoke only Italian, and his son, who knew some French, would sometimes translate for him. During other visits, Pavlova decided to hire an interpreter; but no matter what, Nicolini never seemed to get what she really wanted. The Italian shoemaker was old and seemed to be totally at a loss when Pavlova would explain and explain and then irremediably lose her patience. Nicolini's orders would also always arrive after great delays, probably due to the fact that his small business could not handle large orders. "Sometimes the order would fail to arrive at all, and then all our dancers, whose feet were at all like Pavlova's, would bring her their shoes, from which she would choose a pair or two, or she would go through the rejected shoes of former unsuccessful consignments a second time" (Dandré, Anna Pavlova in Art and Life). One of the problems in finding comfortable shoes was due to the tapered shape of Pavlova's beautiful feet, where all the weight would be on the big toe. Pavlova's life partner, Victor Dandré, used to say, "If all the letters and telegrams sent to Nicolini telling him that the shoes were too long or too short or too narrow or too something else were to be collected, they would fill a thick volume."

Things improved somehow when Enrico Cecchetti moved to Milan. He himself or his wife would go to Nicolini to explain what Pavlova's requirements were and insisting on a quick shipment. Shoemakers from all countries often contacted Anna, offering to provide her regularly with pointe shoes free of charge if she just let them advertise that she was using their brand of shoes. Pavlova particularly disliked machine-sewed pointe shoes; she claimed that "they had no soul" and lacked that "special something" provided by the Italian handcrafted pointe shoes.

Anna Pavlova was often pictured in her dressing room, with dozens of pointe shoes lying on the floor next to her. It is said that she learned how to modify her pointe shoes by inserting a piece of leather under the metatarsal area and flattening the platform to obtain more support and increased balance during her arabesques. She would also darn the tip of the shoes (as all Russian dancers used to do) to enlarge the platform even more and make them less slippery for the stage. In order to disguise these "tricks" that she used, she would carefully have all of her pictures retouched in order to hide the enlarged platform and show a more tapered pointe, similar to the one of Taglioni's as seen in her lithographs. She is thus credited for influencing future shoemakers to produce pointe shoes with a wider box, like the ones we use nowadays.

In 1910, during her first tour in the United States, Pavlova purchased pointe shoes for herself and for her whole company from Salvatore Capezio in New York, thus increasing the popularity of the shoemaker. In her famous solo The Dying Swan, choreographed for her by Mikhail Fokine in 1905, Pavlova immortalizes dancing on pointe by skimming the stage with bourrées for the whole length of her solo.

Pavlova's career was unfortunately too short: she died of pleurisy at the height of fame, aged only forty-nine, at the Hotel des Indes in The Hague, Netherlands. The number of her room was never revealed. It is said that right before she died she asked for her swan costume and her last words were: "Play that last measure softly."

Pavlova was cremated and her ashes were placed at the Golders Green Crematorium, not far from her beloved Ivy House.

"When a small child… I thought that success spelled happiness. I was wrong, happiness is like a butterfly which appears and delights us for one brief moment, but soon flits away."
Anna Pavlova

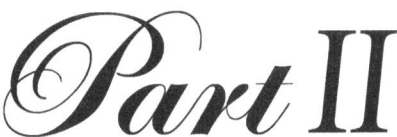

THE PROCESS OF MAKING POINTE SHOES

Chapter 1

Technology Works Side by Side with Art
The New Pointe Shoes Compared to the Old Ones

Going back in time and looking at pictures and descriptions of old ballet shoes, we realize how different they were from today's pointe shoes, crafted using high-technology materials. The demands of choreographers now require a stronger, perfected shoe, able to cope with hours of rehearsals on pointe, providing the ballerina with support and comfort. Freed's pointe shoe expert, Michele Attfield, reveals that Mr. Freed would never have imagined that shoes for men would be made and used in works such as She Was Black for the Rambert Dance Company. Someone making shoes in the 1930s and 1940s would have been shocked by many of the things choreographers like Mats Ek and William Forsythe do nowadays. "The shoes that are made for dancers today," says Attfield, "bear no relation to the shoes made for dancers such as Fonteyn, but then neither does the technique. They may be made in a traditional way, but they have evolved and will always continue to evolve" ("The Evolution of the Pointe," Dancing Times [July 2003], 27).

I was lucky enough to meet and spend some time with Ekaterina Maximova, star of the Bolshoi (suddenly deceased on April 28, 2009) and her husband, Vladimir Vassiliev. It was during their Italian tour with Vassiliev's ballet Anjuta in Genoa. Maximova, Katya as Vassiliev used to call her, had always been my favorite ballerina. That night I had brought a bouquet of flowers from my garden to offer her after the show. She accepted it with a smile and gave me two pairs of her pointe shoes (Vassiliev called her shoes pantofla), which I still keep as a sacred relic.

Maximova's are the tiniest pointe shoes (for an adult) that I have ever seen. I would like to describe them briefly. The brand is unknown, but surely Russian and probably custom-made for her tiny and strong feet. The satin is not pink, but a creamy beige. She must have worn a European size 35 (5 in the United States), and the shoes are so narrow that even my feet (and I have narrow feet) cannot fit in the box! The shank is extremely hard, and looking underneath the sock liner, I can see some sort of double shank of incredibly thick cardboard. There is no flexibility at all in Maximova's shoes; her feet must have been exceptionally strong for her to be able to wear shoes that hard and still show a perfect line of her arch. The tip is absolutely small and round, probably the size of a ruble, or a dollar coin. There is no darning at the tip, but she had removed the satin from the platform and partially from underneath it. Her name is handwritten in Russian (most probably by her), Makcimoba, under the outer sole, which is very rough and scraped with a knife or some other tool to obtain more traction. The shoe has a V-vamp that Katya prolonged by at least two inches with a series of stitches of very thick beige cotton thread. She marked the sock liners with a pen—prava and sleva, which in Russian mean "right" and "left." She prolonged the back of the heels up to the middle seam with an extra inch of grosgrain ribbon, and she slightly lowered down the sides using beige thread. These are amazingly light shoes, but absolutely hard, that she was probably wearing without the use of any type of padding.

In the course of the centuries, pointe shoes have evolved and radically changed.

Marie Taglioni's shoes were nothing more but soft slippers with a simple darning on the tips. Pavlova's pointe shoes were much harder and weighed about half of an ounce more.

The weight of pointe shoes has also changed since the old times: Emma Livry of the Paris Opera used to dance in shoes that weighed 34 grams each (0.074957 lb), and Pavlova's shoes weighed 74 grams.

Today dancers can wear shoes made of high-technology materials by companies such as Gaynor Minden, Capulet, and Flyte. In these shoes, ingredients like polymers, urethane foam, and elastomeric shanks and boxes replace the traditional glue, paper, and hessian. This can be confusing to the young, inexperienced dancer who does not know what is best.

Vanna Porselli, owner and founder of the Italian pointe shoe brand Porselli, says that based on her experience, only pointe shoes built with the traditional materials can obtain the best results. She believes that the ballerina's toes have to adapt themselves to the hardness of the block, and this can only happen through bendable materials conforming to the shape of the foot. Michele Attfield of Freed of London belongs to the same school of thought.

The reality is that dancers have to go through innumerable pairs of shoes before finding the ones that fit their feet perfectly. Professional ballerinas choose to have their shoes specially made in order to customize them perfectly to their feet's requirements. Nowadays, pointe shoes have to cope with the dancers' requirements and hours of rehearsal and dancing on pointe. Several recent types of pointe shoes come with a padded insole (Grishko Miracle), providing the dancer with extra comfort; some are already prearched (Russian Pointe Entrada), or with shock-absorption foam built into the shoe (Gaynor Minden). There is a shoe for each type of feet, and custom-made shoes meet the requirements of dancers with more specific demands.

Chapter 2

The Making of Pointe Shoes and Their Life Span

Although nowadays the technique in making pointe shoes has greatly evolved, many makers still craft traditional "hand-turned" shoes, a system used for all types of shoes until the end of the nineteenth century. But let's explain the meaning of hand turning. The shoes are built on a last, which is a foot-shaped mold. Lasts used to be made of wood, but nowadays wood has almost been replaced by plastic, which is more durable and does not hurt the makers' hands with splints. The shoe is put inside out on the last and hand-turned right side out by hand just for the finishing touches.

Freed's and the Italian shoemaker Gamba's shoes have been the first to adopt this technique, followed by Capezio, Bloch, Porselli, Grishko, and other manufacturers. More recent brands of pointe shoes, like Gaynor Minden, Capulet, and Chacott use different materials and technology-advanced shoemaking systems.

Dancers often hear questions like "How long does a pointe shoe last?"

This is a very tricky question because a pair of pointe shoes can last from several months to . . . a few minutes.

Toni Bentley, a former ballerina with New York City Ballet, believes that a professional dancer can easily use twelve pairs of new pointe shoes a week, and sometimes more. "Under average circumstances," says Bentley, "a pair lasts for fifteen minutes of performing and is then ready to be used in class, [in] rehearsals, [to be] given away with an autograph, or most often, ready to be thrown away. Worn-out pointe shoes cannot be brought back to life (although some dancers think they can); this is why new ones have to be constantly reordered."

Young students taking one or two pointe classes a week might use only two pairs of pointe shoes in a whole school year, including for the end-of-the-year performance. Dancers with strong arches might need three or four pairs, and students in between twelve and fourteen might outgrow their shoes before they wear them out.

Freed's pointe specialist Michele Attfield believes that children beginning pointe work and doing ten to fifteen minutes of pointe at the end of class once or twice a week will outgrow their shoes before wearing them out. In her experience fitting students from the Royal Ballet School at White Lodge, she affirms that by the end of the term, most young dancers outgrow their shoes and have to return the second pair provided by the school. Dancing with "dead" pointe shoes can be extremely harmful to the dancer's feet; the shoes should be replaced as soon as they no longer provide proper support to the feet. This does not mean they have to be thrown away. They can still be used in many ways:

- They can be de-shanked and used in class or rehearsal.

- They can be cleaned or dyed or decorated and kept as mementos.
- They can be autographed and given away or sold during performances and fund-raisers.

Ribbons can be recycled, washed, ironed, and used for a new pair of shoes.

In the chapter called "How to Make Pointe Shoes Last Longer," you will find a lot of useful information about how to take care of your pointe shoes and prolong their lives.

Chapter 3

Visit to a Pointe Shoe Factory: Freed of London

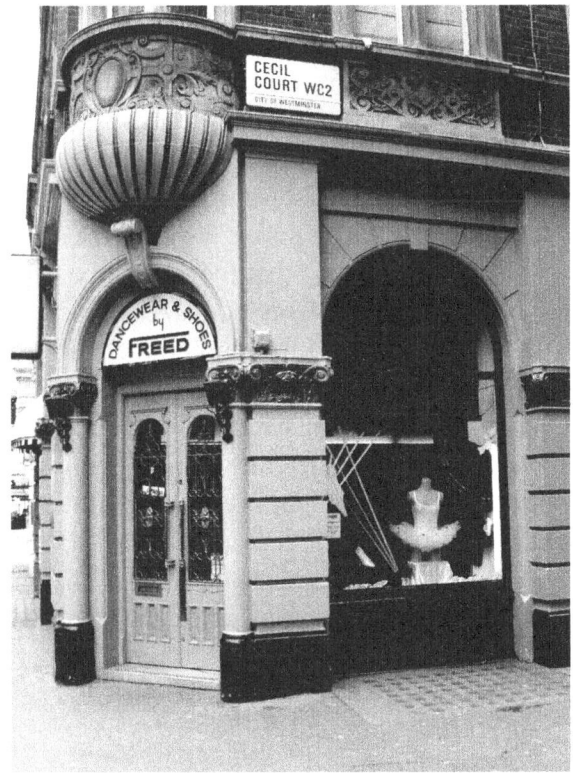

Freed's retail shop in St. Martins Lane, London

I thought this book would not be complete without a visit to one of the most famous pointe shoe factories. The choice was Freed, the oldest and most "traditional" pointe shoe manufacturer on the market. Considered as the leading maker of pointe shoes worldwide, Freed of London started producing shoes in 1930. The factory is located on 62-64 Well Street, in the borough of Hackney, East London. From Bethnal Green, the closest underground station, a short bus ride and a five-minute walk took me to the old Freed building. The visit had been arranged a few months before my arrival; and Gary Brooks, the factory manager, as well as Michele Attfield—Freed's pointe shoe expert—were waiting for me.

Gary Brooks has been working for Freed for over twenty-five years. He welcomed me and guided me through one of the most exciting trips of my life—a detailed visit to the factory, where all the secrets of how pointe shoes are made were unveiled.

Seeing from up close how a pointe shoe is built is a mesmerizing experience. Many dancers do not probably imagine how much work goes into these tiny satin slippers, and how many stages the shoes have to go through before they're finished and ready to be worn and . . . destroyed. Mr. Brooks, a real gentleman with that good sense of humor typical of British people, started our conversation by giving me some important information about the company. "There are about one hundred people working for Freed all together," he explained.

"Mr. Freed was trained at Gamba. That's where he first learnt the art of making pointe shoes. At the time, I believe they had just one last at Gamba."

Frederick Freed and his wife decided to retire from Gamba and open their own shop. They started in the basement of a little store located in St. Martins Lane in Covent Garden, the one that still exists today. The shop has actually changed very little since Mr. Freed started the company; it still looks very old and traditional. "Mr. Freed then invented the 'bespoke' shoe to fit anyone's foot. We created different fittings, so we have X, XX, XXX, all the widths. These individual makers all planted the same seed so that they all make different shoes. The style of a shoemaker depends mainly on the shape of his body. A cobbler with big hands will make hard and heavy shoes with a large platform, while another one with smaller hands will produce lighter shoes with a totally different block," said Gary Brooks.

"The amount of paste they use is not measured, so you might have a maker who is heavy handed, making heavier shoes, and another one crafting lighter ones."

There are now twenty-three makers overall at Freed, each of them having a special symbol or letter that they stamp under the shoe. "A," "B," "D," "E," "F," a key, a club, a crown, an anchor, a bell, a bullhorn, and a Maltese cross, just to cite a few. The only problem with custom-made shoes is consistency. When a maker leaves or retire, the same symbol will not be used by a new maker for a certain number of years.

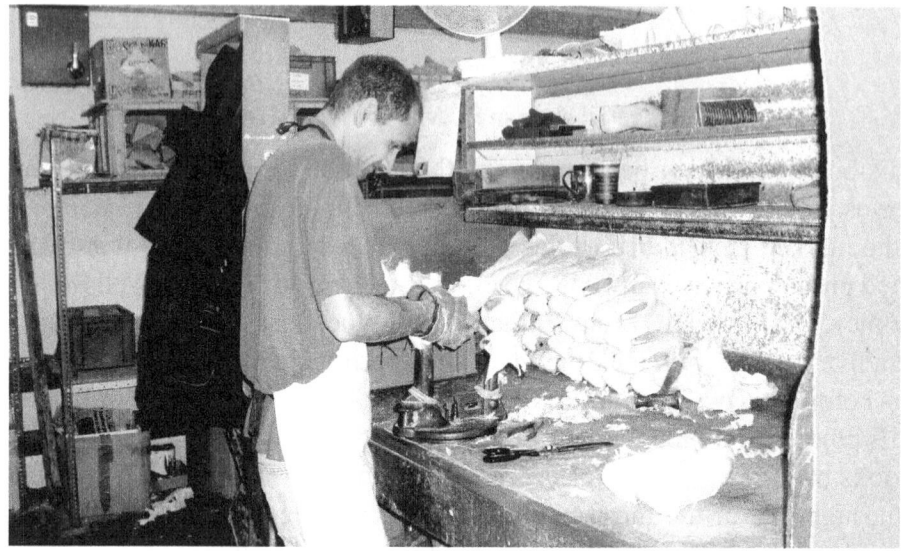

One of Freed's cobblers at work

The Magic of Pointe Shoes

Michele Attfield explained that Freed pointe shoes, although still made in the traditional way, keep evolving in order to meet new choreographic needs and the bodies and weights of the dancers.

"Here in Well Street, there are twelve makers," explained Gary Brooks, "and the rest of them are in the other plants located in Norwich and Leicester. In our three sites, we have more or less 250 people overall working. The biggest factory is this one in Well Street, with about 100 people."

For an experienced pointe shoe maker, it takes about ten minutes to make a pair of shoes, but in order to get to that point, cobblers require at least two years of experience. "Some of the makers only deal with custom shoes due to the huge number of orders, and others do both custom and stock shoes," Brooks explained. "As the makers get older, they make less stock shoes. Some makers have 100 percent order book, very popular, and do not make stock because they have no time and too many orders, and then other makers, maybe less popular, making half and half. Some just make stock because they are new."

All the cobblers at Freed are extremely fast, especially because they are paid per pair of shoes—"piece work," as Mr. Brooks described it—and not per hour. "It's fair for them, and it's fair for us. The more they make, the more they get. It's individual according to their ability and skills and experience. Some makers make forty pairs a day, and some make twenty," Brooks said. "It depends on their skills and ability. It can take a couple of years for a maker to be able to perfect his technique in bespoke shoes. Our most experienced makers make forty pairs per eight-hour day—that's an average of twelve minutes per pair (480 minutes divided by 40 equals 12). However, if you add on perhaps another twelve minutes in the binding room, that's twenty-four minutes, plus the ten hours in drying in our oven."

Crafting pointe shoes is basically a man's job, and the hardness of the work shows on the makers' hands, rough and full of cuts. They looked totally dedicated and absorbed in what they were doing; they did not seem willing to interrupt their work and talk to us. "It's quite very tough," Brooks explained. "We had one lady maker, but she is gone. We have people come for interviews because there are no skilled makers ahead since it's such a special market. Sometimes we have ladies come along, and after, when they see what we do and look at the men's hands, they realize they can't do it. It's very physical.Since it's impossible to make shoes sitting down, the cobblers have to stand all day. "Everything is handmade, you'll see." I can give you a comparison," Brooks told me. He then went on to describe how he saw a video on YouTube showing Gamba making pointe shoes in 1966. "It was exactly the same as we're doing it now, the method is almost identical. We just added a few little things."

The main room where pointe shoes are made looks like a big laboratory with old benches, machineries, shelves, and all the "ingredients" necessary for the pointe shoe making process. Pointe shoes are everywhere, half finished, turned inside out,some still wet, and some having just come out of the oven. In the finishing room, hundreds of shiny, finished, ready-to-ship shoes are scattered everywhere while skilled workers are busy giving them the final touches. It is really loud inside the factory because of the hammering and the stitching machines.

The first two makers at the entrance of the making room are two young men in their thirties. One of the two is Pat Moran, maker Key, an extremely fast cobbler known for making lighter shoes; he has been working at Freed for fifteen years. A picture of his daughter is glued on his desk. His shoes are beautiful and light, but his waiting time exceeds the six months. Freed's makers generally range from young to middle-aged and are of different nationalities. When using the paste, they all wear white latex gloves. One of the things that captured my attention were the shelves loaded with tons of yellow lasts divided according to size and width.

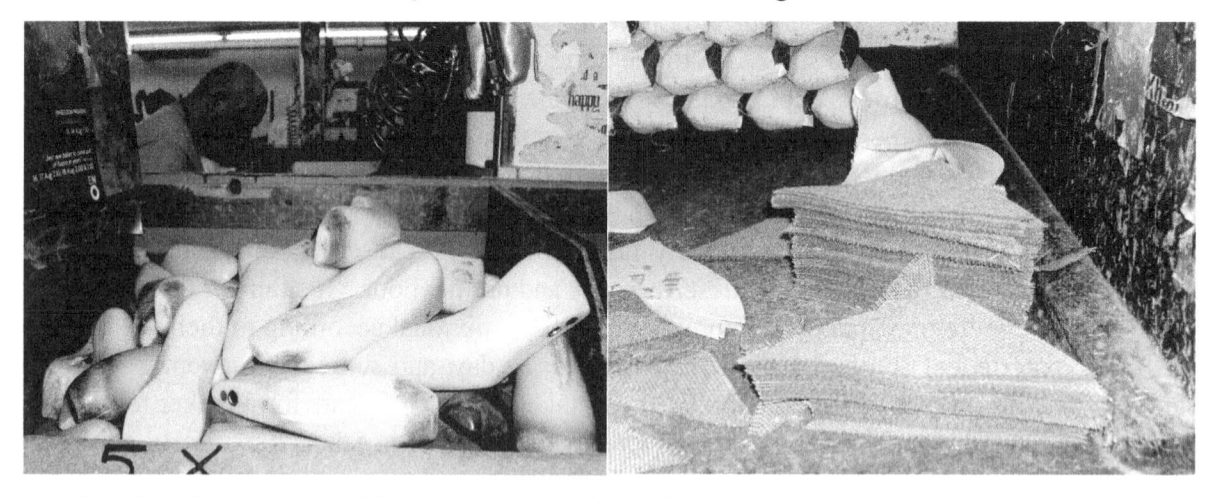

On other desks, one could see pieces of satin cut into the shape of a pointe shoe, triangles of paper and hessian, pots of glue, nails of all dimensions, and everywhere that typical smell that recalls a little bit the smell of bread.

The machines made a lot of noise inside the factory; it was hard to hear, but Gary Brooks patiently kept explaining, escorting me around the factory, carefully describing all the stages of the pointe shoe manufacturing, showing me all the elements that go into a shoe and explaining their purpose in detail.

Every day four hundred shoes are produced at Freed's, for a total of two thousand shoes a week.

Freed uses what they call the "turn shoe" method, which means that shoes are made from the inside out. "From 1930 to 2010," Brooks said," the method is almost identical. This is why we call it classic shoe, because it's original."

Shoemakers at Freed start by tacking the sole into the last; then they fit the upper (which is the satin part already precut and ready to use by the makers) around it, inside out. "So you have the upper, which is all the material" Brooks explained, "the satin part, the sole, after sole, inner sole, upper sole." The makers then tube the shoe on the last with the upper and the layers of material that form the block, and this is made inside out.

The next step is building the block, or box.

The block is formed by hand, using layers of hessian triangles (a brown rough sack material) and paper dipped in the paste made out of flour and water and a few secret ingredients.

"The paste is a little bit like baking a cake," Brooks said. "What we do is we put the shoes in the oven at night and let them dry all night, so that in the morning they will be dry and the block will be hard. For stronger blocks, the maker uses more paste."

After the block is made, with the shoe still inside out, the maker forms the pleats in the satin where the dancer stands, using metal pincers. Pleats can be small or bigger, also depending on the size of the maker's hands. "Small hands will make small pleats, and makers with bigger hands will make bigger pleats," Brooks said.

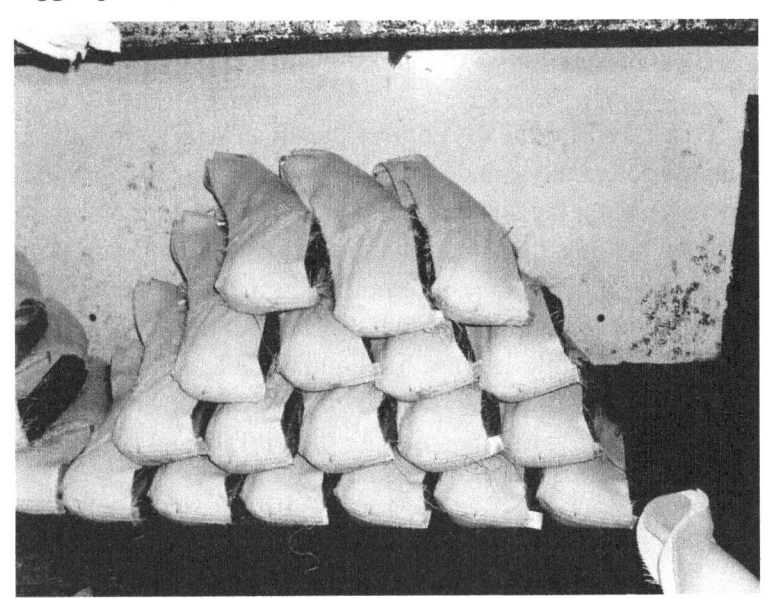

Pointe shoes ready to be "turned"

Then they put a temporary string around the last to secure everything. After this, the shoe is stitched and the sole attached to the upper using a wax thread. Hot wax runs through the stitching machine, so the thread goes into the hot wax in order to hold the stitches together.

The stitching machines used at Freed date back to 1964. Gary Brooks explained that these machines do not exist anymore nowadays, so they take great care of them since they would not be able to replace them. When the shoe is removed from the last, the makers turn it over, using what Brook calls "the secret weapon," basically a wooden stick. Once the shoe is turned, all the excess fabric is trimmed off. The makers then insert the insole and hammer the box, still wet, using a glass-faced hammer. The purpose of this operation is to make the block smooth and to give it the maker's final signature shape. With the same tool, they also shape the platform, which can be round or square. After shaping the block and the platform, the maker stamps his individual symbol onto the sole. "All of our shoes are bespoke, and each maker's shoes are different," explained Brooks.

The shoes, still wet, are placed on peg racks (oven racks where shoes are hung) in a huge oven that holds up to four hundred pairs of shoes at seventy or more degrees centigrade to dry overnight. They need about ten hours to dry. "Before we go home in the evening," said Brooks, "we push a button for the oven, like a washing machine, and the next morning the shoes are dry and ready for the finishing process."

He continued, "Once the shoe has dried, all the measurements are applied, the binding, the elastic, the drawstring, the cutting of the vamp, and the shape of the shoe are all applied, the dressing sock (that goes through a machine lining them with glue) and the packing, checking to make sure that there are no faults."

When the shoes are dry, they are brought into the binding room, where the lasts are removed and the soles marked with their size and width. Each vamp is measured and hand-cut according to the right length for the style required or according to the specifications of the dancer who will wear it.

Then the binding is attached around the edge of the upper with a machine and the drawstring that runs through it is inserted at the same time. "We use a guide," Brooks explained, holding a shoe in his hands, "which we put the shoe into and the binding and the drawstring go through."

Lastly, a canvas liner bearing the Freed symbol (two tiny standing pointe shoes), called sock, is placed into the shoe. Pointe shoes are not made in pairs; they are straight lasted, and this is why there is no right or left and they can be worn in either foot.

The outer sole is made of buffalo leather, hard and thick leather that they keep in big rolls. "All the components are made of raw materials," Brooks explained. "When England had problems with the mad cows, we had hard times finding the buffalo and had to import it from other countries."

More than 75 percent of Freed shoes are made to individual specifications, and the rest are stock.

It is a misnomer that Freed's custom-made shoes are extremely expensive and unaffordable: the extra charge in addition to the regular price of the shoe is only one British pound! The waiting time, though, can sometimes be frustrating. As of March 2010, it ranges up to seven months for certain makers, like in the case of maker Key, or six months for the Anchor and Crown makers. For less busy makers, like D, Y, Q, B, and Bell, the waiting time is two and a half months. J will be retiring at the end of August 2010, so dancers using his services will have to start trying new makers.

Looking around the factory, one would expect to see pictures hanging on the walls depicting ballerinas wearing diaphanous costumes, but in reality, pointe shoe makers seem to be more into pictures of football players, girls wearing a swimsuit, or belly dancers. In the finishing room, images of Princess Diana are glued on the walls, as well as personal mementos and religious images.

The stitching of the shoes is made with thread going through hot wax, so when the wax dries, the stitches are bound together.

The "paste room" looks like a bakery; the machine making the paste is exactly like a machine for making bread, and the smell reminds you of bread too. Freed has a paste maker in charge of making the secret paste that goes into the box. Every day he makes two big bowls of paste (about fifty pounds), and each maker takes a pot of paste or more for his daily use.

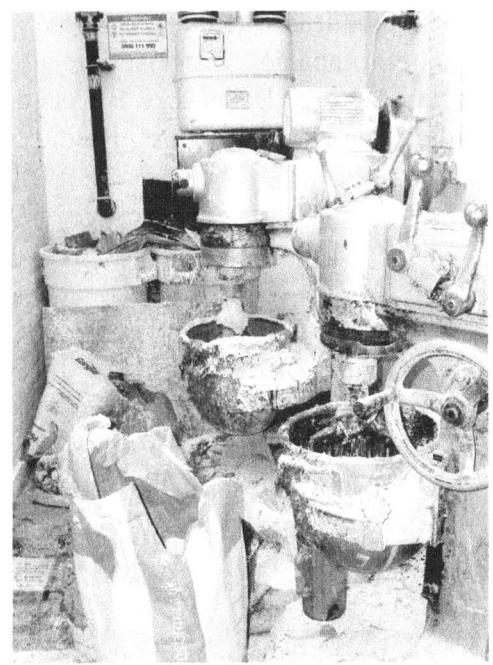

The paste room at Freed's

Another specialist at Freed's is the "clicker," whose task is cutting the leather soles out of a sheet of leather with a special metal instrument.

Since none of the makers was ready to "turn" the shoe yet, Gary Brooks took me to the finishing room, which is separate from the makers' room. This is a quieter and better-lit area where about a dozen people work, mostly women. Here the material is cut to size, the binding stitched on, and the soles stamped. The binding is hand-finished, the makers making sure that the drawstring is running freely. Hundreds of brand-new shoes lie in big trays nesting inside each other, shiny and featuring Freed's typical peach color.

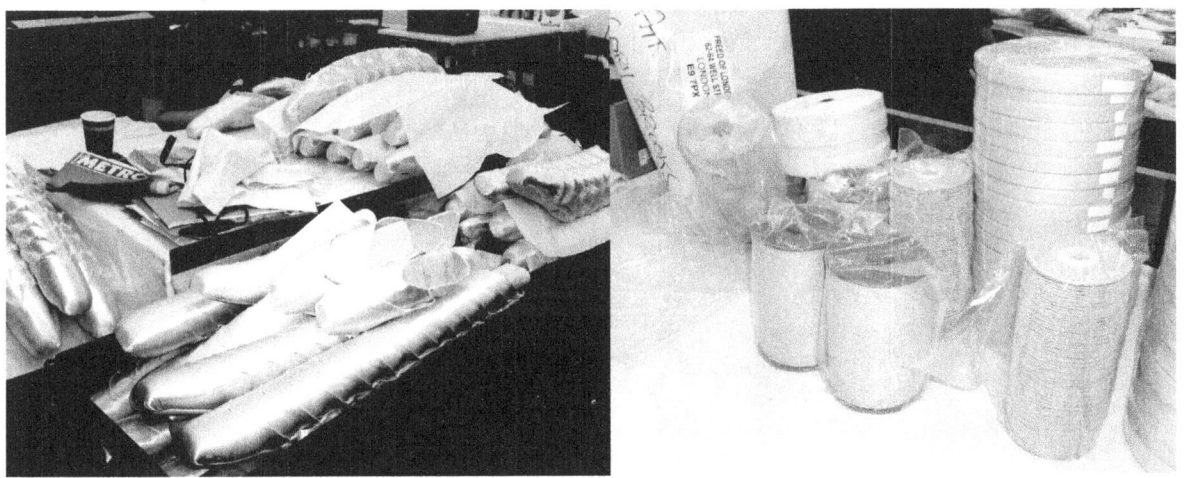

The shipping room comes next, and it is where the shoes are put in bags and boxes to be sent worldwide to dancers and ballet companies. Big boxes are aligned, bearing names such as Royal Danish Ballet, Stuttgart Ballet, Royal Ballet, Les Ballets de Monte Carlo, Les Grands Ballets Canadiens, Carolina Ballet, Pennsylvania Ballet, Pacific Northwest Ballet, San Francisco Ballet, and many others.

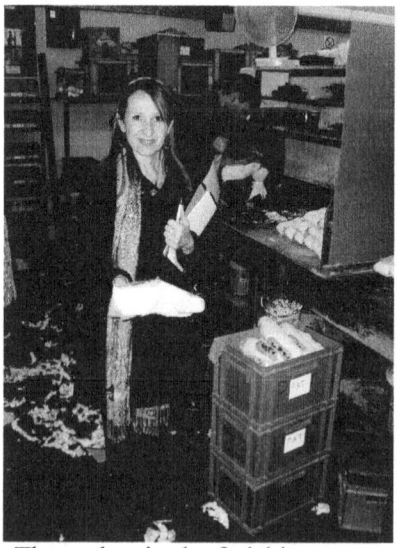

The author in the finishing room

Dancers send in their specifications about size; width; hardness of shank; size of platform, which can be tapered, medium, wide, or square; height of the sides, width of the heel; length of vamp; and much more. Thinner insoles can be fitted, and a layer of hessian can be omitted to give the shoes a less acute angle. Four widths are available in stock, and the "heel pin" system fits feet that are in between sizes, when the full size is too small and the half size is too big. The heel pin is a little piece of leather inserted when the shoe is still on the last, filling just that little extra space when half of a size can be too long.

At Freed's pointe shoes always go through a final inspection before they are put in a bag and sent.

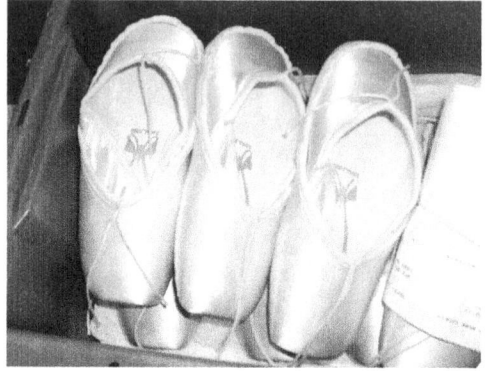

Pointe shoes ready to be sent

We finally headed back to the making room, where a couple of cobblers were ready to turn the shoe. This procedure happens really fast, and the makers use a wooden stick to help the shoe turn.

Besides the pointe shoe department, Freed also features a theatrical department making all other types of shoes, from ballroom shoes to tap shoes, jazz shoes, soft ballet shoes, character, as well as leotards (all the RAD regulation uniforms are manufactured and endorsed by Freed), ballet tights, etc.

The visit ended with a tour of the administrative offices upstairs and afterward in Gary Brook's office.

After visiting the factory, I feel that I have more respect for my pointe shoes. I don't want to destroy them anymore because I have seen how much work goes into them. I have also seen from up close how much tradition goes into Freed's pointe shoes and how high is the quality of the materials they use.

Chapter 4

Meeting a Pointe Shoe Maker: Ushi Nagar

It is a relationship of love, the one between Ushi Nagar and his pointe shoes. He puts his heart and soul in the shoes he makes. "Ballet shoes are in my blood," he says with a big smile, "and what makes my shoes different is the love and care that I put into them. And all the detail." Ushi is definitely a man out of the ordinary, and talking to him is like reading through the pages of a book.

He welcomed me to his retail shoe shop in Norbury, London. Shoe Avenue is not a ballet shop or a pointe shoe store, like one might think, but just a regular shoe store like many others, selling purses, handbags, sandals, and all types of street shoes. His laboratory is located a couple of streets from there. Ushi is a very friendly man, and his eyes sparkle when he talks about pointe shoes. I immediately felt a bond with him.

Born in Nairobi to Indian parents, Nagar came to England from Uganda in 1961. His father and his grandfather were both shoemakers. He came with the intent to join the air force, but destiny had something else in store for him. A friend took him to the Jobcentre, who directed him to Freed, back then located on Mercer Street, Covent Garden, where more than one hundred people were working.

"Once I started working for Freed in 1960," he recalls, "I was trained by Bill Boots, who was the foreman at the time. I was first trained on making soft ballet shoes of leather and satin. It is necessary you first learn how to make these types of shoes for the pleating. After a week of training on basic shoes, you switch to pointe shoes, and you get to make two pairs a day, for a couple of days. Then you start making ten pairs of stock shoes a day."

He recalled that when he started making pointe shoes, he looked at a pointe shoe and thought, "This is something unique. Manufacturing pointe shoes is something unusual and unique, and I said to myself, if I ever had to do something, I would do this!"

His face lightened up as he remembered the early days at Freed. I admit I have never seen anyone loving his profession the way he does! "Mr. Freed," he continued, "took me under his protection and loved me as a son, because he saw I was honest, although a little bit of a troublemaker! He felt I was the right man."

Nagar speaks with a light voice, and looking at his hands, I could see his cracked fingers, witnessing fifty-five years of making pointe shoes! He shared with me that Margot Fonteyn's shoes were crafted by a maker who worked next to him. "He was a Greek guy."

In 1983 Nagar left Freed, having decided to establish his own pointe shoe business, making only custom-order shoes for most European and American ballet companies. Ushi doesn't keep any shoes in stock. "All the shoes we make are shipped out. We don't keep any in the store. Everything is custom-made. There is no stock shoe. The stock system is not good for me. You need to have thousands of pairs of shoes, and what if you don't sell?

My wife comes from a family of shoemakers too. Between me and her, it's eighty years of making shoes!"

Nagar explained that when he makes shoes for a ballerina, "the most important thing is to establish the correct fitting. The fitting has to be 100 percent correct!"

Nagar makes pointe shoes following Freed's same system—the turn shoe technique. "Everything is done by hand," he explains, "apart from stitching and drawstring binding, sole and back seam, which are machine done. Turn ballet shoes are, from my point of view, the oldest traditional ballet shoes. Nobody can beat that."

The process of making a pointe shoe is quite complex. Ushi starts by cutting the fabric for the uppers; he cuts eight or sixteen pieces into size. The soles and the insoles are cut to the same sizes, the soles are grooved and channeled and then put on the lasts, while the upper is placed inside out. He continues lifting the top layer of the lining ready for forming the block and starts pasting the inside layer of the block with one hand or with the fingers using hessian. He puts two layers of paste and then the glue. The hessian is put layered, not one right on top of the other, otherwise it would make a big bump. He basically follows the same procedure as Freed's.

"Once I form the block," he continued, "I cover it with the lining ready for lasting [making the pleats].Once lasting is made, the shoe goes to the stitcher, and after, we trim off all the excess materials on the soles. The stitches go through the channel and through the upper. It's called a chain-stitch with hot wax, and the thread goes through it. When the hot wax dries out, all the stitches are bonded and will not fall apart, so the satin stays on the shoe. No matter what happens with the thread, it will not break or cut. I believe that the stitching is one of the most important phases in the making of a pointe shoe. When the dancer is on the stage, and there is something like five thousand people watching, and you can see the shoe falling apart because of the stitching, the performance can be ruined. The dancer might have to leave the stage."

Once the shoe is stitched, it is ready to be turned. "When turning the shoe, you have to do it in a certain way. If you don't turn it evenly, one side of the shoe may be stronger than the other. We push all the materials into the pointe and then put the shoe on the last. The next stage is forming the shape by hammering and gradually shaping the block and the platform. At this point, the shoe is basically done and ready for the shank to be inserted. Shanks can be of various strengths according to individual requirements. Shanks are made of fiber, leather board, or anything special to the dancer. You can use different strengths of fiber. I don't like cardboard shanks because they break."

Nagar patiently showed us how his shanks are made. They are actually made of two parts: an insole with a smaller centerpiece glued on top. The central piece without the insole would break, and the insole gives flexibility. He personally prefers fiber shanks to cardboard ones. "Because a fiber shank is very flexible, it does not matter what you do, it comes back. You can bend it, it will never break! You can even cut it narrower to make it more flexible. Anything can be done."

All of Nagar's shoes are bespoke, which means they are made after the requirements of the dancer. He does not sell ready-made pointe shoes, and you cannot find his shoes on the market. He does not have a website and does not like too much publicity.

He made shoes for many famous ballerinas, including Dame Antoinette Sibley, now President of the Royal Academy of Dance.

He believes that the measurements, the shanks, and the squareness of the tip are the most important things in a shoe.

"For girls with bunions," he explained, "we make the shoes wider. Everything is possible. During my leisure time or the weekends, I make a lot of experiments, and I love this!"

Ushi Nagar often travels to other European countries and makes shoes for dancers for many companies like Ballet du Nord in France, Göteborg Ballet and Malmö Ballet in Sweden.

"When I go to the ballet companies, like New York City Ballet or San Francisco Ballet, all the girls come to me. What I do, I establish the size, and if they wear Freed shoes, I know immediately what they want. Capezio has a different last. Gamba and Chacott too."

His first trip to America was to Reno, Nevada, and then to the San Francisco Ballet, Kansas City Ballet, Richmond Ballet, Atlanta Ballet, Royal Winnipeg Ballet, Ballet Met, Milwaukee Ballet, and the New York City Ballet. He likes to work with American ballet companies. "Every time I visit, I am welcomed like at my home," he says with a huge smile. "I supply San Francisco Ballet, Kansas City Ballet, Ballet Met, and Richmond Ballet."

When he visits a ballet company, he generally only accepts orders from five to ten girls, only the ones already wearing Freed. "I don't do shoes for someone who doesn't have a Freed to compare," he says. "It is essential for the fitting, since my shoes are made on the same last as Freed's. When they wear Freed, it's easy for me. I write all the details down, and I look [at] what type of shoe the dancer needs or what type of requirements," says Nagar. "Some other shoemakers do not care for the shoes. They do a mass production, and they don't even look at it. With me, every pair I make, I make it exactly the same, from the platform to the cutting and all the rest."

The most important thing, according to Ushi Nagar, is to establish the correct fitting of the shoe.

I asked him if he enjoys watching ballet performances. "I like watching the ballets," he said. "I especially like being backstage observing the dancers' feet."

It takes Ushi Nagar about half an hour to make a pair of shoes, and he does not dry his shoes in an oven, like most big companies, including Freed, do. He lets them dry naturally, and this process takes about a week. "There are secrets when making a pointe shoe," he says, smiling, "that I cannot disclose at this time."

I asked him what he thought about new technology shoes, like Gaynor Minden. "It's a good shoe, but you see, this is a matter of taste. It's a very expensive shoe. But the beauty of these shoes is that they last a long time."

I visited Nagar twice during my stay in London, and before I left, he kindly gave me . . . a pointe shoe kit. Pieces of hessian, a satin upper, a sole, and a shank. "Now you can build your own shoe!" he said with a smile.

It was hard to say good-bye to Ushi. I felt I wanted to spend more time with him. I could never be tired of hearing the fascinating story of his life. There is so much history in what he lived and saw, so much tradition and love. He is not only my pointe shoe maker now. I consider him a friend, and one of the kindest souls I have ever met. He promised that the next time I am in London, he will craft my shoes in front of me, showing me all the stages. So I look forward to my next visit to London; I look forward to seeing Ushi again. He is a man with a passion deep in his soul, putting his love and, as he says, "his blood" into the making of a pink silk slipper.

Chapter 5

The Anatomy of a Pointe Shoe
The Parts of the Shoe

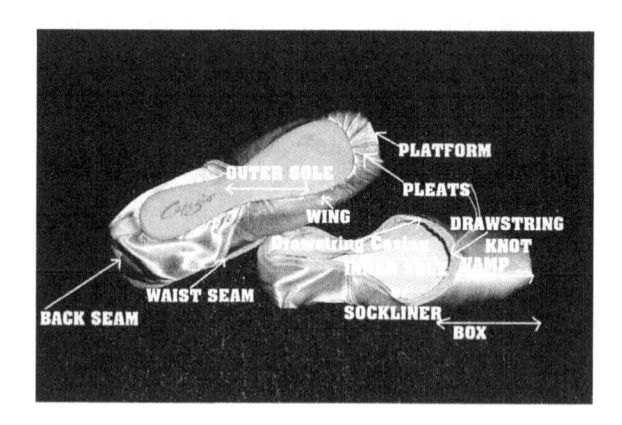

The upper

The word upper refers to all the fabric parts of the shoe. In traditional pointe shoe factories like Freed or Gamba or Capezio, just to name a few, uppers are assembled at another location and stored at the factory till needed. Uppers are actually made from one layer of satin—a mix of cotton and viscose—and two of cotton canvas, all stitched together.

The vamp

It is the portion of the shoe that surrounds the block covering the forefoot, and this is where the drawstring casing comes out. It spans from the platform to the U or V cut, or to the drawstring. The length of the vamp is generally determined by the length of the dancer's toes, to give support when dancing on pointe without limiting movement.

If the vamp is too long, it will make it very difficult for the dancer to roll through demi-pointe, or even prevent the dancer to reach full-pointe. If the vamp is too short, the dancer would not have enough support and would go too far forward on the pointe. V-shaped vamps can also be ordered instead of the popular U-shaped vamp, but they should always be long enough to cover the joint at the base of the big toe.

The box (block)

It is the hard part of the shoe that covers, protects, and supports the toes. It is made with different layers of fabric and paper, dipped in glue. All makers have their "secret" recipe, of which they are very jealous and which they never reveal. The blocking is thick at the tip of the toes near the platform and thinner as it extends over the sides of the wings. There are different degrees of hardness, varying widths (known by the use of different letters), shapes (square, long, flat, oval, or curve), and also different lengths (three-quarters, which is from toe to drawstring and half boxing).

A "winged box" is a toe box with extra-hard and stiffened sides. According to pointe shoe maker Ushi Nagar, the block is the most important part of the shoe, because that is where the ballerina dances and balances.

The platform (tip)

This is another important part of the shoe. It is the round (or square or oval) part at the bottom of the shoe where the dancer stands when on pointe. Platforms come in different shapes: round, oval, or square. Bigger platforms offer the dancer more balance and stability, especially in turns and balances.

The crown

It is the vertical height between the sole and the vamp that determines the fullest of the toe box. Higher crowns accommodate fuller toes. Dancers with shallower feet usually prefer lower crowns. When the crown is too low, it squeezes the toes too tightly, while when it's too high, we are able to put a finger in between the foot and the shoe.

The throat

We call throat the open area on top of the shoe, which can be V-shaped or round. It is the part of the upper meant to show and highlight the arch of the dancer's foot.

The shank (insole)

It is one of the most important parts of the shoe. The shank is the spine of the pointe shoe; it's the part that keeps the dancer up on pointe and is usually placed in between the outer and the inner soles. The centerpiece extends from just under the ball of the toes to the middle of the heel, creating the dancer's arch. Shanks can be made out of leather, fabric, cardboard, or fiber and can be ordered in different strengths.

Nowadays pointe shoe manufacturers offer the option between a full and a three-quarter shank for more flexibility.

Professional dancers cut their shank to the desired length in order to achieve more flexibility in the shoe and show a better line of the foot.

The binding (drawstring casing)

It is the fabric channel that runs all the way around the shoe and contains the drawstring. Drawstrings can be made of cotton or elastic.

The sock liner

The sock liner is the fabric situated right underneath the foot and runs the length of the shoe.

The pleats

They are found at the back of the block where the satin is folded into the sole. They are important for the sense of feeling on the floor. They can be ordered longer, with a shorter or longer outer sole. Some brands of pointe shoes, like Gaynor Minden, produce shoes without pleats. The length of the pleats can range from one half to one inch in length.

The outer sole

It is the leather or suede sole situated underneath the shoe. It covers the shank and provides traction. It generally also gives a lot of information about the size, the width, and the brand and type of shoe. It is most often made of thin leather, which allows flexibility and contact with the floor. The end of the outer leather sole should cover the rounded portion of the heel so that the shoe stays in place when the dancer is on pointe.

The inner sole

See sock-liner.

The side quarters

Side quarters are those sections of satin going from the side seams to the back of the stay.

The stay

The stay is the portion of fabric covering the seam in the back of the shoe at the dancer's heel. The term stay refers to the sections of satin from the side seams to the back of the shoe.

The edge of the pleats (feathers)

The feathers are the pleats under the toe.

The waist seam

The term refers to the seam that divides the wings from the quarters and keeps the front and the back of the shoe together.

The heel section

The heel section is the satin part corresponding to the dancer's heel.

The wings (support)

The wings are the stiff parts of the block on either side of the shoe that prevent the dancer from sickling and provide lateral support while the dancer is on pointe.

The side quarters

They consist of the sections of satin from the side seams to the back of the stay.

The drawstring knot

The back seam

The back seam is the seam behind the heel of the shoe that connects the quarters and keeps the two sides of the shoe together.

The feathers (pleats)

We can call feathers the pleating under the toes, resulting when the last layer of satin is added to the outside of the pointe shoe.

The hessian

Hessian, otherwise called burlap, is a brown coarse-looking jute fabric. Layers, or hessian triangles, are dipped into the special paste to form the block of the pointe shoe.

Learn to Read Your Shoes

On the outer sole, you will be able to find all the information about your pointe shoes, from the brand to the size, width, and much more.

The brand

The name of the brand is generally stamped on the outer sole.

The size

According to the manufacturer, the size will be given using the European, British, or the American numbering system.

For example, a British size 3.5 corresponds to a European size 36 or to a US size 4.5!

The width

The width of the pointe shoe is generally indicated by X. You can find X, XX, XXX, and sometimes even XXXX. Other brands use letters like S, M, and W; and other brands use A, B, C, D, and E.

The maker's symbol

Each maker has a special sign or symbol, and this is also stamped on the outer sole, especially when shoes are custom-made.

What's Inside a Pointe Shoe?

This is one of the most common questions students and parents ask. They all wander what is inside the block of a pointe shoe, and what makes it so hard. Some think there is wood, some plaster, and some . . . cement! Well, none of the three. So which are the "secret ingredients"? In traditional shoes like Freed, Gamba, Bloch, and Capezio, blocks are made of layers of hessian triangles, white-and-gray paper and cardboard in decreasing sizes, dipped into a special paste. The basic ingredients of the paste are flour and water, to which each manufacturer adds some "secret ingredients." Every pointe shoe maker is very jealous about the secret of his paste and will never reveal how it is really made.

New technology shoes like Gaynor Minden, Capulet, and Flyte are made of high-technology polymeric ingredients, promising shoes that last five times more the traditional ones and molding to each dancer's foot, without any break-in period! Capulet Juliet D3o pointe shoes are crafted with special material from D3o in the box, vamp, and midsole, giving the shoe maximum flexibility and shock absorption. D3o is a patented shock-absorbing material containing "intelligent molecules." The material is soft under general conditions, but during impacts the molecules lock together, providing shock absorption and preventing injuries.

These shoes are advertised to last for twenty full performances . . . and more. New types of sophisticated, high-technology pointe shoes appear on the market every year, making pointe work painless and separating us more and more from the times of Taglioni's rudimental first pointe shoes.

Chapter 6

Demi Pointe Shoes and Soft Slippers

Some call them shankless, but they are especially known as three-quarter pointe, demi-pointe, or soft-block pointe shoes. Research has shown that they are an excellent way to prepare and strengthen dancers for pointe work.

Freed is one of the first manufacturers who created the satin soft-block shoe—called Freed demi-pointe—for demi-pointe work, to be used as a transition shoe or for RAD vocational levels.

At the Royal Academy of Dance, ballet students use them as a transition between soft shoes and pointes. This type of shoes helps tremendously in strengthening feet and ankles by working against the resistance of a harder sole and harder block. They also improve the dancer's balance with the harder and thicker outer sole, which requires much more stability when working at the barre or in the center.

Starting from RAD Intermediate Foundation level (and mandatorily at Intermediate level), students wear demi-pointes instead of regular soft slippers. Demi-pointes also help strengthen the muscles around the ankles and the muscles that support the arches of the foot, called the longitudinal and transverse arches. The three longitudinal arches run from

1. The center of the heel to the joint at the beginning of the big toe
2. The center of the heel to the beginning of the second toe (the center of the foot)
3. The center of the heel to the beginning of the little toe

The transverse arches run across the foot from the beginning of the instep to the beginning of the toes.

Toronto's renowned National Ballet School (NBS) also utilizes shankless shoes in pre-pointe training.

Dancers need to use more strength if they have to stay up without wobbling and get the feeling of wearing pointe shoes. However it is good to alternate them with the soft ballet shoes, to enable students to feel the floor more freely.

But how do demi-pointe shoes look like? From the outside they look exactly like a regular pointe shoe, although they are not built the same way. A pointe shoe has six layers of material in the vamp, while a demi-pointe shoe has only four layers. The sole is also not as thick as in a pointe shoe, but still thicker than in a "flat" leather or canvas ballet shoe. The wings are also slightly smaller, and the platform is smaller. The most important difference is that the demi-pointe has a leather sole, a thinner inner sole, but no shank. Demi-pointes are cheaper than regular pointe shoes, but more expensive than soft slippers.

If you cannot afford to buy demi-pointe shoes, you can make your own out of an old pair of pointe shoes, by de-shanking them and thus obtaining a "homemade" demi-pointe shoe. All you need to do is remove the shank, and you will get a pair of soft pointe shoes to use in class or rehearsal, although the feeling is not totally the same. You might need some help in order to remove the tacks, and also a pair of pliers. Once you have removed the tacks, you will remove the shank and replace the sock liner—or glue it—on top. It is really hard to de-shank Grishkos or Russian Pointe, though, due to the way they are made. Freed, Bloch, Capezio, Gamba, Repetto are very easy to de-shank.

My students generally start wearing demi-pointe shoes at RAD Intermediate Foundation level and continue through all the vocational levels. They are allowed to wear "flat" shoes for free classes and rehearsals (when not on pointe), but for syllabus classes they are required to wear demi-pointe shoes, also in preparation for their exams where soft shoes are not accepted (at Intermediate foundation level the use of demi-pointe shoes is still optional). It is also a good idea to start wearing demi-pointe shoes one or two years before starting pointe work, and use them as a transition, or pre-pointe, shoe.

I truly think demi-pointe shoes are an excellent stepping-stone leading to real pointe work. Children are excited to get to wear "satin shiny hard shoes," and they slowly and safely get the feeling of working with pointe shoes. They also become more familiar with how to sew and tie the ribbons in preparation for real pointe shoes.

A soft-blocked shoe has to be fitted as tight as a pointe shoe and the foot has to start getting used to work in a more restricted space. You can purchase demi-pointe shoes at your local ballet store or order them if they are not in stock at the moment. The best brands available are Sansha, Freed, Bloch, Capezio, and Grishko.

Soft Slippers: Leather or Canvas

Many students are at a loss when it comes to buying ballet slippers. They do not really know what is best for them, and why. The choice is generally guided by the shop assistant, the parents, or by economical reasons. Both leather and canvas shoes are available on the market, but which is the best one, and why?

This is quite a big debate between teachers. Personally, I advise my younger students to use leather full-sole soft shoes instead of canvas split-sole. The full sole makes the foot work harder, and the shape of leather shoes is more flattering to the foot than canvas, which makes all feet look alike and very wide. Leather also offers more support to the feet.

Canvas shoes tend to get dirty very fast and last less longer than leather, which is more durable. The type of floor can also affect the choice of shoes. If the floor is marley and very sticky, canvas can be a better option, especially during the summer when the floor gets hot. On a slippery wooden floor, I would definitely have my students wear leather, which provides more grip. Split soles are good for more advanced dancers and for rehearsals. Carol Beevers, shoe specialist and manager of the Shoe Room at the National Ballet

School in Toronto, explains, "One school of thought is that the full sole works the intrinsic muscles of the foot more than the split sole. In other words, you have to work your foot harder."

I also advise full soles for beginners in order for them to develop more strength in their feet and ankles.

At the Royal Academy of Dance, we encourage students from grade 3 up to sew satin ribbons to their soft shoes, in preparation for future pointe work. Ribbons help holding the whole foot and ankle better than elastics and show a nicer line of the foot and the leg.

Part III

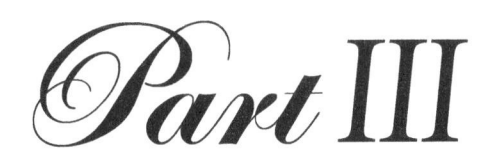

EVERYTHING A DANCER NEEDS TO KNOW ABOUT FEET

Chapter 1

The Anatomy of the Foot

Feet are a fascinating part of our body. As a dancer and a teacher, feet have always been so important to me. Podiatrist Elizabeth H. Roberts, author of On Your Feet, describes feet in a very expressive way that I would like to quote.

Feet are a magnificently well-engineered part of your body. They carry the weight of your entire body. They help to hold your body in a stationary, upright position. They coordinate to maintain your body's balance as you walk. They allow you to accelerate your pace as you run. They have the precision that permits you to leave the ground completely and return in an upright position as you jump.

Celia Sparger, author of the famous book Anatomy and Ballet, is convinced that ballet makes unique demands on the foot.

It has to become strong, very supple and as sensitive as the hand, and it is used in positions and movements quite outside its natural range. For this reason the original shape will be either an asset or a handicap but it will certainly not remain unchanged and therefore a detailed understanding of its structure is important," she says. (p.32)

The foot is made up by 28 bones, 107 ligaments, 33 joints, 28 muscles, and several tendons. The foot is composed of three parts:

- The tarsus, which consists of seven tarsal bones corresponding to the carpal bones of the wrist
- The five metatarsals corresponding to the carpal bones of the wrist
- The fourteen phalanges corresponding to the digits of the fingers

The seven tarsal bones constitute the hard part of the foot. They are separated from each other by cartilage and bound firmly by ligaments that allow some degree of movement between the bones. The two largest bones are the calcaneous, or the heel bone; and above it is the talus, or the astragalus. The heel is a projection of the calcaneous.

In her book Chaussons de pointes, Christine Jeannin explains that in Chinese medicine the foot is considered a vital part of the human body, where all the other organs are reflected.

Although it is often said that there are twenty-six bones present in a foot, there are actually twenty-eight bones in each foot.

Chapter 2

Types of Legs

After many years of teaching, I came to the conclusion that most young students are not aware of the shape of their legs and the type of their feet. Knowing your body is very important, especially when starting pointe work. This knowledge is crucial for teachers in order to guide students in making the right choice of a pointe shoe.

If dancers learn how to recognize their type of legs and feet, they will also learn how to deal with their problems and make the best out of what Mother Nature gave them. Dr. Thomas Novella is a podiatrist who sees over two hundred dancers a year, besides working side by side with some of the major ballet companies. He strongly believes that the fit of the pointe shoes is much more important than the brand.

Knowing your type of feet will be extremely helpful in finding the right shoes and accessories and in working on the right placement and weight distribution.

Hyperextended legs (Sway-back knees)

This type of leg is very often seen in dancers. On one side it has a very pleasant look, perfectly straight, with the knee totally disappearing; but on the other it is extremely difficult to train.

This condition exists from birth and in many cases is inherited from one of the parents.

Michelle Arnot, in her book Foot Notes, claims that dancers with hyperextended legs "must develop firm muscle control of the joint in order to keep it stable and avoid a sway-kneed posture."

But why the term hyperextended? Because in hyperextended legs, the ligaments of the knee are long, and the muscles passing over the back of the knee are overstretched. This can affect and upset the whole balance of the body. Children with this type of legs–generally presenting very loose ligaments-will tend to put a lot of weight on their heels and will most of the time present an increased lumbar lordosis. Corrections must be given in order for these students to bring the weight over the front of the foot, pull up their quadriceps muscles at all times, and avoid locking back the knees.

Celia Sparger, in Anatomy and Ballet, says that "the result is disastrous from the point of view of training, since the 'placing' of the body is completely upset, the weight falling on the heels and any pulling up of the thighs increasing the trouble." According to UK osteopath Dr. Margaret Papoutsis, hyperextension can be corrected using a combination of therapeutic exercises and corrective teaching.

"I find that the main difficulty to overcome is the lack of motivation in the dancers themselves," Papoutsis claims, "particularly if previous teachers have encouraged/ordered them to 'pull up their thighs' or 'fully straighten their knees.'"

Dr. Papoutsis says changing such habits can be difficult and physically hard, and that many dancers go back to their old habits when they are tired or bored. She believes that early corrections will be more useful if the dancer has naturally lax ligaments in the knees. In this case, she will need to learn how to correct muscle usage in order to maintain stability for the whole length of her career.

Knock-knees (Genu valgum)

The condition called knock-knees is characterized by an exaggerated slope inward of the lower leg, making it angle outward. In Anatomy and Ballet, Celia Sparger explains that the shape of the pelvis and the position of the thigh are important elements in determining the shape and straightness of the legs. A child with knock-knees, when standing with parallel feet and legs fully stretched will show a gap of about two inches between the heels while the knees will be touching.

A slight degree of knock-knees is generally present in young children up to the age of three, but they should generally straighten out by age five or six. In some cases, however, knock-knees continue or get worse after this age and can be a problem for a future dancer's career. Celia Sparger suggests that knock-knees are generally always accompanied by rolling feet and people with knock-knees are more prone to injuries and knee problems.

Bow legs (Genu varum)

Bow legs cannot be changed, because it is a skeletal condition. It can be frustrating for students wanting to achieve a "particular look," and their training is going to be harder at times. There are basically two types of bow legs. The first is the one where the femur is normal but the tibia is curved outward. In the second type the bowing also involves the thighs and when the feet are together there is a gap between the knees. Students with this type of legs have by nature a restricted amount of turn-out that intreferes with technical accomplishment, besides being not attractive from the aesthetic point of view. Training will not correct the bowing, even after many years of training.

Chapter 3

Types of Feet

This is a really large topic for discussion. In my career as a teacher, I have seen millions of feet—highly arched and flat feet, long and short toes, feet with bunions, flexible and stiff feet . . . All of them are different, and fascinating at the same time. It is very important for teachers and dancers to be able to recognize the different types of feet and to train the dancer accordingly.

We can say that there are two main factors determining feet type:
- The arch, or cou-de-pied in French
- The length of the toes

Based on toe length, we recognize five different types of feet:

Egyptian feet

The big toes are generally the longest, and the rest of the toes are tapered.

Greek feet (Morton's feet)

The second toes are the longest, the big toes shorter than the second, and the other toes are generally tapered.

This type of feet is less stable in relevé (rising from any position to balance on one or both feet). Peter Marshall, physical therapist at the American Ballet Theatre, affirms that dancers presenting this type of feet tend to shift their weight to the inside of the foot, and that relevé in this winged position can cause injury. Shoes should fit the length of the second toe, which is the longest, not the big toe.

Dr. Novella, a consultant with New York City Ballet and the American Ballet Theatre, suggests using padding such as a one-eighth-thick felt or a few layers of moleskin to relieve pain when on pointe and even out the weight. He advises dancers with this type of feet to put small pads under the first, third, fourth, and fifth ball joints but not under the second. Judy Weiss, who has been fitting pointe shoes in New York for over thirty-five years, explains that such feet are very hard to fit. "You have to compensate and fill the box of the shoe with lambswool or other padding," she says.

Peasant (Giselle feet)

This is the ideal feet for pointe. In this type of feet, all the toes are the same length. The shape appears square and gives the dancer an excellent wide base to stand and balance on, on pointe.

Simian feet

This type of feet generally presents a bunion, mostly coming from a genetic predisposition. Dancers with bunion-prone feet should avoid narrow shoes and use a spacer in between the big toe and the second toe for better alignment. Bunion surgery should not be considered by dancers since removing the bunion would result in decreased motion in the joint and difficulty in relevé.

Compressible feet

The compressible feet generally look thin and fine boned. The metatarsal area is usually very compressible with toes that easily overlap.

Compressible feet generally become smaller on pointe. Dancers with this type of feet need to wear slightly tighter shoes or use heel pads.

High-Arched Feet

All dancers long for feet with high arches. In medicine a foot with a very high arch is called pes cavus. Most ballerinas use all sorts of tricks in order to improve the look of their feet. Unfortunately, the natural arch can be only slightly modified, through hard work and constant exercise.

Feet with very high arches are generally soft and flexible and need more careful training than feet with smaller arches. Highly arched feet are also more prone to injury as well as to sickle in or out. They do look beautiful, but they are usually weak because when on pointe, the toes tend to curl under, thus forcing the instep and the forefoot downward and forward from the ankle, which is also generally weak. Esther Juon, pointe shoe fitter and ballet teacher, noticed that dancers with a high insteps or arches have, as a rule, weak feet and a shallower plié. This is because without trying very hard to point their feet, they can still achieve a beautiful look.

Consequently, these dancers don't build very strong feet, and the lumbricles muscles, which are found under the arch of the foot, are not used properly. Drs. Stephen F. Conti, MD, and Yue Shuen Wong, MD believe that "excessive plantar flexion through the midfoot can lead to strain of the dorsal structures of the foot while en pointe." They describe the cavus foot as "relatively stiff and poor at shock absorption," thus more prone to shock injuries ("Foot and Ankle Injuries in the Dancer," Journal of Dance Medicine & Science 5, no. 2 [2001]).

Low- or Medium-Arched Feet

A great percentage of dancers have low- or medium-arched feet. Most of the time, these feet are not as beautiful as feet with high arches, but much stronger and less prone to injury. Through exercise and hard work, the arch can be improved to become more prominent.

Medium-high to low arches often belong to dancers who have strong lumbrical muscles. These dancers work much harder with their feet to get some sort of an arch, and consequently these are the dancers with the "stronger" feet.

Flat Feet

Flat feet, or pes planus, have a deeper plié but are more subject to tendonitis because of their tendency to roll in and their hypermobility. Flat feet are not really suitable for the demands of classical ballet. The debate is, can these students still go on pointe?

Dance physiotherapist Lisa Howell, BPhty, believes there are two types of flat feet.

Anatomically or genetically flat feet

These feet present a flat longitudinal arch from birth.

In this case, the look of the foot on pointe will not be flattering, but pointe work is still possible, as long as the dancer meets all the other requirements necessary to be on pointe.

Flat feet with very mobile ligaments and poor muscular support

These feet generally have a better look but are too weak for safe practice on pointe.

Only a specialized medical professional can determine the true nature of any flat foot.

Feet with Longer Second Toes

Feet with longer second toes can sometimes give the dancer a small amount of trouble when on pointe.

You should always fit the length of your second toes when choosing pointe shoes.

Linda Reid-Lobatto, Grishko professional fitter of Dance Laines Ballet School and Pointe Shoe Fitting Center in Brighton, England, shares her ideas about feet with longer second toes. "I come across this very frequently, and I have never found it to be a problem. Firstly, I usually pop a little toe sock on the end of that toe. I only use tape and toe socks. It's very difficult to explain, but because of the way I fit shoes—tight—the foot is supported around the metatarsal and heads and so moves nowhere. That way, the foot is held in the shoe and does not slip down at all, and the long toe is held firm.

Chapter 4

Taking Care of Your Feet

Five Ways to Make Your Feet Feel Better

Be kind to your feet and they will be kind to you!

Feet are extremely important for a dancer, so you need to take great care of them to make sure they will offer you long and painless years on pointe!

Ballerinas are obsessed with feet, and spend a long part of their career caring for them, working on them, pampering them, and, finally, healing them.

In a recent interview, Royal Ballet artist Darcey Bussel claimed that feet should be as expressive as hands. But in order to be expressive, feet must be, first of all, in good condition.

Most of the time, dancers' feet can be . . . not really pretty to look at, but we have to understand that they are the primary tool for their dancing, and they are exposed to a huge daily demand. George Balanchine said something totally right regarding this subject. "Women who dance have ugly feet. Their feet aren't pretty anymore, but they're professional."

Here we list a few ways to efficiently take care of your feet after a long day of rehearsing on pointe.

- In order to avoid ingrown nails, never cut your nails too short, but nails that are too long can also cause severe pain and bruising.
- In her book On Your Toes, Thalia Mara claims that the skin of the toes and foot should always be kept soft and moisturized. She suggests bathing and drying feet every night and to massage them with Vaseline until it is totally absorbed by the skin. She also advises dancers to put a little Vaseline in the space around the toenails using an orangewood stick in order to prevent calluses between the nail and the skin. Also, according to Mara, the skin at the back of the heels should never become too dry or crack.

  "During the massage," she says, "take hold of each toe individually, pull it and stretch it a little, and move it around. Knead the metatarsal arch with the thumb, particularly around the big-toe joint."
- Esther Juon, in her book Pointe Shoe Secrets, believes that dancers should spend a few minutes after class massaging their big-toe joint. She suggests sitting on the floor, placing one foot across the lap. This simple exercise simply consists of holding the foot with one hand, gently pulling the big toe out in a straight line, and then making slow and graceful circular movements with it. This, according to Esther, should help to relax the ball joint after it has been carrying most of the body's weight during class.

- Soak your feet in warm water and Epsom salt before you go to bed. Use a couple of cups of salt and let your feet soak for fifteen to thirty minutes. This will make your feet feel soothed and relaxed after a day spent dancing.
- Indulge with arnica gel. This homeopathic pain rub, used for centuries, is made with the arnica plant, which grows in the Pacific Northwest. It speeds up the body's natural healing process and reduces inflammation in conditions like plantar fasciitis, internal tissue damage, swelling, and bruising.

Exercises to Strengthen Your Feet and Ankles

Do hundreds of relevés in the first and second position—they are invaluable in strengthening your feet and ankles. Take care to fully stretch your knees while you're up on pointe and lift your weight off your waist.

Battements tendus and battements glissés (dégagés) are also excellent. Anytime you do tendus, remember you do it for your feet; articulate your foot in tendus and glissés pointing hard all the way to the tip of your toes. Also try relevés just from demi-pointe to full-pointe, keeping your weight lifted off the hips. When you get stronger, start relevés from one foot to another, with one leg in cou-de-pied, retiré (side, front, or back) or even in arabesque and attitude.

Thera-Bands (resistance bands) are excellent to work your feet and strengthen them. These elastic bands generally come in three different types of strength: soft, medium, and hard. The color varies according to the band's strength. Use a strong band if your feet are strong or very arched, and use a soft to medium band if you are still building strength in your feet. Here is a simple exercise: Wrap the ball of your foot in the band (keeping the toes inside the band) and start pointing and flexing from the ankle. Then do the same, but using only your toes. The more you pull the band toward you, the stronger you will have to point your feet.

Here is a lot of good advice and a few very useful exercises suggested by Dianne M. Buxton, a graduate from the National Ballet School of Canada, who also taught ballet at the National Ballet School, York University, George Brown College, and Harvard University.

"For ankles, if you are wobbly going up and down in slow relevés, in soft shoes, you are not strong enough to be in pointe shoes. You must check your overall posture, use of the core muscles, turnout, and how your feet rest on the floor when flat. Wobbling can be for many reasons."

According to Buxton, if you get corrections for sickling in and your weight goes toward the outside of your foot, you should do this exercise: Sitting, legs straight, loop the band around your right foot at the metatarsal area. Hold the band ends with your left hand. Pull the foot outward, and you will feel the muscles on the outside of the foot-ankle area working. Pull and hold for ten seconds, ten times. Repeat on the other side.

If you go up onto demi-pointe or pointe and your weight leans onto your big toe, you would loop the band and pull your foot inward, working the muscles on the inside of the foot-ankle area.

Another strengthening exercise is, while sitting with legs straight out in front, to slowly stretch the feet, splaying the toes apart and stretching them long. You can use the Thera-Band around the metatarsal area for resistance, except for one instance. If you have highly mobile ankle joints, repetitive pointing and compressing a pointed position can irritate the back of your ankles. You need to increase strength in the soles of the feet and to control slow rises with no loss of ankle control.

Relaxing the foot muscles is important. You can roll your foot over a tennis ball, or better yet, use a rubber ball that has a little give.

Here's a stretch suggested by Deborah Vogel, dancer, author, and master teacher.

With a soft rubber ball, kneel down on the floor and put the ball under one of your legs, under the shin. Let your weight press into the ball, inch by inch, and it will relax the tibial muscles. Go all the way down to the ankle area, kneading and stretching the muscles.

Then put the ball under the top of the metatarsal area, and pressing into it, you will get a stretch down the top of the foot and over the ankle, increasing the curve of your point.

Jean Nuckey, a vocational examiner at the Royal Academy of Dance, suggests that "simple exercises teaching an articulation of the feet and flexion and extension at the metatarsal arch are correctly executed battements glissés and petits retirés."

Gloria Govrin, former NYCB ballerina and currently running the Dance Institute at Minnesota Dance Theatre suggests, "Point all the way to the tips of your toes, so that there is energy in the foot and you don't just have these appendages hanging at the end."

Dr. Remy Ardizzone, a consultant with San Francisco Ballet, recommends picking up marbles with the toes or putting a towel on the floor and scrunching it toward you.

According to Dr. Chris E. Chung, MD a sports medicine specialist at South Bay Sport & Preventive Medicine Associates Inc. in San Jose, California, this is an excellent exercise to strengthen the muscles of the foot and the ones supporting the arch of the foot. "Building muscles in the foot provides shock absorption. In the long run, increased muscle in the foot helps prevent injury to bone, to muscle, and to joint."

Doing fifteen crunches on each foot for two repetitions per foot is the source of good daily work. According to Kim Gardner, lead dance medicine specialist at South Bay Sports & Preventive Medicine Associates Inc., foot "doming" over a tennis ball is another excellent exercise to reinforce the intrinsic arch muscles. Simply hold the arch over the ball for five seconds at a time and repeat about fifteen times a day. She suggests practicing it with one foot and then with the other.

Gardner, who used to be a professional ballet dancer, describes another exercise called "pushing sand," which is especially good for pre-pointe students. It involves stretching the arch of the foot and the muscles along the sides of the ankle and calf to build and increase ankle stability. Gardner explains that these muscles "attach under the foot like stirrups, but you don't want one pulling up tighter than another. The inner stirrup muscles help avoid pronation while the outer stirrup muscles help avoid supination." She suggests imagining standing in wet sand scooping sand to the side with the sole of the foot. This exercise, according to Gardner, can be practiced in a sitting position, imagining yourself scooping sand toward the center of the body and then pushing it away from the center and toward the outside of the body. It can also be practiced using a Thera-Band.

Chapter 5

Arches

Very High Arches: The Pros and Cons

First of all, let's explain the difference between arches and insteps: the arch is that pronounced curve that we see in the underside of the foot, between the heel and the forefoot, while the instep is the bony structure on top of the foot. So basically, a dancer can have a high arch without much of an instep, or the other way around, or both of these attributes can be found together. In a battement tendu à la seconde seen from the front, we are normally able to see both the arch and the instep. Highly arched feet, pes cavus in medical term, are what all dancers dream of. Some are born with them, and others struggle throughout their career to achieve a higher instep, and some even use tricks to make their arch look bigger.

Nowadays ballet companies tend to prefer dancers with aesthetically beautiful feet, which show a better line on pointe. However, besides the aesthetic look, high arches present a few problems. The mid part of these feet is generally quite rigid, and there is very little shock absorption when landing from jumps. Pes cavus are also very vulnerable to fasciitis, stress fractures, and ligamentous strain.

According to Dr. Thomas Novella, a consultant with New York City Ballet and the American Ballet Theatre, if you have a very arched foot, pointing your foot too much can cause painful pinching in the ankle. If the pointe shoe is rounded, rather than squared off around the top of the block, the dancer will tend to roll too far into pointe. A square shoe instead will give a little "stop" when you get up there.

Jean Nuckey explains that a very high arch may show a beautiful classical line but it can be weak and not easy to train. She believes that dancers with this type of feet might have trouble sustaining their line on pointe, resulting in strain to the ligaments of the foot and ankles and in loss of balance.

"A dancer with a high instep needs the toes to be a little straighter to the floor so she doesn't fall forward," says Suki Schorer, former dancer with Balanchine and now teacher at School of American Ballet.

Joan Lawson writes that dancers with very high insteps are extremely difficult to fit because they generally have weak ankles and arches. "To overcome this problem, most manufacturers can provide a V-vamp, or if the little toe protrudes, a wing block. Both styles help the metatarsal arch to retain its shape and prevent the dancer sinking too far into the block." Lawson also believes that these dancers need to exercise their feet more than all others.

"Many hours of slow, careful strengthening exercises will be needed to overcome the natural tendency to 'roll' either inwards or outwards, instead of maintaining a straight line through the middle of the stretched foot," says Richard Glasstone in his article "Some Thoughts on Pointe Work."

Low-Arched and Flat Feet: Ways to Improve your Arch

This type of feet generally tends to put stress on the muscles supporting the arch so the dancer tends to roll in, which causes strain on the inside of the foot and knee. Flat feet (pes planus), which are often hypermobile and fatigue easily, can absorb shock better than high-arched feet. However, very tight feet might limit the capacity to place the weight properly and prevent the dancer from achieving correct balance. Such feet should be sometimes considered not suitable for pointe work.

According to Suki Schorer, a dancer without much of a natural arch should try to push more over the shoe, but not too far as to lose all the strength.

Flat feet are not ideal for ballet, especially for dancers aiming for a professional career. However, it does not mean that dancers with flat feet cannot enjoy classical ballet or even go on pointe.

Professor Stephen F. Conti describes the flat foot as "one that is ligamentously lax and tends toward pronation. This overworks the plantar flexors and predisposes the dancer to tendinitis, shin splints, and plantar fasciitis."

In my career as a dancer and later as a teacher, I have seen many dancers with very little arch achieving a decent, if not beautiful, "cou de pied" just by working hard and exercising their feet daily.

Always practice your battements tendus and glissés (or dégagés) very carefully, using the floor and articulating the feet through demi-pointe and pointe, and your feet will become stronger and your arch will look better. Remember that even a grand battement starts and finishes like a battement tendu and requires the same attention and footwork. Try to always "shape your foot" when doing battements tendus and battements glissés. Always close with the feeling of "polishing the floor," articulating through the demi and the pointe.

Thera-Bands are also very valuable instruments to strengthen your feet and improve your arches. I always have at least one in my dance bag that I use before performances (before I put on my pointe shoes) or before class to warm up my feet.

Chapter 6

Different Ways of Rising Up to Pointe

In "Some Thoughts on Pointe Work," Richard Glasstone quotes Nora Roche saying "When you relevé, only leave the floor just enough to pass a piece of tissue paper under the foot."

Glasstone continues, saying that there are two different ways of rising up to pointe. "This can be done either with a smooth rise through the foot, or with a very light spring onto a completely stretched foot. In both cases, it is essential to engage the whole leg, ensuring that it is fully braced."

According to the Royal Academy of Dance, a dancer can rise on pointe by performing either a "rise" or a "relevé." Rising on demi or on pointe does not involve any movement of the toes. The movement is achieved by lifting the heels off the floor while the weight is adjusted farther forward. The dancer should feel like pushing the floor away with the feet while pulling forward and upward with the body. Rises are normally taken without the use of plié and can be executed in all the positions. A rise correctly executed should go through the quarter-pointe, the demi-pointe, the three-quarter pointe up to the full-pointe. The descent should be controlled, coming down through the quarters.

The Dictionary of Classical Ballet Terminology, published by the Royal Academy of Dance and compiled by Rhonda Ryman, describes the rise as "an ankle action in which the legs are straight and the heels are released gradually from the floor until the ankle is fully extended" (London: Royal Academy of Dance, 1995).

Relevés are different in quality and always start from a demi-plié or fondu. It is a stronger movement to the full-pointe or position achieved with a slight withdrawing of the dancer's toes toward her center. According to The Foundations of Classical Ballet Technique, published by the Royal Academy of Dance, the toes should be retracted by a distance equal to the length of the toes (London: Royal Academy of Dance, 1997).

The rules regarding the descent change slightly from school to school, but the quality remains the same. The weight of the dancer in relevé position should ideally be over the first three toes, and the descent should be controlled and through the foot, maintaining the turnout and pushing the heels forward. This movement is described by the Dictionary of Classical Ballet Terminology as a leg action which begins in one of the five positions of the feet en demi plié, arrives en pointe/s with a strong and speedy stretch of the legs, and finishes again in one of the five positions of the feet en demi plié.

Part IV

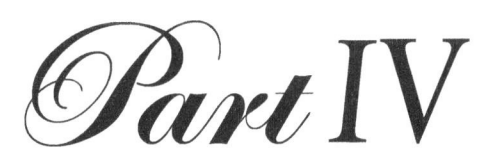

POINTE WORK

Chapter 1

Beginning Pointe Work

Pointe is a French term meaning "tip," "extremity," or "point." It became the term to indicate dancing "on the tips of the toes."

How to approach pointe work at the beginner's level is the responsibility of the teacher. If students are carefully trained in the beginning, they will eventually develop into strong dancers on pointe, but if the initial training was poor or incorrect, it will reflect in their future as dancers. Schools allowing students to go on pointe before they are ready or before the age of eleven do not realize how much damage can be done to children's still-soft bones.

Pointe shoes are not to be used at home as toys, and not without the supervision of a ballet teacher. Many young dancers get injured just by "playing" with their new pointe shoes at home.

According to Dr. Heather Snyder, a well-known podiatrist in Virginia and a member of the International Association for Dance Medicine & Science, not all ballerinas meet the physical requirements for dancing on pointe. She also claims that this is regardless of how many years they have been taking ballet classes or of their age. "Adequate bone, tendon, and ligament structure in the lower extremity (hips, knees, ankles, and feet), as well as maturity level and knowledge and execution of proper ballet technique must all be prerequisites to safely dancing on pointe," she says.

I strongly believe that all exercises in the initial stage of pointe work should only be practiced working with two hands facing the barre. Simple exercises to soften the backs of the shoes but without putting weight on both feet should be attempted in the beginning. Also, smooth rises in parallel position are very good to start, and slowly students can progress by performing them in the first and second positions. Care must be taken, when working in the second position, to use a shortened second: too wide a second could make it really hard for the young dancer to rise on pointe. Lowering down should always be executed with a clear articulation of the foot, going through the three-quarter and demi-pointe and with a feeling of resistance. When the heels come down in first position, they should maintain the turnout at the end of the movement.

Talar Margarosyan, junior school coordinator at the National Ballet of Canada, says that "in order to successfully move in a pointe shoe, you must learn how to use your feet in the shoes. Your feet must be very active, they must easily articulate. So to successfully dance in pointe shoes, you need very strong feet."

Here is how Anna Pavlova described the efforts of going on pointe for the first time.

One of the first problems to be faced by the future dancer is that of learning to keep the equilibrium when standing on the tips of toes. At first a child is unable to stand in that position for even a minute, but gradually sufficient strength is developed in the muscles of the toes to enable a few steps to be taken, uncertainly at first, as in skating, then with more and more assurance, and finally, without any difficulty at all. (Dandré, Anna Pavlova in Art and Life)

Chapter 2

The Right Age to Start Pointe

This is a very large subject for discussion, and opinions vary according to types of training and types of bodies. I personally believe that children should not start pointe work before the age of twelve, exception made for students with extremely strong feet, legs, and backs who train intensively at least three to five days a week. In newborns the bones are soft and not yet formed, and as the child ages, they begin to ossify and become harder. It has been proven that the long bones in our toes usually begin to ossify between the ages of eighteen and fourteen and continue until the age of twenty-one. This is one of the main reasons why young children should not be allowed to wear pointe shoes before at least the age of twelve.

Going on pointe prematurely can result in future injuries to the child's feet, legs, and back. Dr. Heather Snyder, a podiatrist with Albemarle Family Foot and Ankle in Charlottesville, Virginia, believes that some common dance injuries that can occur from beginning pointe training too soon are bunions, hammertoes, neuromas, bursitis, Achilles tendonitis, ankle sprains, and foot fractures. She also stresses that several of these conditions can end a dancer's career and lead to chronic disabilities as an adult.

Physicians like Dr. William Hamilton (consulting orthopedist for New York City Ballet and the American Ballet Theatre) and Dr. David Weiss (orthopedist at the Harkness Dance Center in New York) recommend a minimum of four years of pre-pointe training.

Dr. Hamilton suggests that "the first consideration should be the shape of the student's toes." Hamilton believes the "peasant," or Giselle's foot, is the most suitable for pointe work, while Grecian feet (where the second toe is longer than the first) or Egyptian feet present some handicaps. "However," says Hamilton, "even a poor foot has never prevented anyone from standing on it."

Daniel D. Arnheim, professor at California State University, states that the young student who dances on pointe before her feet are strong enough to maintain the foot, ankle, and leg in proper alignment may develop deformities of the toes, in particular the big toe.

Most teachers and ballet studios agree on age eleven to twelve being the suitable one for starting pointe, but the age range can vary according to the strength, placement, and physical structure of the young dancer. I firmly believe that going on pointe before age eleven can be harmful to the still-soft bones.

Celia Sparger wrote her book Anatomy and Ballet in 1949. In 1970, in the book's fifth edition, she writes,

It cannot be too strongly stressed that pointe work is the end result of slow and gradual training of the whole body, back, hips, thighs, legs, feet, co-ordination of movement and the "placing" of the body, so that the weight is lifted upwards off the feet, with straight knees, perfect balance, with a perfect demi-pointe, and without any tendency on the part of the feet to sickle either in or out or the toes to curl or clutch." (p. 74)

Sparger continues to explain that not all children will be ready to go on pointe at the same age. All will depend, she stresses, on the training they have received and on their body type.

The bones of the tarsus do not ossify and become true bones until the child is at least seven to eight years old, and for many years after they continue to become harder. Before that age, bones are still soft and easily distorted.

Joan Lawson, author of The Teaching of Classical Ballet and many other books on ballet training, says that there are two main factors to consider when placing girls on pointe for the first time. The first is to make sure that their ankles, knees, metatarsals and longitudinal arches are strong enough and that they can control and distribute their weight properly over the center line of balance. The second important factor to consider, according to Lawson, is the choice of the right shoes (p. 120).

The child starting pointe work at age twelve is supposed to have had at least three to four years of serious classical ballet training. Her feet and ankles should be strong, with good control of the trunk and pelvis. I normally start my students with at least six months of pre-pointe classes. During this time frame, I focus on rises, relevés from two feet to two feet and then from two feet to one foot and échappés facing the barre and in the center, with the aim of strengthening their feet and ankles. If the result is satisfactory, students can be fitted for pointe shoes. In the beginning, their pointe class would last only about fifteen minutes, concentrating on slow barre work (rises, relevés, and exercises to soften the back of their shoes). Students should also be taught how to articulate their feet, jump, walk, and run in pointe shoes.

Luana Poggini, a professor at the Accademia Nazionale di Danza in Rome, Italy, stresses how important it is for the student to go through some years of preparatory exercises to reinforce the instep, such to obtain a good muscular development that enables complete control of the body. For this reason, at the Accademia Nazionale di Danza, teachers tend to match the beginning of pointe work to the ten or eleven years' time when the skeletal development is done and where children start acquiring both technical control and alignment of the body.

Dr. Justin Howse, author of Dance Technique and Injury Prevention, states that several famous dancers did not start pointe work until the age of sixteen, but this did not affect their career. We should not forget that the dancer's body will also determine whether pointe work at a later stage will be possible or not. As described in The Progressions of Classical Ballet Technique by the Royal Academy of Dance, "not every female dancer can perform pointe work, even with the best instruction and the most sincere motivations."

Here is a very interesting excerpt from an article entitled "When Can I Go on Pointe?" by Dr. Richard Braver (a sports medicine podiatrist and medical consultant to Capezio):

The dancer must be able to go onto the center floor and be able to relevé and hold passé position and must be able to stand balanced up on the ball of one foot with minimal shaking for a period of 15-30 seconds. She should also be able to walk in the relevé position without problems. When the child is in the barefoot relevé position, the fat pad on the bottom of the toes should be in contact with the ground. The toes should not be curled downward or knuckled. The weight should be centered on the ball of the foot as well as to the bottom of the toes.

Suki Schorer stresses the importance of having the weight between the big toe and the one next to it when on pointe.

Esther Juon, author of Pointe Shoe Secrets and a qualified ballet teacher and pointe fitter in England and New Zealand, affirms that the strength in the muscles of the foot is crucial to pointe work. "The foot," she writes, "does not finish hardening and growing till the age of twenty-one. Therefore, the bones can be deformed when put on pointe." According to Juon, only dancers with strong muscles in the feet and good body placement will be able to avoid bone injuries and painful pointe work.

Lisa Howell, a physical therapist based in Sydney, Australia, and the author of The Perfect Pointe Book, claims that in Australia many dance teachers have each girl individually assessed before letting her go on pointe. They advise every student to undertake an assessment with a special dance physical therapist to assess readiness for pointe work. This will take much off the responsibility of each teacher in deciding who is able to go on pointe and when.

George Balanchine used to say that it takes at least fifteen years to acquire the necessary technique of pointe work!

At Miami City Ballet, as at the School of American Ballet, girls in the advanced levels wear pointe shoes for all classes, both at the barre and in the center. The principle is that their feet must become accustomed to the feeling of a hard shoe as a preparation for the stage. Once students are admitted into the ballet company, they are going to be on pointe all day, so they have to be trained from the beginning.

Jean Nuckey says that "in the context of the Royal Academy of Dance's syllabus, the answer is at Intermediate Foundation level, with its minimum age of eleven" (Nuckey, J. 1997).

According to Nuckey and the RAD system, simple exercises at the barre like slow rises or simple relevés in fifth position and échappés to second are performed, as well as a barre preparatory exercise for courus (or bourrée). The same applies for center work, where all the steps are very basic and their purpose is to build strength for the next level, which is Intermediate and has a much larger pointe section. Nuckey stresses the importance of strength and control of the torso. She also claims that the sides of the body must be stabilized in order for the weight to be correctly held and lifted up and off the feet. According to her, weakness in the upper body causes overarching of the spine, throws the shoulders back, and forces the rib cage forward.

Massimiliano Scacchi, who graduated in classical ballet technique from La Scala in Milan and from the Accademia Nazionale di Danza in Rome, believes that the choice of the right shoes should always be guided by the teacher.

I would like to end this chapter by quoting what Wendy Neale had to say about pointe work in her book Ballet Life Behind the Scenes.

A girl's feet take the most excessive abuse during her years in ballet. From the beginning she must build up calluses for protection when doing pointe work, and there will be very few moments while she is dancing that her feet are not sore."

Chapter 3

Buying the Right Shoes

The First Fitting: A Big Day in a Dancer's Life

Getting fitted for the first pair of pointe shoes is a great event in the life of a dancer. It's always a magic moment to wear pointe shoes for the first time, and the young dancer should make the most out of this unique experience.

The big day has come. You are finally going to buy your first pair of pointe shoes, those "magic slippers" that have been making you dream since you were a child. This day will be part of your ballet memories for a long time, so enjoy it! Once your ballet teacher decides you are ready for pointe, be sure you go to a store where they have a good fitter to help you with the choice of the proper shoes, or have your teacher meet you at the store if possible. The choice of a specialized shop or fitter is crucial to the way your shoes will feel and how you will work on pointe. Ask your teacher if she has a preference in brand and whether or not she is against the use of toe-pads.

Do not buy your first pair of pointe shoes online, especially your first ones! You will eventually be able to do this once you know exactly what type of shoes you want. I generally set up a day for my students' first fitting, and I meet them at the dance boutique and fit them one by one; but unfortunately, this is not always possible. Ballet teachers are busy people, and each student normally goes though ten to twenty pairs of shoes before finding the right one or a compromise at least! It generally takes between thirty and forty-five minutes to fit a student with the first pair of pointe shoes.

Joe Kaplan, vice president of sales and marketing for La Mendola, manufacturers of dance and gymnastic footwear, has been lecturing on the correct fitting of dance shoes for more than twenty years; and according to him, "fitting the first shoe requires that the salesperson knows from experience how to evaluate the feet nature has given the student; be able to determine if the student is in a growth pattern; and be able to see, almost at a glance, how much training the student has had for pointe work."

Make sure you go to a store with an experienced fitter and not just a simple clerk helping you to try on shoes, or just trying to sell shoes! Furthermore, parents' belief that pointe shoes have to fit a little wider to accommodate the child's growth is certainly incorrect. A pointe shoe should be snug and fit like a glove, and there should be no room to grow in. Kaplan stresses again that parents and teachers should "never, never permit a child to wear a shoe with more width than necessary. In ballet shoes, the toes may wiggle a bit, but not in pointe shoes. If the toes look bumpy, however, the shoes are too tight. As for length, no more than one-fourth inch should be allowed for the growing foot." Kaplan further says, "It's dangerous to wear a shoe so wide that it moves when the child tries the shoe on the floor."

According to Freed's pointe shoe fitter Michele Attfield, "A correctly fitted shoe is the safest shoe for the dancer."

Linda Moran, a tutor at Central School of Ballet in London, says that parents should know that there should be no growing space in the shoe. In order to protect toes from the friction, Moran recalls she was putting methylated spirit on her feet, but now she thinks it's better to keep the skin moisturized.

Do not forget to trim your nails a few days before you go to the fitting. If your nails are too long, they are going to dig into the skin and eventually get bruised. Do not cut them the day of the fitting, though, to avoid tenderness and soreness in your toes. Nails should not be too long because they might become ingrown, but not extremely short either; they should at least cover the nail bed. If it's not your first pair of pointe shoes, take with you the type of toe pad you generally use to help with the sizing. Also bring your ballet tights: even the thickness of your tights can affect the size of the shoe. So prepare to be patient and don't feel frustrated if you have to try on so many shoes. The fitter will, first of all, measure your foot with a Brannock device (sometimes one foot is bigger than the other) and evaluate your arch and foot type.

There are a few important things to look at when you get fitted for pointe shoes.

- The length of the vamp is a very important factor in the choice of the right shoes, and it is normally determined by the length of the dancer's toes. If the toes are long, a long vamp should be chosen, while shorter toes will require a shorter vamp. Vamps that are too high will not let the dancer roll up through demi and three-quarter-pointe; however, they should be long enough to cover the top of the toes and prevent them from going too far on pointe.
- The length of the shoe is also very important.

If the shoe is too short and the heel is dropping down, there will be a lot of trouble keeping the shoe on when going on pointe.

If the heel is too high and the drawstring sits where the Achilles tendon joints into the heel and actually digs into it, the dancer could experience a lot of tension and inflammation, and eventually Achilles tendonitis.

Pointe shoes are not going to feel like regular shoes, so it is normal to experience some discomfort at first. Pointe shoes have to be harder to give proper support when a dancer is on pointe. Carol Beevers of the Shoe Room at the National Ballet School of Canada and fitter for thirty-five years stresses that shoes require expert fitting, since "every pair of feet differs from every other."

She suggests making an appointment with a qualified fitter, or buying educational videos, such as Patricia Barker's On Pointe Shoes. Beevers also suggests reading informative books and articles about pointe shoes. "The first fitting should be an enjoyable experience, and such an exciting time for the dancer!"

Beevers encourages parents to take videos and photos. It should not be underestimated that feet change shape with age, work, or injuries; this is why it is important to frequently check the fit of pointe shoes. "It's just about getting a fitter to spend time with a dancer and asking the dancer what she needs from a shoe, and where her problems lie, and then working together."

Professional British fitter Linda Reid Lobatto agrees that different tries are necessary in order to find the right shoes. "I often make dancers try all sorts of things before we find the perfect shoe," she claims. "Trial and error is the only way it works, and feedback, lots of feedback!"

In order to check the length of the shoe, the fitter will have you do a demi-plié in the second position; if the size is correct, you should feel the tips of your toes just touching the edge of the shoe. If the toes are already knuckling, it is a sign that the shoe is too short, and you would develop a lot of blisters across the top of your toes. While you're standing flat, the first and fifth toes should be just touching the sides of the shoe. You can also check the length of the shoe on a pointe position: stand in first position and go up on pointe with one foot without putting any weight or pressure on it. There should be a pinch of fabric left at the back of your heel if the size is right. If there is no fabric at all left, it means the shoe is too short. Also check if the sole of the shoe is in alignment with the foot. The foot on pointe is slightly shorter than when on the ground, but if when on pointe the sole extends beyond the foot, then the shoe is too long.

- The width of the shoe is generally determined by the width of the dancer's foot in the metatarsal area. The shoe should hug the foot firmly and smoothly, without gapping or squeezing.

It is recommended to also try and stand in fifth position, on pointe, and do some relevés to discover eventual gaps or movement in the vamp. The final choice should be lightweight and flexible shoes, to continue the strengthening of the feet as only pointe work can do. The shank should follow the dancer's arch and "hit the arch" rather than lie at a distance from the instep in order to provide the dancer with adequate support.

Lynn Wallis, artistic director of the Royal Academy of Dance, emphasizes the fact that "students need to be taught how to prepare their shoes, to darn the toes and stitch the ribbons so that they may be correctly tied and kept securely in place."

Before ribbons or elastics are sewn onto the shoes, be sure the shoes have your teacher's approval. Bring your new pointe shoes to class and ask your teacher to check their length, width, and type. Joan Lawson, in The Teaching of Classical Ballet, claims that "even if teachers do not fit themselves, they should be able to explain why a shoe is not right."

Brands of Pointe Shoes and Eternal Debates

I often hear my students or their parents asking me, "What brand of pointe shoe should we buy? Do you have any preference?" It is sometimes hard to make them understand that all the brands are more or less equally good; it is just a matter of finding shoes suitable to the student's feet and strength. Only through personal experience can a dancer assess which shoes are the best for her type of feet. The shape and strength of the feet, the level of training are factors that will affect her choice of type of shoes. It sometimes takes years to find the "ideal" pointe shoes, and some dancers have to opt for custom-made shoes in order to finally have what they want. The huge selection of brands and types of pointe shoes on the market nowadays makes the choice easy and hard at the same time. Soft, medium, or hard shanks, elastic or traditional drawstrings, wide or narrow boxes and platforms, V-shaped or round vamps, cardboard or fiber shanks, traditional materials or polymers—all these can be extremely confusing. Without the guidance of an expert, finding the right shoes could be a long and stressful procedure.

"All I want to see when I fit is a beautiful line, where the shoe and the leg become one, not a leg with a shoe," claims UK-based pointe shoe fitter Linda Reid-Lobatto. The choice of the right shoe should always be dictated by the anatomical features of the foot. In my experience as a ballet teacher, I advise beginners to buy shoes with a soft and flexible shank to have an easy roll up and down from the pointe. I believe beginners should start pointe work with "traditional" pointe shoes; by traditional I mean shoes with a cardboard shank that molds to their feet when working, and I would leave the more technology-advanced shoes (like Gaynor Minden) for later on in their training.

"There are shoes sold today," says Joe Kaplan, "that would not have passed over the counter years ago. The best shoes still have handmade boxes. Some manufacturers, however, use preformed plastic boxes that do not permit the dancer to rise through quarter-, half-, or three-quarter-pointe until the final spring to the tip because of the rigidity of the box."

After a few years of practice, the dancer should start knowing what she wants from her shoes. What she likes and what she doesn't. This is very important when shopping for a new pair of pointe shoes. If you still do not know what is best for you, always rely on your teacher's advice, unless you are fitted by a professional fitter, like Mary Carpenter, Judy Weiss, or Zoe Cleland in New York; Michele Attfield of Freed in London; or Carol Beevers of the Toronto National Ballet School.

Hard or Soft Shoes, Very Tight or Loose

George Balanchine used to say that "a pointe shoe has to be like an elephant's trunk: strong and yet flexible and soft!"

It all depends on your type and shape of foot and on the strength you have. Pointe shoes should fit snugly and not allow for growth. The toes should be able to spread slightly sideways and the tips should just feel the block when the dancer is standing with flat feet in first, second, or fifth position.

Never buy shoes that are too big thinking, I will be able to wear them next year. Your feet always change, and generally your second pair of shoes will need to be different—different size, width, or shank—and your pointe shoes will have to fit you snugly, like a glove on your foot. Anaïs Chalendard, first soloist at the English National Ballet, claims that "the preparation of the shoe is one thing, but of course the basic shape of the shoe is extremely important." Chalendard believes that it takes ballerinas years and years to find the perfect shoes and is convinced that pointe shoes have to look and feel like gloves. "They have to look like they are part of the leg," she says. "It is just a thin extension. So I prepare my pointe shoes with this in mind."

There are different opinions about buying hard or soft shoes for the first time. Some teachers want a soft shoe to enable the student to roll through the demi- and three-quarter pointe and build strength in the foot; other teachers prefer a hard shoe to have students build strength by working against the shoe. I prefer to have my students fitted with a light and flexible shoe. I like to see them being able to articulate the foot in their new shoes and going up on pointe without struggling too much. I don't like seeing the shoe commanding the foot; in my opinion, it should be the other way around. Once feet and ankles get stronger, the second pair of pointe shoes can be harder. At this point, students are able to make the decision themselves.

After six months of pointe work, they already know what they want from their shoes; and when they get fitted a second time, they know what to expect based on their first experience. I sometimes encourage them to write their impressions on a piece of paper, so they will not forget when they go for the second fitting.

Young students outgrow their pointe shoes very quickly, and will probably need at least three pairs in a school year. Christine Jeannin, in Chaussons de Pointes, reports that in a specialized medical magazine, a doctor claimed that shoes become too small in less than four months in children aged eight to twelve, in less than five months for children aged twelve to fifteen and every six months between the age of fifteen and twenty. The same also applies to pointe shoes, of course. I had cases of students wearing their pointe shoes just a couple of times and already complaining that they were too small. Of course, parents might be upset because of the high cost of pointe shoes, but it is important to stress that wearing shoes that are too small can severely damage the feet. Ballet is an expensive activity, and all these factors have to be taken into account before the child gets enrolled into a ballet programme.

In the article "Evolution of the Pointe," Freed's pointe shoe expert Michele Attfield gives her enlightened opinion on how heavy a pointe shoe should be.

There is no correct weight for a pointe shoe, because this is exactly what you need at the time you need it. At Freed, the integrity of the block is very important, and the fact that they can be worked through to become softer is essential to the dancer. If a dancer is doing pas de deux or 32 fouettés, then they'll need a strong new shoe with a firm block. However, if they're running down the stairs in Romeo and Juliet or dancing one of the white acts either in Swan Lake or Giselle, then they'll need a soft, silent shoe that has been worked through. (Dancing Times [July 2003], p. 27)

Professional Grishko fitter Linda Reid Lobatto believes that harder shanks can sometimes be easier to work with. "In my experience I have found that the softer the shoe the more core stability you need, the harder the shank the more support it gives a dancer."

Lobatto states that too many dancers think that a soft shoe is an easier shoe to dance in, but it is not always true. "When you look at the platforms, you will see that the satin is not completely worn away, showing that the dancer is not over the box, and proving she does not have the strength to wear a softer shoe and push the feet, but because the roll through breaks quicker, she thinks the shoe is easier to work in. With a harder shank, you have to work your foot correctly.

You also build the strength in the feet required for pointe work, making it easier . . . softer shoes sadly mean softer feet. Of course this all has to do with the way I think, and I am not saying it is 100 percent correct. I just work with what I am presented with and what I see."

Chapter 4

Toe-Pads
Which Are the Best Toe Pads to Buy? Are They Really Necessary?

This is really a very personal choice. I am not a fan of toe pads, and I believe that the more you put into the shoe, the less you are going to feel the floor and dance properly. I generally advise my students to try Bunheads Ouch Pouch Jr.; the pads seem to work very well, can be washed, last for a very long time, and do not take up much room in the shoe.

Remember that toe pads generally add one half to one inch size to your foot, so it is crucial to get fitted wearing the toe pads you are going to use.

Many students are now switching to new brands of gel toe pads like Gellows. They feel wonderful to the touch, but I think they are too thick, especially under the metatarsals, where you actually do not need any padding and should feel the floor. I tried them myself, and after trimming off a small section underneath the toes, they felt much better, allowing me more freedom and better contact with the floor. The Royal Academy of Dance, in The Progressions of Classical Ballet Technique, stresses that "while some padding may be necessary, the sensitivity of the toes and the ball of the foot should not be disturbed by anything too thick or constricting."

I find gel pads very bulky, but some dancers seem to like them. I prefer the ones that are made of very thin gel on the outside and fabric on the inside, like Danztech ToeSavers Skinny Dips toe pads. The best thing would be getting used to no toe pads at all. It might sound painful, and it is in the beginning, but only without toe pads can you build the calluses you need to be able to work without pain or blisters.

RAD examiner Michele Pearson discourages her students from using toe pads. She believes it is best just taping the toes and using a little bit of tissue paper around them to protect the skin. As an alternative, she thinks very thin gel pads are good for students wanting more protection.

Some dancers rub surgical alcohol on their toes every night (not if you have blisters!) to make the skin harder and eventually less prone to blisters. Lisa Howell, physiotherapist and author of The Perfect Pointe, suggests using a foam inner insole (very cheap from any drugstore) and create a little pad to sit up in the front of the shoe to create some cushioning, so that the toes are not pressing directly on the canvas.

If you have a problem with a single toe, you can wrap it in different ways and with different materials. You can use a dishcloth cut into fine strips, just wrapping it individually around one toe and then securing it with a fine piece of masking tape. It is very effective, and it also helps absorb the sweat. If there is some rubbing, it will rub through the layers of the cloth rather than cause friction on the toe itself. Lamb's wool is excellent for protecting the toes against blisters; it does not take too much volume inside the shoe and is not made with plastic or chemicals.

Ballet teacher Joanne Morscher kindly gave the "recipe" for comfortable homemade lamb's-wool toe pads.

How to Make a Toe Pad with Saran Wrap

Supplies: Saran Wrap and Lamb's wool

1. First roll out and remove a 4- to 6-inch-long piece of Saran Wrap from its container.
2. Fold the Saran Wrap until you make a square piece that will fit comfortably over and cover all your toes.
3. Remove the Saran Wrap after checking the fit.
4. Place a small amount of pulled lamb's wool over your toes, covering just the tips and nail beds. You can adjust the amount of lamb's wool for your comfort.
5. Place the Saran Wrap over the lamb's wool.
6. Put your pointe shoes on.

Addendum:

1. Any type of Saran Wrap will suffice.
2. You do not need to tape or glue together the Saran Wrap and the lamb's wool. Eventually, the Saran Wrap will break down to a very light floaty substance. Many dancers will remove the lamb's wool when the Saran Wrap breaks down. The time it takes for the Saran Wrap to break down varies from dancer to dancer. It depends on the usage, amount of sweat, and whether the dancer is wearing tights or barefoot.
3. You can wear the Saran Wrap toe pad without lamb's wool.

What is most exciting about this toe pad option for dancers is that the lightness and thinness of the toe pad allows for a beautiful feel of the shoe, while offering comfort.

Chapter 5

Fitting Help from Grishko Pointe Shoe Expert Judy Weiss

This chapter is intended to be a guide for pointe shoe retailers or dance boutiques that are not familiar with the fitting of pointe shoes.

Judy believes that the most important thing is getting the right size and style for the customer's foot. Once that is done, the fitter should explain how the foot should feel inside the shoe.

- All the toes should be totally flat. They should feel the end of the shoe. The toes should not be pushed back or crossed over.
- When on pointe, the foot should not fall down into the box. A wide second position demi plié is a good test. This is the longest the foot will be. It should lie flat in this position.
- The shoe should fit like a glove without being too tight. The snugger the shoe, the more support it will give. There might be some discomfort, but never any pain."

Ballet stores should keep a file of each dancer they fit, in order to facilitate future fittings. Here is some information that should be kept on file for each fitting:

- Name of the student, address, and telephone number
- Age, height, and weight
- Type of foot (narrow, wide, square, compressible, tapered toes, longer second or first toe, etc.)
- Particular problems like bunions or other
- Type of arch (low, medium, high)
- Regular shoe size, specifying if one foot is longer or wider
- Brand of pointe shoes she was fitted with, including size, width, model, vamp, eventual maker

The above information will help the fitter in finding new suitable shoes, or just refit the dancer with the same shoes, maybe just altering size or width.

Chapter 6

Teachers' Guidelines: Step-by-Step on How to Check the Fit of a Pointe Shoe

The importance of a student's readiness to be on pointe will never be stressed enough. If a young dancer is not physically ready, as discussed in previous chapters, the result can only be disastrous for the child's health. Teachers should never allow a student on pointe just to "please the parents," "make the child happy," or because some other student bought pointe shoes. The young dancer's safety is the responsibility of each educator, as well as injuries brought about by poor or careless teaching.

When a beginner student buys a new pair of pointe shoes, she generally brings them to class, so that the teacher can check the fit and approve them before sewing the ribbons on.

This check is crucial: if the store did not fit the dancer properly, it is up to the teacher to detect what is wrong with the shoes and give suggestions about a different size, width, vamp length, shank strength, or brand. Ballet teachers are not supposed to be fitters, but they should be able to tell if the shoe fits right or not. This will save the parents a lot of money: if the shoe does not fit and has not been used yet, it can still be returned and exchanged with another brand, type, size, or width.

Here are step-by-step directions on what to check for:

1. Look at the dancer's feet; check for width, length of toes and eventual bunions or bunionette. Have the student wear the shoe and look at the foot flat on the floor in a demi-plié position: the shoe should feel like it's "hugging" the toes, but with no pressure. Toes should not be overlapping or cramping.
2. Have the student fully point one foot without putting weight on it. Check the length: there should be a little extra pinch of fabric at the heel.
3. Control the width: if the sole twists away from the foot, it means the shoe is too narrow.
4. Check for the length of the vamp. This is generally determined by the length of the dancer's toes. Students with high insteps should generally be fitted with longer vamps.

It's important to hold a class where students are taught how to sew ribbons and elastics. During that class, teachers will also explain how to take care of feet and how to prolong the life of the pointe shoes, as well as how to break them in.

Kyra Nichols, former NYCB ballerina, stresses the importance of pointe work in class. She thinks students do not use their pointe shoes long enough; according to her, the fifteen minutes at the end of each class are definitely not sufficient to build strength, especially for students aiming for a professional career. She remembers that Mr. Balanchine wanted his dancers to wear pointe shoes all the time, even if they were not going on pointe, so that the shoes would become "part of the feet." The role of the ballet teacher is of the utmost importance in the choice of a student's pointe shoes, and dancers should always listen to their teacher's advice.

Chapter 7

Bringing the Shoes Home

Pointe shoes are the jewels of the body. Something you cannot explain can be expressed on pointe.
—George Balanchine

This is such a special event! You can't wait to take your brand-new shiny shoes out of the box and try them on. I still love the smell of new pointe shoes, and it always brings back memories of stage performances, or just happy days of class and rehearsals. Trying your new shoes on is fine, but do not play with them at home. Without the supervision of your teacher, you might injure yourself. Also, do not sew the ribbons or make any other alterations to the shoes before you get them approved by your ballet mistress. If the shoes get dirty, it will be impossible to change them in case they do not fit or are not approved. One thing you can do at home is just walk around the house wearing your new pointe shoes. You will get accustomed to the new feeling of the hard blocks, and they will mold your feet.

How to Prepare Your Pointe Shoes
Ballet Stars Share Their Secrets

Every ballet teacher should give students very precise guidelines on how to prepare their first pointe shoes. The shiny pair of pointe shoes is finally in the young dancer's hands, but does she know what to do with them? A special introductory class is necessary, where the teacher explains to both students and parents the necessary steps to "prepare" the shoes and get more familiar with them. Professional ballerinas can sometimes be hard on their pointe shoes, but this is only because they know exactly what they want from them. This knowledge can only be acquired after years of practice. Let us have a look and see what some famous ballerinas do to their shoes.

Christie Sciturro of Miami City Ballet uses paper towels to protect her toes. She wraps 4 or 5 layers over her toes before she puts her pointe shoes on.

Darcey Bussel, former Royal Ballet principal, applies plasters on three toes in order to prevent blisters and puts a gel cushion on her big toes to protect her nails.

Caroline Duprot, Corps de Ballet member at American Ballet Theatre, reports that preparing her shoes takes her more than an hour. She starts by cutting the satin at the ends of the shoes; then she darns them and sews on ribbons and elastics. After this, she squeezes the shoes and cuts the soles with a Stanley knife, and then cuts some parts of the insoles. Tamara Oughtred, first soloist at Birmingham Royal Ballet, uses forty-five minutes to prepare her shoes, which includes darning the tips to enlarge the platforms and sewing elastics on the backs. After her workload increased when she became a first soloist, she just sews the ribbons on and shaves the soles with a Stanley knife. Now her shoes are ready in five minutes!

Adrienne Schulte, first artist with English National Ballet, used to wear her shoes really hard, so she basically just sewed on ribbons and elastics, put some superglue in the tips, made them a bit malleable in her hands for a minute or so, and then used them in class or straight on during a performance. Now she prefers wearing her shoes a bit softer, which means she needs to bend them a lot more with her hands and wear them down rather well in class and rehearsals before going onstage.

Elizabeth Harrod, first artist with the Royal Ballet, wears Gaynor Mindens. Since Gaynors are much harder to sew than a regular pair of Freeds (the material and satin are tougher), she usually ends up with cuts and blisters on her fingers! First she unpicks the drawstring on the heel; she believes this stops it from digging in. She reveals that this procedure is quite long and usually takes about an hour per pair. She then sews on her ribbons, followed by crossed elastic from where the ribbons are sewn to the back of her heels. She is happy that Gaynor Mindens last for a long time; otherwise, she would have to come up with a much quicker system!

Anjuli Hudson, artist at English National Ballet, wears handmade shoes by Freed, which molds really well to the shape of her feet even after she has worn them only once. She starts by darning the ends of her shoes to make them last longer. She sews the ribbons on, and she burns the ends with a lighter so they don't fray. When the backs of the shoes begin to get soft, she uses shellac to harden them. She usually prepares about three or four pairs at the same time so she doesn't wear them out too quickly.

Tracy Jones, dancer with Corella Ballet in Spain, starts by cutting the backs so that they are three-quarters in length. She then darns an outer ring on the tips of the shoes and then sews on elastics and ribbons. She breaks her shoes in over a few classes and bangs them against concrete so as to eliminate the sound.

Ruth Brill, artist at ENB, wears custom-made Freed pointe shoes. She starts by darning around the edges of the blocks; then she sews on elastic and ribbons, puts the shellac inside, bends the backs, and squashes the fronts.

Alexandra Fern, dancer at Ballet Theatre UK, practices at least five minutes of relevés from half-pointe to full-pointe before wearing her new shoes in class. She also executes slow rises in parallel and in first position to have the shoes mold to her feet.

Rym Kechacha, apprentice with Northern Ballet Theatre, starts by cutting the satin off the toes, to give a better grip on the floor; and then she sews ribbons and elastic on each shoe. Then she'll take the top nails out of the shanks so that the shoes bend with her feet and work the soles with her hands to make them a bit more flexible. It takes about forty-five minutes for a pair. Then she uses shellac on the inside of the soles to make them keep their shape longer.

Adela Ramirez, first soloist with English National Ballet, first cuts half of the soles. Second, she sews the elastics and ribbons on; and third, she sticks a piece of tape in each sole. Afterward, she sews the front of the pointe shoes to have more balance; and to finish, she puts some glue inside the pointe shoes.

Hayley Forskitt, artist at the Royal Ballet, starts with sewing the elastic and ribbons on, and then she darns around the edge of the tip of the shoe to get a better platform. With a Stanley knife, she evens out the sole of the shoe to make it easier to balance in adage. Then she stands on the vamp of the shoe to soften it before she tries them on. It usually takes about forty minutes a pair.

Celisa Diuana, artist with London's Royal Ballet, likes to cut the satin off the ends of her pointe shoes after sewing on her ribbons and elastics. Afterward she shaves and scratches the outer soles with a Stanley knife. It takes her half an hour. If she doesn't have the time to do all that, she says, she can still dance in them, but it doesn't feel as good!

Tempe Ostergren of Boston Ballet wears Freed Wing Block. She usually softens the blocks by standing on them, and afterward she continues bending the shanks. She also hammers the shanks right at the balls of the feet to have them mold to her demi-pointe. She also glues the shanks with Jet Glue. Tempe likes to customize her shoes according to what she will dance. She prefers harder shoes for pas de deux, where there is a lot of balancing and turning.

Anne Marie Melendez of Ballet Austin wears Sansha 202S. She doesn't wear any type of padding; she just tapes three toes on each foot and uses a jelly toe for protection if she has a bruised or cracked nail. She removes the nails from the shanks of the shoes in order to achieve more flexibility, and she cuts part of the shanks then softens them using rubbing alcohol. She removes the satin from the tips using a pair of scissors, and she steps on the boxes to make them wider and softer.

Nadia Iozzo of Kansas City Ballet wears Freed, Maker J. She wears masking tape on most of her toes and thin lamb's-wool toe pads. Sometimes she uses spacers to avoid having corns. She flattens the box by standing on it, and although her shoes already come with a three-quarter shank, she cuts it down even further.

My Personal Experience with Pointe Shoes
How I Prepare them for Class or Performance

Preparing my pointe shoes is a long procedure, but I love doing it. My dancing will largely depend on this, and I try to do it as meticulously as possible.

My first pointe shoes were Porselli. Of course, since I am Italian! I cannot say that I loved them, but I was very young and with very little experience, so I followed my teacher's advice. In the years that followed, I tried other brands and types, in my continuous quest for something better. I tried Freed but did not feel comfortable with them at the time; I did not like the block, and my toes were always sore. Then I switched to Gamba Turning Pointe (this type of shoes has been discontinued), which I liked and found very good for my feet.

Once these shoes disappeared, totally by chance, I found my dream shoes, my magic slippers, in a small dance boutique in Nice, France. The brand was Contin-Souza, and I just couldn't believe my eyes when I tried them on and found they were exactly the way they should have been. The shoes were ready for performance just as they were! The only thing you needed to do was sew the ribbons on, and that was all! The best thing about Contin Souza pointe shoes was that they were extremely light and flexible. They would mold to your arches perfectly and would not need any breaking-in at all. The outer soles were different from the traditional ones; I recall they looked more like they were made of a resin material, but very soft and pliable. I think even the box must have been made of a different material, maybe some sort of plastic. Unfortunately, none of these shoes survived in order for experts to analyze the way they were made. The magic shoes disappeared a few years later. The factory went out of business, and this was the end of my dream shoes. In the years to follow, I used Repetto Bayadère 207 LM, XX size 17 (or 37½). They were comfortable, but still did not make my feet look as pretty as I wanted them to look. I tried Bloch Alphas, but they did not really work for me, their vamp was too high. Then I found Gamba 93, which are the shoes that I have been wearing for many years. My size in Gamba is 4 1/2, while in Freed it's 4 1/4 –4 and a heel pin. I love Gamba shoes, and I wear them for class and performance. The shanks are made of cardboard and mold to the feet when the shoes warm up, but then return to their original shape when they cool down. The block is really comfortable, and I could wear them even without toe pads and straight out of the box. Their particular type of block keeps me up and well lifted, and there is no pain or rubbing. I also tried Gamba 97, which has three-quarter shanks, but I did not like them as much as the 93, so I switched back to the 93s.

I recently tried new shoes made by Grishko called Miracle. They are wonderful pointe shoes, really light and very soft and cushioned on the inside. They have a full shank, but it is a very pliable one that gives the foot a lot of flexibility even without breaking the shoes in. The only bad thing about them is that they are on the market only for a limited edition, so I don't want to become addicted to these shoes because I know that one day—probably soon—they will disappear!

I was lucky enough to be fitted by Michele Attfield at Freed's shop in London. I found wonderful shoes called Classic Pro that I immediately liked. They are shoes ready for the stage. They have very wide platforms and graduated flexible shanks that push you forward when you're on pointe. They are pointe shoes worth trying, beautiful to look at, very good for taking pictures and for performance if there is no time for breaking-in. If I wear Classic Pro, I insist to have Maker Key, since this cobbler makes really lightweight shoes. In order to have my Classic Pro last more than two or three rehearsals, I pour Jet Glue inside the blocks and let them dry overnight. This procedure extends their life and re-hardens the blocks.

Ushi Nagar recently custom-made shoes for me, to my requirements. He is my shoemaker now, and the shoes he crafts for me are totally made to my specifications. Graded shank for more flexibility, round vamp, extra room in the right shoe to accommodate my bunion, special anti-slip outer sole, lowered-down sides and heels, wide platforms for more balance, and, as he promises, the lightest shoes you could ever find. If I am in London, Ushi makes my shoes while

I am there; otherwise he sends them through the mail. It is a totally different feeling to have custom-made shoes; they really fit your feet, and you can ask anything you want. You know that they were specifically made for your feet and they are not just another pair of stock shoes waiting on a shelf. It doesn't take much to prepare your shoes then, because they have already been made to your specifications.

I use thin toe pads that are gel on the outside and fabric on the inside, but sometimes I prefer lamb's wool or other types of toe pads. I generally tend to get a blister on the outside of my right big toe, so I tape it before I start rehearsing. If I feel I am getting a blister, or my skin is getting thinner and red in a certain spot, I rub it with a stick called Blister Block, which is excellent. I also use a toe separator between my big toe and the second toe to align my bunion.

Preparing my shoes is a ritual I just love. Dancers should take great care in preparing their shoes for performance. The quality of their dancing will largely depend on how their pointe shoes feel on their feet, and if the shoes do not fit well, this will greatly affect the quality of their dancing. I always want to have at least two to three pairs of pointe shoes prepared and modified to my feet's requirements before I go onstage. If one pair breaks or gets too soft, I want to have at least another pair in my dressing room or backstage. This is what I do with stock shoes: I start by cutting a portion of the shank in order to make my shoes more flexible and show more of my arch. I lift the sock liner and remove the tacks from the back of the heel.

After that I use my Exacto knife to cut the shank until I reach the degree of flexibility that I want. Then I glue the sock liner back in place and let it dry. I use Freed's pointe shoe Ruffer, and I scrape the outer sole in order to make it less slippery, especially if I have to perform. Sometimes stage floors can be extremely slippery, and rosin is not always allowed, so I make sure that the back of my shoe will allow me to have a good amount of traction with the floor. Before I sew the ribbons on, I start marking my shoes where my arch is and where I need more support. I like to sew them right where my foot breaks, so I put a pencil mark right at the spot where I want my ribbons. I also decide which is my right shoe and my left shoe and mark the backs with "R" or "L." Since my arches do not break the same way, I always like to wear the right in the right and the left in the left. This way my ribbons fit perfectly and I don't have either too much ribbon or not enough, like I would if I wore them interchangeably. I like to sew my ribbons in a whole piece, down at the bottom of the sock liner. (See "Ways of Sewing Ribbons" for a complete description of this procedure.) This way they really hold the whole foot and not just the sides.

In order to do this, I just cut the whole piece of ribbon into two equal parts. Then I wear the shoe and I put my foot on top of the ribbon and pull up the sides. I pin the ribbon at the bottom of the shoe in order to be able to sew it without having it slip away. I use a Bunheads stitch kit for my sewing. The thread is so exceptional; I can sew a pair of shoes in less than ten minutes! It's thick and waxed, so I am sure my stitches will never break. I sew my ribbons slightly angled forward toward the block with straight (horizontal) rows of stitches from side to side, going up toward the drawstring without sewing into it. I like to have at least seven or eight rows of stitches, and I want them to look nicely sewn and straight. Even if nobody sees the inside of the shoe, I don't want it to look messy, or to know it is messy.

Once the ribbons are sewn, I tie my shoes on and cut the excess ribbon off. I generally leave only a maximum of three inches of extra ribbon, and I cut out the rest. After this I burn the edges to be sure my ribbons won't fray. I personally like Freed's ribbons. They are very soft and have a good grip against my leg.

I would never let anyone sew ribbons on my shoes! This is a special ritual for me, and I want to be the only one responsible if a problem occurs or if the shoe doesn't fit well because of the placement of the ribbons. I do not need to alter my shoes now because they are custom-made and they come exactly as I want them.

If I use stock shoes, I lower down the sides with a few stitches, in order to see more of my foot when I dance. It takes only a few minutes, but the result is worth the time spent sewing. I generally do not lower the sides too much, though, because the shoe tends to slip off my heel if it goes down too low. The sides should be just low enough to make my arch look a little bit better and show more of it.

I do not do much to the block. I like to have a soft shank and a hard block. I only soften the sides of the block by gently pressing them down with my hands. I don't like to "destroy" my shoes. I know how much work goes into them, and I try to be as kind to them as possible. I just make them a little bit kinder to my foot, but only if I wear stock shoes. And this happens when my bespoke shoes cannot arrive on time from London.

I always darn my pointe shoes, even the custom-made ones. This is a long procedure (about an hour each shoe!), but it gives them a beautiful finish and makes them last much longer. It also makes them less slippery onstage and gives them a better grip on the floor and a wider base to balance on. I use a special crochet thread imported from England and a curved needle. I remove the satin from the platform and start darning from underneath the block, at the bottom right-hand corner, and start darning in a circle, anticlockwise. I put the needle through the satin (on the pleats), and pull through, right at the base of the platform. I repeat the same procedure about one-half centimeter to the right, but this time leaving the needle halfway. I take the thread hanging from the previous stitch and wrap it tightly and clockwise around the needle. I hold the thread down with my left thumb as I pull the needle through. It creates a sort of loop around the stitch I have just sewn. I continue with the same technique all around the edge of the platform. This is the easiest type of darning, excellent if I do not have time to darn all the tips. The result is more or less the same, and it still looks good. Please see Part V, "Darning Your Shoes: A Long but Rewarding Procedure."

I generally sew elastic around my ankles to prevent the heels from slipping down. I always measure how stretchy I want my elastics to be before I cut to the right size and start sewing. I sew it on the outside of the shoe, near each side of the back seams, making a loop around my ankle and reaching the other side of it, right by the other back seam. Sewing elastics on the outside prevents friction on my Achilles' heel, and if sewn properly, it doesn't look messy. I prefer one-inch elastic; I don't want it to be too thick or showy onstage. The color should match my ribbons, so I choose a light pink or beige elastic that I generally order in a big roll from England.

I use calamine lotion to cover the shine of my shoes during performances. I rub the lotion on the whole shoes and ribbons using a cottonball, and immediately after, I stuff the shoes with newspaper and put them into a plastic bag, so the shoes keep their original shape instead of shrinking. One of my ballet teachers used to say the pointe shoes need to "age" once you buy them. She believed that the glue and the different components of the shoes need a certain time to "settle down" before the shoes can be worn. So her advice to us students was to hang our new shoes in a ventilated place and let them "age" for at least a week after purchasing them.

One of the last procedures before my shoes are ready is pulling the drawstring tightly until the shoe conforms perfectly to my foot. I tie the drawstring in two knots and cut the excess off. I generally do not buy shoes with an elastic drawstring because it makes it very difficult to sew the ribbons on. It also creates a funny, wrinkled look on the shoes! Since I use many pairs of pointe shoes at a time, especially for performances and rehearsals, I like to give a name to them, so I can recognize the pairs I like the most. Sometimes I just write underneath them "good," "very good," "not so good," "Sugar Plum Fairy," "Pas de Deux," "White Swan," and so forth.

When I perform, I always have at least three pairs of pointe shoes in my dressing room. I normally use two different pairs when I dance a full-length ballet, plus I want to have a spare pair just in case something happens. Carla Fracci, the world–famous Italian ballerina, always used to have an extra pair of shoes in the wings, in case of an emergency!

For partnering, I generally prefer harder shoes, especially if there are a lot of pirouettes and balances. Ballets like Sleeping Beauty or Swan Lake (black swan) require hard shoes, due to the large amount of balances and pirouettes; while for ballets like Napoli, Giselle Act II, or White Swan, I wear softer shoes, which are better for jumping and achieving softer and noise-free landings.

I tie my ribbons in the traditional way, starting with the inside one and finishing with a knot at the inside of my ankle. I roll the excess very meticulously and tuck it in into the crossing. Once I've tied my ribbons on, I spray them with hairspray "strong hold" to prevent them from coming undone while I am dancing. I clean my shoes (if they have time to get dirty) with rubbing alcohol on a cottonball, but I do not insist too much on the block because alcohol makes it softer.

My pointe shoes are very important to me. The way they look, the way they feel—they are an important part of me, an extension of my feet. They affect my dancing and the way I feel onstage. In a way, they represent the image of the dancer I am, and they have to look as perfect and professional as possible. When I teach, I dedicate a lot of time inspecting my students' shoes and giving them guidelines on how to make their shoes look or feel better. I always ask them what they like and what they don't like and try to solve their problems, which are most of the times very simple ones. Students should be aware of the importance of a well-fitted and carefully prepared pair of pointe shoes, especially before they go onstage. Carefully prepared pointe shoes are also an indication of good training and reflect the image of a professional school.

Is There a Right or Left in Pointe Shoes?
Are You Supposed to Always Wear Them on the Same Foot?

There is no right or left in pointe shoes, and since they are handmade, all pairs are slightly different.

Some dancers mark their shoes with "R" and "L" and always wear them on the same foot; others prefer to wear them interchangeably, although this will affect the length of the ribbons. In cases where one foot is much stronger than the other, it is best to switch the right and left shoes, to prevent one shoe from being really worn out while the other is still in good condition.

Esther Juon, in Pointe Shoe Secrets, stresses the importance of putting on the shoe with the foot in a straight line instead of twisted, in order to achieve proper alignment when on pointe. Some dancers believe that switching shoes might make your feet look sickled, since the shoe will take the shape of either the right or the left foot.

In my own experience, I believe that wearing a shoe always on the same foot is the best option, as each shoe molds to the shape of each foot, and the correct length of the ribbons can be calculated. In case both feet are totally identical, the issue does not really exist, and shoes can be worn interchangeably; however, the length of the ribbons could still be a problem.

Chapter 8

Ribbons and Elastics
How to Sew Them On and the Best Ways to Tie Your Ribbons

Choosing suitable ribbons and elastic is an important part in the preparation of your pointe shoes. There are endless types of ribbons and elastics on the market, and sometimes choosing can be really hard.

Ballet stores generally supply ribbons free of charge with the purchase of the shoes, and certain shoes already come with their ribbons. This does not mean that you will be totally satisfied, and most of the time, you will use different ribbons.

Ribbons

Most dancers spend half of their free time sewing: ribbons, elastics, and sometimes mending their tights; even boys have to know how to sew their elastics. It is a special ritual, very important and time consuming. Pointe shoes generally come with ribbons, or they are provided by the store where you buy the shoes. If you are not satisfied with the ribbons available at the dance boutique, you can buy your own, either online or at the dance store, paying them extra. You can find polyester, nylon, and satin ribbons, single or double faced.

Ribbons normally have two sides: one is shiny, and the other is dull. The non-shiny side should be in direct contact with the leg for more traction, while the shiny side will face the outside. I generally use a 1" (2.5 cm) wide ribbon.

When I was a ballet student and a dancer later on, I liked the grosgrain ribbons. They are easy to find in Europe, but not very popular in the United States. Grosgrain is not as shiny as satin, but has much more grip on tights, and is less prone to coming undone.

Bryony Brynd, former principal with the Royal Ballet, shared with me that she used to sew her ribbons to her tights for performances. She suggests "folding the ribbon down and tucking it up."

Many ballerinas, like the Italian Elisabetta Terabust, use rosin on the tips of their ribbons to prevent the knot from becoming untied.

I think most students underestimate the importance of well-sewn ribbons and most of the time do not do the sewing themselves. It should be stressed how essential this procedure is, since it largely affects the way the shoe feels and "stays" on the foot. I would never imagine someone else sewing my ribbons for me; it is something totally personal, and no one else but the dancer herself knows how to do it the right way.

Keri Gorman--pointe shoe specialist; owner of Spotlight Dancewear in Lewisville, Texas; and co-owner of Suffolk Pointe USA--believes that every ribbon placement can help the shoe mold to the foot and "make the instep look bigger." Instead of using the well-known system of folding down the back of the shoe to determine ribbon placement, Gorman suggests to tendu devant, and therefore mark the shoe at the center of the curve of the foot.

The length of the ribbons also depends on the circumference of the ankle.

Moira McCormack, head physiotherapist for the Royal Ballet in London and ex-principal dancer with the Sadler's Wells Royal Ballet, suggests that "the knot should be tied on the inside of the ankle, in the soft depression behind the anklebone." McCormack says it is only there that the knot can be tucked away comfortably and nowhere else would it be invisible enough. She also explains that the ribbon attached to the inside of the shoe has to be slightly longer than the other since it has to go around more.

When sewing the ribbons, remember to keep the stitches into the lining and do not sew through the satin. If you see your stitches on the other side of the shoe, it means you went too deep inside! Never angle your ribbons back, but slightly forward toward the front of the shoe in order to allow more movement when the ankle flexes.

Patricia Barker, former principal with Pacific Northwest Ballet, likes to sew elastics and ribbons together on the front section.

She folds the edge of the ribbon twice over, and she makes a little casing into the ribbons for the elastic to go in. She sews her shoes in a crisscross fashion. "I like to see as much of my foot and my arch as possible," she says. "Sewing elastics and ribbons together makes it look like a classically sewn shoe," continues Barker, "and nobody knows that I have a lot of elastic there, helping my shoe to stay on."

Megan Fairchild, principal at New York City Ballet, uses crochet thread to sew on her ribbons. Before she goes onstage, she sews a couple of stitches (like a big X) in the knot of the ribbon to tuck the ends to be totally sure her ribbons will not come undone.

In Suzanne Farrell's autobiography, she reveals that she always used twenty-nine stitches to sew on her ribbons. Why twenty-nine? The stairs at the School of American Ballet had twenty-nine steps, that's why!

Once the ribbons are sewn on and trimmed at the right size—remember to cut them at an angle—don't forget to burn the edges (using a match or a lighter) to avoid fraying. With the edges burned, the threads will melt together, thus preventing unraveling. Another way of doing it is by painting the edges of the ribbons with clear nail polish. Wider ribbons offer more support, especially in the case of dancers with big ankles. The color should match the color of the shoe's satin. I personally like Freed's ribbons: they are very light colored and have a particular good grip on the dancer's leg; they are also extremely soft to the touch and perfectly adhere to the leg. I also highly recommend Bloch Elastorib; this ribbon has an elasticated section, and it has been created to reduce pressure on the Achilles tendon.

Always keep an old ribbon to use as a length sample; this will spare you time when you're preparing new ones. You can also recycle ribbons from other pointe shoes that you do not use anymore. Make sure you handwash them in mild soap and iron them, and they'll look like new!

Elastics

In my opinion, elastics should be used only if strictly necessary, but not as a routine.

Moira McCormack suggests that extra elastics are often used to compensate for ill-fitting shoes, or shoes that are too hard, whose heels constantly slip off.

There are many ways of sewing elastics, and I believe that they should always be personalized. There is no standard way to do it since all feet are different and you want to have your elastics exactly where you need more support. Some dancers crisscross their elastics across the instep, some sew them around the ankle, other ballerinas use them to keep the heel from slipping down and sew them at the back of the heel, other dancers like to have them across the vamp, and some sew elastics into their ribbons to have more elasticity at ankle level.

As Moira McCormack stresses, tight elastics across the front of the ankle should be avoided. They would cause constriction over the extensor tendons and block blood circulation. Crystal Brothers, dancer at Ballet Memphis, likes to crisscross two pieces of one-inch-wide elastic. She places one end at her heel and one end at her arch. In order to avoid tendonitis, she sews a good inch of elastic into each ribbon to make it give and conform to the movement. This way she can achieve a better plié and have more flexibility at ankle level.

As a general rule, you never sew elastics on the inside of the shoe: the stitches might bruise your tendons, so you always want to sew elastics on the outside. No one will notice it from a distance!

You can also sew a wide piece of elastic across the vamp for added support if you have weak ankles or a strong arch. It should not be too tight, however, or it could prevent the blood from flowing properly. If the elastic is placed across the top of the foot, I suggest using wide elastic. If the elastic is to be sewn on the heel of the shoe, then you will need thinner elastic, between 3/8" to 5/8" wide. Always keep a piece of old elastic to use as a length sample; this will save you time in preparing a new pair. Do not forget that elastic stretches, so you have to stretch it when you measure it before you sew it.

RAD examiner Michele Pearson thinks elastics sewn around the ankle (sewed on either side of the back seam) can be a lifesaver, keeping the shoe on the foot during performances, in case the ribbons would come loose.

For better results, try to choose elastics matching the color of your pointe shoes, and do not forget that even the edges of the elastics have to be burned.

Here are a few ways to sew elastics:

- Criss cross across the instep
- Across the vamp
- As a loop at the back of the heel if the shoe slips down

Which Is the Best Way to Tie the Ribbons?

There are two ways to tie ribbons. Both ways are correct, it's just a matter of what you feel more comfortable with. Do not tie your ribbons sitting down on the floor; you need to kneel on one leg with the other leg bent in front of you, with the other foot flat and fully flexed on the floor. This way you are sure that your ribbons are not tied too tightly, leaving your ankle more freedom to move.

1. Always start with the ribbon toward the inside of your foot.

Draw the inner ribbon in front of your foot, wrap it all the way back and back to the front in a straight line, and hold it there with one hand.

Take the outer ribbon and cross it on top of the other, making an X in front of your ankle.

Wrap all the way to the back and all the way to the front, right on top of the first ribbon, then tie a knot on the inside of your ankle. Carefully fold the excess ribbon by rolling it in toward the shoe.

Tuck the excess underneath the ribbon, either from the top or from underneath it.

2. Cross both ribbons in front of the instep, wrap them around the foot and bring them back. Bring the outside ribbon across the Achilles tendon to meet the ribbon on the outside of the foot and tie a knot between the inside anklebone and the Achilles tendon. Fold and tuck the excess ribbon from the top (some dancers do it the other way around) under the ribbons wrapped around the ankle.

Chapter 9

Padding

Padding in general is not a good idea. Some teachers are even against toe pads. It is true that the more you fill the shoe with padding, the less you are going to feel your foot and the floor. Your foot will eventually go numb if there is too much padding. Some dancers do not use padding in their shoes. Dame Margot Fonteyn used to say that she liked to "feel the floor" when on pointe.

Joe Kaplan makes no allowances for padding into the shoe—lamb's wool, toe pads, heel grips, or socks. "You're not fitting the shoe," he says. "You're fitting whatever you stuffed into it. Feet will toughen up. If you pad to avoid friction, the shoe has not been properly fitted, and the foot cannot work through the pleats."

Personally, and as a ballet teacher, I allow my students to use some type of thin toe pads (Ouch Pouch Jr., for example)—lamb's wool or the new type of toe pads that are thin gel on the outside and soft fabric on the inside. I believe that a dancer's first experience on pointe should be something special and not necessarily associated with excruciating pain. I check my beginner students' feet after class, and if they start having blisters, they are not allowed to go on pointe until the blisters have healed.

Nowadays there are so many types of toe pads, and some of them are a real blessing because they can help reduce some of the pain and pressure, without making the dancer feel too padded. When I was a student, toe pads did not exist, and we used cotton or paper, or nothing at all.

When you put too much padding, the foot is unable to tell when the shoes are broken, or if the correct level of support is lost. Also, you will not be able to feel the floor, and this is very important when you dance. If there is room for padding in a pointe shoe, then the pointe shoe is almost certainly too big; so if you are planning on using toe pads, you have to buy your shoes half a size, or even one size, bigger. I don't particularly like gel or foam pads—they are too bulky and can take up over a size's space in the shoe. I prefer to use lamb's wool or Bunheads Ouch Pouch. You can also individually tape your toes with surgical tape or with special ballet tape sold online or at your local dance store.

There are many types of padding available on the trade:

1. Lamb's wool

    It is generally sold in a one-ounce bag at any dance store or online. This is the most common and widely known padding that dancers wear. Wool has wonderful properties—the fibers breathe naturally, absorb and take moisture away. It's natural and healthy, it doesn't get dirty, and you can reuse the pads endless times. It is very "cushiony" to the skin and doesn't cause blisters. It is also more hygienic than toe pads. Carrie Jensen, dancer at American Ballet Theatre, wears loose lamb's wool because "I can form-fit it around my toes." Unlike toe pads, whose shape cannot be altered, lamb's wool gives the dancer more choice in shaping the padding where she really needs it.

2. Toe pads

    Toe pads are the most common type of padding between dancers and students. There is a great variety of toe pads on the market, from gel to silicone, fabric to nylon; they all offer some comfort in the toe area and relief from blisters.

    However, wearing toe pad affects the size of your shoe by at least a half size, so always be sure you get fitted with the toe pads you are going to wear. Gel toe pads can take up to a size in space, and jelly or silicone pads are generally very thick and take a lot of space inside the shoe. I believe the thinner the better, so if you really want to use this type of toe pads, you should trim them underneath so that you will still be able to feel the floor. Heather Ogden, principal at the National Ballet of Canada, prefers toe pads over lamb's wool or paper towels, since you do not need to arrange them as you would do with lamb's wool. She wears toe pads made of light foam.

    Don't forget that toe pads need to be washed at least every two to three months, and yes, even toe pads have a life span, so try to allow at least two pairs of toe pads per school year, and more if you dance professionally.

3. Paper towels

    Tempe Ostergren of Boston Ballet likes to use paper towels to protect her toes. "It's quick and convenient. And it's consistent, because you always start with a fresh sheet."

4. Socks

5. Paper towels, toilet paper

Chapter 10

Softening Pointe Shoes and Break-in Techniques

How to Make Pointe Shoes Feel More Flexible in 8 Steps

There are hundreds of ways to soften pointe shoes. Every dancer develops a secret ritual to perform with each new pair of pointe shoes. However, some systems are very extreme and reduce the life span of the shoe, so I do not advise anything too radical. Here are some:

- Using a hammer to make them softer
- Shutting them indoors
- Jumping on them
- Putting them in the oven

Here is what you can do without damaging your shoe:

- Delicately bending the soles back and forth a few times and wearing your pointe shoes at the barre while doing rises, relevés, and échappés. A couple of times should be enough to soften the shoes and have them mold to your feet. Some dancers wear them at home and just walk around with them to have them conform to their feet.
- Other dancers rub the block and the wings with alcohol or slightly dampen the front of the shoes by spraying it with water. Then they wear the shoes for a few minutes, walking or performing rises or relevés to have them conform to their feet.

Anjuli Hudson, dancer with English National Ballet, says that her custom-made Freed shoes mold well to her feet after she had worn them just once.

Freed pointe shoes

If you are wearing Freed pointe shoes, remember that they are entirely made with natural ingredients, and therefore they are more delicate than other brands. Freed pointe shoes need very little breaking-in, if anything at all. Check out my interview of Freed's pointe shoe expert Michele Attfield, where she describes in detail how to take care of Freed pointe shoes. Break-in systems can sometimes vary according to the brand of shoes and the paste they are made of.

Traditional paste shoes like Freed, Gamba, Repetto, Capezio, and Bloch do not need much breaking-in. They are made of a special paste that automatically molds to the feet when it gets warm. Any other extreme way used to soften them would reduce their life span by at least 50 percent.

High-technology pointe shoes like Gaynor Minden come already prearched and can be molded by heating the soles with a blow-dryer. For more details, see the next chapter, "Breaking-in Techniques."

Physiotherapist Lisa Howell, in her book The Perfect Pointe, describes an interesting and easy way to soften the back of the shoes:

1. Turn the satin of the heel out, as much as you can to allow you to see the sole.
2. Slide your foot into the shoe (wearing your usual toe pads or any other protection).
3. Place your foot en pointe and press down a little, without putting all your weight on it.
4. Put your finger inside the shoe and find the spot where your arch ends and your heel begins.
5. Turn your finger over and find the same spot on your shoe.
6. Take your foot off the shoe and gently, pushing on the floor, bend the back down to this point
7. The remaining part of the shank should still be straight and the shoe should bend and conform to your arch.

Most dancers cut portions of the shank in order to achieve more flexibility and show a better line of their feet.

Other ballerinas use a pair of pliers to remove the nails from the shank, in order for the shoe to mold with the foot. There are many shoes on the market already offering a ¾ shank, but some dancers still need to adjust the length of the insole to their own tastes by cutting it down even shorter. Make sure you do not cut it too short or you will lose all the support provided by the shank.

Different Break-in Techniques

The way you will break-in your new pointe shoes will largely depend on the brand and the paste they are made of. Always check with the manufacturer or with your fitter if there are special guidelines about the breaking-in of the shoe, in order to obtain good results without damaging the shoe permanently.

This is why we should divide pointe shoes in three categories:

- Traditional paste pointe shoes (otherwise called English paste pointe shoes)
- Modern paste pointe shoes
- High-technology or new-material pointe shoes.

The first category includes brands of shoes such as Gamba, Freed, Bloch, Capezio, Repetto, Suffolk, Bob Martin's Innovation, Grishko, and Ushi Nagar.

Anna Blackwell, an apprentice with Northern Ballet Theatre, has her own special ritual to prepare her pointe shoes: she stands on them to flatten them a little, bends them, and pours superglue into the blocks. She sometimes shaves the soles of the shoes, so they have less of a ridge. She sews ribbons and elastics on, and if the shoes are looking a little worn, she darns the platforms to try to make them last longer.

Bloch Break-in Technique A

This technique is to be used with the following types of Bloch pointe shoes:

S0131L Serenade and S0131S Serenade Strong
S0105L Aspiration
S0130L Sonata (three-quarter shank)
S0132L Suprima and S0132S Suprima Strong

A little extra time needs to be taken to break in these shoe types. They are made with a harder paste than shoes requiring Technique B, and are therefore susceptible to "snapping" if treated roughly at first. Once broken in correctly, they have a long life span. Doing barre is the best way to break in a pointe shoe. The shoe needs to be prepared for barre in advance, by gently softening the shank and the box by hand. Concentrate on the demi-pointe area of the shank, being careful not to crush the box. Then work your way up to the heel, gently massaging the shank until it is at a point where tendu and relevé to demi-pointe is comfortable. Softening the box is not always necessary and is left up to the individual dancer. If softening is necessary, then concentrate on gently softening the sides of the box by using your fingers. Lots of dancers stand on the top of the box in order to soften and widen it. We advise that if you stand on the box, you need to concentrate the pressure on either side of the box center. This is important because the top centre of the box is the weakest point and prone to damage if stood on.

Once the shoes are ready for barre, one to three barres will be a sufficient time to shape them to your feet. At this point, the shoes will be evenly softened, with no weak points resulting from an incorrect breaking-in technique.

Bloch Break-in Technique B

This technique is to be used with the following types of Bloch pointe shoes:

S0101L Synergy three-quarter shank
S0111L BPS (Bloch's Professional Shoes)
S0104L Alpha
S0168L Signature Rehearsal and S0168S Signature Rehearsal Strong
S0100L Synergy Full Shank

Bloch shoes are made from a paste that is designed to soften with moisture or perspiration. Follow all steps in break-in technique A. After working at the barre two or three times, the shoes will become moist and shape themselves to the dancer's feet. Once the shoes have broken-in to your liking, allow it to dry thoroughly for twenty-four to forty-eight hours. When the shoes have totally dried, they will have molded in the shape of the dancer's feet. At this point, it is possible to apply a hardener such as Jet Glue or lacquer sizing to the inside of the block and shank. This will not only harden the shoes in their current shapes, but it will also keep any more moisture from entering the shoes. So you are left with strong shoes, molded in the shape of the individual dancer's feet on the inside, and leaving a quiet exterior.

Break-in System
The Break-in Process

This process is a real ritual for most ballerinas. It can take hours of patient and careful work to sew ribbons and elastics, cut the shanks, darn the platforms, scrape and roughen the soles, soften and sometimes mattifying the satin. At the end of this long procedure, the result is a new pair of personalized shoes ready for class or a performance. Every dancer uses a different system when preparing her pointe shoes and even ballerinas ordering custom-made shoes will sometimes still need to make changes and alterations.

Toni Bentley, a former dancer with New York City Ballet, says that a brand-new pair of pointe shoes presents itself to us as an enemy with a will of its own that must be tamed. "With the combined application of door hinges, hammer, pliers, scissors, razor blade, rubbing alcohol, warm water, and muscle power," says Bentley," we literally bend, rip, stretch, wet, flatten new shoes out of their hard immobility into a quieter, more passive casing for our feet."

Chapter 11

How to Take Care of Pointe Shoes

This is a very important subject: taking good care of your pointe shoes will save you money and will make your feet look better onstage.

Here are many things you can do to keep your shoes nice and clean, and to prolong their life! First of all, pointe shoes should be kept free from stain. If they get very dirty, a light-colored Pan-Cake or calamine lotion can be used to cover the marks. Dirt and dust can also be removed just by gently brushing a nailbrush along the grain of the satin. I used to clean my pointe shoes with rubbing alcohol, and that works fairly well, although this contributes to the melting of the glue in the block. Calamine lotion is also a good option and works as well. (See directions for getting pointe shoes ready for performance). Ballet is based on discipline and grooming, and your shoes reflect your approach to your work, and even your self-esteem and respect for your teacher. Pointe shoes should never look messy or dirty.

One of the most important things to remember is that your shoes need to dry after class. After practice, never put your shoes with wet toe pads inside your dance bag and forget them there until the next lesson. This is for a very simple reason: your feet sweat a lot during pointe work, and all the moisture gets into the shoes. If you do not allow your shoes to dry, all that moisture will make the box incredibly soft and reduce your shoes' life span.

Mesh bags are a wonderful invention: thanks to their little holes, they allow the shoes to dry until your next class. Before mesh bags existed (or if you do not wish to buy one), dancers used to stuff the inside of the shoe with paper—or tissue paper—wrapped in plastic. You should do this immediately after class; then hang the shoes in a ventilated place and let them dry for at least twenty-four hours. Also keep ribbons tidy and clean. If you use the same pair of shoes for several months, you will probably need to change the ribbons, or at least wash them. Do not forget to always burn the edges to avoid fraying and a "messy look." Darn the tips of your shoes—if you are good at sewing—for a perfect finish; otherwise cut the satin off the tip. "I do loads of darning," says Ksenia Ovsyanick of English National Ballet, "so that every inch of the shoe fits my foot perfectly."

Do not leave fragments of frayed satin on the edge of the shoe platform. This would make the shoe slippery and look very untidy. Maintenance of pointe shoes include the use of shellac (Jet Glue is another option), which is a clear varnish normally used for sealing wood. It can be bought from most dance suppliers. Poured into blocks that have become too soft, it will dry out and harden the shoe to prolong its life.

Here is what Joe Kaplan suggests you do to make your shoes last longer: "When your perfect shoes no longer look presentable onstage, line the inside of the box with shellac or Fabulon, a hardening liquid made by Pratt & Lambert and available in any hardware store. Cut the loose threads on the tip of the shoe and darn it again. Use powder or cream stick on the outside of the box to restore color. If there are nails in the shank, remove them and slip out the shank, replace the lining, and wear the shoes to rehearsals. Every now and again, rise up on pointe in a shoe that can still make your feet stronger."

Life is so much easier now with all the new products available on the market. Patricia Barker, principal at Pacific Northwest Ballet, says: "It's very important to become a part of your shoes and have your shoes become a part of you."

Chapter 12

Some Sample Exercises for the First Week on Pointe

At the barre:

Stepping up on pointe

Facing the barre with feet parallel, place arms on the barre.

Lift and bend the right knee, with a fully pointed foot looking towards the floor. Step up onto pointe with the right foot then step up onto the other foot. Roll down slowly through the three quarter and demi pointe. Repeat 8 times alternating feet.

Facing the barre, in 1st position.

Demi plié in first, roll up to the pointe, stretch knees, lower down in two counts. Repeat 4 times. Then reverse it. Rise, demi plié on pointe, down the heels, stretch the knees. 4 times. Repeat in 2nd position.

Feet together

R foot demi-pointe, pointe, demi-pointe, lower down. Repeat with the same foot. Cross the R foot over and bend the supporting leg so that you push the R foot forward bending the sole, release parallel in front of you slightly off the floor, and brush close in first.

When Can You Safely Start Dancing in the Center?

Students should not begin pointe work in the center unless they have gained strength in their feet, ankles, and backs. I generally have my students spend at least three months working exclusively at the barre doing rises, relevés, échappés, mainly from two feet to two feet. There is no rush in leaving the barre and starting exercises in the center. When the dancer is stronger, center work can be attempted without fear of injury and obtaining better results.

Placing the Foot Correctly on Pointe

When you're standing on pointe, your instep should be fully stretched with your toes forming a perpendicular angle with the floor. Your teacher should always see an imaginary straight line that could be drawn through the hip, knee, and ankle joint though the block of the shoe, or between the second and third toes. By no means should that line get distorted and that alignment lost.

Part V

HOW TO SOLVE PROBLEMS WITH POINTE SHOES
AND HOW TO MODIFY THEM

Chapter 1

What to Do If the Shoe Is Slipping Off the Heel

Do not panic if your heels are slipping down, especially when you roll down for a rise in first, second, or fifth position. The heel of the shoe is probably too high compared to your own heel. I have been seeing more and more students with a very thin heel having a lot of trouble with their pointe shoes. Here are a few things you can do.

- You can sew a little elastic loop at the back of your heel. Choose thin elastic and always sew it on the outside of the shoe. If sewn on the outside, the elastic won't rub against your Achilles tendon and cause damage. Position the elastic on each side of the back seam and sew it using strong thread (like Bunheads) or dental floss. You will then tie your ribbons, crossing them into the loop, and this will prevent your heel from slipping down.
- You can also buy a heel gripper and stick it inside the shoe at the back of your heel; it will create some extra thickness and keep the heel of the shoe in place. My advice is to cut the heel gripper in half and to place the two sections about one-half inch apart, on either side of the back seam, so that it doesn't come directly in contact with your Achilles tendon.
- Rosin is also a very good compromise if you do not like elastics. Rub your heel in the rosin bucket and wear your shoes after this.
- If the heel of the shoe is too high, you can "lift your heel up" by cutting the back part of an insole (they are cheap and you can find them at any drugstore) and placing it in your shoe, under your heel.

Noisy Shoes: 4 Ways to Reduce the Noise

Squeaky Shoes

Pointe shoes that are too noisy can affect the outcome of a show. They can ruin that sensation of lightness so typical of classical ballerinas. Noisy shoes can also be distractive for the audience and take the attention away from the choreography, or even interfere with the music. The great Anna Pavlova used to say that noisy pointe shoes were "a sin"! Landings and running must be kept as quiet as possible; this is why most dancers spend a good amount of time trying to make their shoes less noisy onstage. The way the floor is constructed and the materials used can also play an important role.

Although you can find shoes on the market promising quietness and shock absorption (Gaynor Minden, Grishko Pro Quiet 2007 etc.), there are many ways to make your shoes less noisy.

- Alcohol and water
  Prima Ballerina Gelsey Kirkland wanted her pointe shoes to be totally quiet. In the book Dancer's Shoes by Daniel and Stephanie Sorine (pp. 78-79), Kirkland describes how she would put alcohol around the pleats under the box to take some noise out of the shoe. You can rub the block with alcohol on a cottonball, or lightly spray the block with water, taking care not to get the shoe too wet.
- Darning
  Darning the platform will reduce the noise without ruining the shoe.
- Scraping the soles
  Former Royal Ballet principal Darcey Bussel used a Stanley knife to scrape the back of her soles in order to make her shoes less slippery, and less noisy.
- Hammering
  You can gently hammer the block with a wooden mallet, but remember that hammering could reduce the life span of your shoe if you do it too hard.

Another issue a dancer might deal with is squeaky shoes. It is very common for pointe shoes to squeak sometimes. I often have to deal with students coming to me and complaining that their shoes squeak! It is quite normal, and it does not mean that the shoe is coming apart. This is due to a movement of the shank, which is situated between the outer and the inner soles; and there is no need to worry.

How to Make Shoes Less Slippery

Shoes can sometimes be slippery, especially if you're dancing on wooden floors or on stages not specifically designed for ballet.

There are many ways to reduce slipping, sometimes just by creating more friction.

I generally use Freed Pointe Shoe Ruffer (see description in "Pointe Shoe Accessories") or a shoe scraper to rough up the bottom of my shoes and increase traction. You can also use a pair of scissors or an Exacto knife to score the outer sole with diagonal or wedge-shaped lines.

Rosin is, of course, the most traditional way of making shoes (and floors!) less slippery. Be sure you do not use too much, since rosin packs up under your shoes, and these deposits will eventually make your shoes more slippery.

Darning the platform is another excellent way to reduce slipping and increase traction. It takes quite a while, but the results are rewarding (see "Darning").

The Solution to Baggy Ribbons

Baggy ribbons can be due to different factors. This problem is mainly related to the way the ribbons were sewn or tied.

- The ribbons are sewn too far backward.
- The ribbons are sewn too far forward.
- The ribbons were not angled forward before being sewn.

- The ribbons are not tied tight enough.

In Part IV, you will find useful information on how to sew ribbons and elastics and on how to tie your ribbons properly.

Different Ways to Protect the Platform

The easiest way to protect the platforms of your pointe shoes is to cut the satin off the tips and underneath, where the pleats are. It is best to wear the shoes a couple of times before you start cutting. You can eventually cut a piece of moleskin in the shape of your platform and stick it on for a better finish and more grip on the floor. Ready-made suede or crochet toecaps are available in dance stores, online, and through the major companies like Freed or Capezio. Place the rounded edge of the toecap on the platform, then fold the remaining part under the shoe and over the pleats. Use superglue or any other strong type of glue available, and make sure the toecap is perfectly glued, so that it will not make you trip while dancing.

However, the best and most traditional way is to darn the shoe. (See below for instructions on how to darn a pointe shoe.) If you want to save hours of darning, Porselli makes the right accessory for you: it's called Point2Point, and it is a self-adhesive ready-darned pointe shoe protector. You can find it online through www.dancewear.co.uk.

Darning Your Shoe: A Long but Rewarding Procedure

What is darning? Darning is a very classic way of finishing your shoes. It is a long but very useful procedure that makes your shoes last longer and makes dancing easier. In the past, all dancers, especially Russian dancers at the Vaganova School in St. Petersburg, used to darn their shoes and would spend most of their free time doing this. Here are some of the benefits of darning:

- It protects the satin and prevents it from fraying.
- It improves grip on slippery floors.
- It creates wider platforms and provides the dancer with increased balance.
- It gives the shoes a nicer look.
- It allows you to modify the shape of the platforms.

Crystal Brothers, dancer at Memphis Ballet, uses what's left after she has tied and cut the drawstring to darn the tip of the shoe. It gives her a flatter, more solid platform and helps the shoe hold its shape. According to Brothers, you have to sew deep up to the canvas; and although it takes a long time, it's worth it at the end.

I will pass on the precious tips given by former Australian ballerina and Cecchetti examiner and teacher Valrene Tweedie (sadly, deceased in 2008) on how to darn a pointe shoe.

To darn, hold the shoe upside down with the toe facing you. Start on tip of the block, nearest the underneath of the shoe and darn toward the top of the shoe. Make two or three long stitches across the width of the tip, then sew across this base, using buttonhole or blanket stitch. If you find it hard to get the needle through the satin, spit on the satin and the needle will go0 through, it's amazing what the spit will do! When the tip of the block is covered, repeat the same from the edge of the darning underneath the shoe to the start of the sole. ("Make your Shoes Last," Dance Australia [February/March 1994])

Ms. Tweedie, who danced side by side with ballerinas like Anna Pavlova and Irina Baronova, recalls that during Pavlova's time, dancers used to darn all around the sole, anywhere the shoe would be in contact with the floor, not only the tip.

How to Darn a Shoe

There are several darning techniques, and you might get a little discouraged if you are not good at sewing. Anyway, with some practice, you will be able to darn your pointe shoes and get the best out of them.

This is how I darn my pointe shoes: First of all, I use very thick pink cotton yarn and a big, long needle. You might want to use a thimble since the satin is very stiff and you could have trouble pushing the needle through the fabric.

Thread your needle and make a knot at the end of it. Insert the needle at the bottom right part of the platform and pull the thread through. Repeat this operation half an inch (one-half centimeter) over to the right. This time do not pull the thread all the way through. Wrap the thread left from the previous stitch clockwise around the needle and keep it down with your left thumb. It will make a loop around the previous stitch. Continue all around the edge of the tip.

In order to reinforce the darning, pass your thread through the stitches—just under the thread, not under the satin—all around the platform, and pull tight.

This is one of the quickest ways to darn your shoes, if you are short of time. It does not require any particular sewing ability and makes a difference in the way your shoe will feel and work for you.

4 Signs Your Shoe Is Getting Old and Needs to Be Replaced

- The box feels soft
- Sinking at the metatarsal area
- The shank bends too much or feels broken
- The satin on the shoe tip is torn and you can almost see through the shoe

If all of the above signs are present in your shoe, you should stop doing pointe until you buy a new pair of pointe shoes. This does not mean you have to throw your shoes away. You can still de-shank them by removing the nails and the inside shank and wear them in class or during rehearsals. You can also recycle ribbons and elastics for a new pair of pointe shoes. Wash and iron them, and they will be like new!

How to Make Pointe Shoes Last Longer

the Re-hardening Process

Taking good care of your shoes is surely one of the best ways to make them last longer and save money. When pointe shoes start feeling too soft in the block and in the shank, it is a sign that they are "dead" and need to be replaced. However, there are ways to temporarily "revive" the shoe.

Gluing

Glue is very effective for re-hardening dead pointe shoes. It will not make them brand new, but it will certainly give them a few extra hours of practice! Aesha Ash, dancer at Alonzo King's Lines Ballet, says that glue makes her shoes last for at least two more shows. She also uses glue to reinforce the shank inside and out and adds a little bit to the shank just under the arch. You can apply the glue straightaway to the new pointe shoes, or—as some dancers prefer—you can wear them a couple of times to have them mold to your foot before you apply the glue. If you do not have a specific brand of pointe shoe glue (like Jet Glue or Daniel's Glue, for example), even Crazy Glue, Gorilla or any strong glue can be used. For more support in the toe area, pour the glue into the inside of the block (use gloves to avoid getting the glue on your fingers!), move the shoe around to make the glue cover the inside of the platform evenly, and let your shoes dry in a ventilated place for at least a few hours. According to Pamela J. Pribisco, ballet mistress for Les Ballets Trockadero de Monte Carlo, one bottle of Jet Glue can reinforce up to five pairs of pointe shoes. Pribisco also suggests using glue to get more support under the arch by lifting the insole and gluing the shank area.

Fabulon

Another good hardener is Fabulon, a kind of wood varnish similar to shellac generally found at hardware stores, or even at certain dance stores. Let your shoes dry for about thirty-six hours after your last class, and then pour a little amount of Fabulon into the block and smooth it around using a small paintbrush. If you wish the wings to be stiffer, continue brushing the Fabulon up the sides of the box. If you want the wings to remain soft, then stop brushing where the metatarsals bend the block. Apply thin layers and let the shoe dry in between applications. This procedure will re-harden the shoe for one to three more wearings, depending on the amount of pointe work and on the dancer.

Minwax

Another good product is Minwax. Found at any hardware store, Minwax is a wood hardener that works very well to restore the hardness of your blocks. Available in two consistencies; be sure you buy the thinner one. Pour about two tablespoons inside the block and move the shoe around to have the wax coat the inside of the block evenly. Let the shoes dry for a few hours in a ventilated place before wearing them again.

Rotating the shoes

According to some dancers, rotating the shoes is also a key to making them last longer.

Drying

Rule number one: it is extremely important to let your shoes dry between classes. One of the most common mistakes you can make is to put your pointe shoes in the ballet bag straight after class and forget them there until the next lesson or rehearsal. The sweat coming from your foot (often up to half a pint!) when you dance softens the block and shortens the life span of your shoes. At the end of each class, remove any padding from the box; take a plastic bag and stuff it with newspaper or tissue paper. Stuff the bag into the block of your pointe shoes and let them air in a dry place for at least twenty-four hours. This will help your shoes last longer. Try to carry your pointe shoes in a mesh bag, not in your ballet bag.

Darning

Darning the tips of the shoes is also a very good way to make them last longer. (See chapter 7.)

Wearing tights

Do not wear pointe shoes without tights. Tights help absorb some of the moisture when your foot sweats and prevent the moisture from getting directly into the shoe.

In Italy some of my colleagues mix rosin with alcohol, then brush it in each shoe and leave them to dry on a hot radiator. They swore it was prolonging the life of their shoes.

Pan-Caking the Shoes

Many choreographers and teachers like all their dancers' pointe shoes to look alike during performances, so they ask the dancers to "pancacke" their shoes. This procedure mattifies the shoes so that they all look alike and don't reflect the lights. Pan-Caked pointe shoes also blend better with pink ballet tights without showing too many different shades of pink.

There are several products on the market you can use to Pan-Cake your shoes.

- Max Factor Pan-Cake
  To be applied evenly on the shoe and ribbons using a wet makeup sponge.
- Calamine lotion
  It is generally used to soothe the skin after insect bites, and it's found at every drugstore or grocery store or pharmacy. It's a pink liquid that makes shoes pink and look similar to the ballet tights (if the color used is Theatrical or Ballet Pink).
  Just pour some calamine lotion on a cottonball and start rubbing it evenly on the whole shoe, even on ribbons and elastics. Once you have finished, stuff the shoe with paper to prevent shrinking and let dry for at least a couple of hours before wearing it.
- Kryolan Professional Make-Up
- Rosin
  Some dancers rub a little amount of rosin on the top of the shoe in order to take the shine off and tone down the color.

Three-Quartering the Shoe

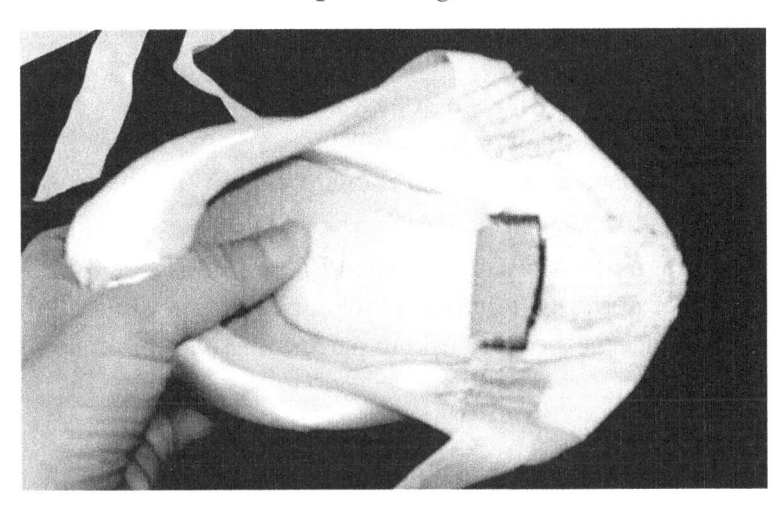

Three-quartering the shoe basically means cutting portions of the shank in order to make the shoe more flexible. How much you cut is entirely up to you and to the degree of flexibility that you wish to obtain.

You can start by cutting just a small part of the shank (the heel portion), and then try how it feels. If you want more flexibility, you can keep cutting a little farther, until you reach the degree of flexibility you want. Just remember that if you cut too much your shoe will lose all the support the shank provides, and you might permanently damage your shoe. If you are not very experienced, you can try at first with an old pair of pointe shoes. Cardboard shanks are easy to cut, while shanks made of other materials like resin will require more sophisticated tools or the help of an adult.

Rosin: One of Dancers' Best Friends!

What Is Rosin?

Rosin is also known as colophony or Greek pitch and is a kind of solid resin obtained from pine tree. It presents itself in the form of crystal-looking tiny rocks of a yellow, semi-transparent color. It is very brittle, and when you smash it with your foot, it breaks into small particles. It is also very sticky, so be careful not to put your hands in it. In all ballet studios, you will always find the traditional "rosin box" in some corner, where ballerinas go and rub their feet in before they start pointe work. It is part of the tradition, and dancers cannot do without it, especially when working on wooden or slippery floors. Pay attention not to overuse rosin because it will create a solid deposit under your shoes and will eventually make them more slippery. If this happens, use a penknife to scrape the excess rosin off the shoes.

Rosin is an invaluable companion and lifesaver for dancers. It also has multiple uses. Slippery floors and stages can ruin a whole performance and can also be the cause for main injuries. This is why rosin is used in order to make floors sticky and create more traction.

Here are some effective ways to use rosin:

- Some dancers put rosin on their tights, on the bottom of the heels, and at the edge of the heels. This allows the shoes not to slip off the heels and allows better use of them.
- If you are trying to get your shoes to look a little bit less shiny, you can rub some rosin onto the satin. Use a cottonball or paper towels.
- Another way to use rosin is to put a little amount on the knot of the shoe ribbons to prevent them from coming undone.

I always carry a package of rosin with me when I perform, especially if I am dancing in a theater where I have never performed before. Floors always tend to be a little slippery, and I don't want to take any chances, especially if I am performing a lot of piqués or pirouettes!

Part VI

BRANDS AND TYPES OF POINTE SHOES

Chapter 1

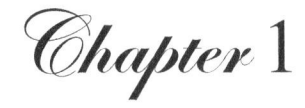

The Pointe Shoe Market

I tried to provide as much information as possible on all the brands of pointe shoes available on the market. The choices are endless, and I am sure that your dream shoes are somewhere out there.

Bloch
1170 Trademark Drive, Suite 112
Reno, NV 89511
Phone: 800-94-BLOCH
Fax: 775-824-2551
www.blochworld.com

Bloch is one of the highest producers of pointe shoes in the world, making more than ten thousand shoes a week. Bloch shoes are manufactured in Thailand.

The founder is Jacob Bloch, who arrived from Europe and settled down in Australia in 1931, starting his handmade-shoes business in his own home. Bloch liked to visit ballet studios, and one day he met a dancer having trouble standing on pointe with her own shoes. He offered to craft a better pair for her. It was back in 1932, and it would mark the beginning of Bloch's career as a shoemaker. His reputation grew quickly, and when foreign ballet companies started to tour Australia, Bloch started making shoes for the dancers. When Colonel De Basil's Monte Carlo Russian Ballet (formerly Ballets Russes) came to Australia, Bloch crafted shoes for Irina Baronova, Tatiana Riabouchinska, Olga Spessiva, and Tamara Toumanova, as well as for the male dancer David Lichine. Today Bloch's company, managed by his grandson David Wilkenfeld Bloch, is one of the largest in the world, producing ballet shoes, leotards, dance accessories, and fashion shoes. David Wilkenfeld, owner of Bloch, recently introduced TMT (Thermo Morph Technology) in some of the pointe shoes. Thanks to the new technology materials, these pointe shoes can be molded to the shape of the dancer's feet just by warming them up for forty seconds with the heat of a blow-dryer. Bloch's last addition to the pointe shoe collection is Amélie, a new shoe created for beginners.

Russian Pointe Shoes by Bloch

These are extra-quiet shoes with shorter vamps compared to most traditional Russian V-vamp shoes.

Balance

This shoe features a wide box to give toes extra room and a wide platform for easy balance, an elastic binding, low-cut sides to show a better arch, a thin outsole, and a heel seam cushion. This particular shoe is also available in Balance European, which is similar but with a more tapered box.

Alpha

This shoe features a three-quarter outer sole, a large platform for balance, and a high-cut vamp. Suitable for advanced students or professionals.

Amelie S0103

This is a beginner shoe offering a graded shank and a wide platform.

Amelie Soft S0102

This shoe is the latest addition to Bloch's pointe shoes. It's a shoe designed with the young beginner dancer in mind. It features a graded shank, a large platform for increased balance, and a softer insole.

Aspiration

Beginner's shoe built with a flexible but supportive shank.

Axis S0190L

This shoe offers a TMT box and shank. It is a tapered shoe built on a curved last, promising quietness, and is suitable for the advanced student/professional dancer.

B Morph

Another shoe built with the TMT technology. It features a very wide platform and block and is suitable for advanced dancers.

Balance ES150

This shoe is suitable for both beginners and advanced students. It has a very wide block to help dancers with a wide forefoot or bunion to spread their toes. It also offers a very wide platform for more balance.

RAD Demi-Pointe S0165

Demi-pointe shoe suitable for RAD vocational exams.

Serenade

This pointe shoe features a narrow heel, a wide platform, and a strong shank, ideal for high arches.

Suprima S0132

This shoe is very well suited for a narrow foot. It offers a very small platform and a tapered box.

Sonata S0130

This very popular shoe has a wide box and a tapered heel and suits both beginners and professionals.

Bob Martin, Innovation

Dance Workshop 2000

Bob Martin wass another cobbler who started learning how to craft pointe shoes at Gamba's. His factory, named Dance Workshop 2000, opened its doors in 1995 and closed in 2010. With over forty years of experience, he created the Innovation pointe shoe to suit the needs of each individual dancer.

> Capezio
> One Campus Road
> Totowa, NJ 07512
> Phone: 800-982-33997
> Fax: 800-522-1222
> www.capeziodance.com
> E-mail: info@balletmakers.com

Salvatore Capezio (1871-1940) was born April 13, 1871, in the town of Muro Lucano, Italy. His father worked as a construction engineer, but Salvatore eventually became a cobbler specializing in dance shoes. Salvatore immigrated to America in 1887, when he was only seventeen years old. In New York, he opened a little cobbler shop on 39th Street and Broadway, near the old Metropolitan Opera House. The name of his store was the Theatrical & Historical Shoemaker.

Salvatore began his new business as a simple cobbler, repairing theatrical shoes for the Met. His life was meant to change the day he made an emergency pair of shoes for the Polish tenor Jean de Reszke. He quickly became a shoemaker, an art that he loved, and started to produce ballet and pointe shoes for the dancers at the Metropolitan House. Capezio's reputation grew, and dancers would regularly stop by his store and order custom-made shoes. He also met an Italian dancer, Angelina Passone, who became his wife. In 1919 the famous Anna Pavlova, while touring the United States, ordered shoes for herself and for her whole company and claimed that Capezio's shoes were the best she had ever tried. His fame was established at this point, and dancers from all around the world wanted shoes crafted by him. Capezio taught the art of making pointe shoes to his family, who joined him in his successful business; and the

Capezio Foundation was established in 1953. Nowadays, third- and fourth-generation family members continue Salvatore's tradition and commitment to serve the arts, and still produce handmade shoes.

Capezio Pointe Shoes

Tendu I

This shoe has a #2 lightweight medium shank for easy break-in. It molds easily to the foot.

Capezio Tendu II

Same as Tendu I, but offers a wider box and a larger platform.

Capezio Aerieal

This shoe offers a narrow heel, a tapered box, a low vamp, and a cotton drawstring.

Capezio Aria

This features 1/4" lower sides and a 3/8" lower back. For this shoe, Capezio used a new satin color, named petal pink, with matching satin binding and elastic drawstring. It features the special So Suede lining, promising to be moisture absorbent to reducing foot odor and fungus growth.

Capezio Contempora

Shoe with a wide box and platform, a long U-throat vamp, and an elastic drawstring.

Capezio Elan

Crafted by one single maker according to the dancer's specification, this shoe features a 1/4" lower back and sides, a wide hand-molded box and a U-shaped vamp. This shoe is available in any size and color.

Capezio Glissé (style 102)

This shoe features a wide box and a platform, a long vamp, and an elastic drawstring. Also available in Style 102ES and Glissé Pro 115 and 117.

Capezio Pavlowa

This is a Russian-styled shoe offering a tapered box, a wide platform, and a long vamp, with a prearched shank.

Capezio Plié 1

This shoe has a slightly tapered box with a medium vamp and an elastic drawstring.

Capulet
PO Box 3435
Barnet EN5 9FG

United Kingdom
Phone: 44-845-060-3190
Fax: 44-700-594-2803
www.capuletworld.com
sales@capuletworld.com

Cecilia Kerche

The brand Cecilia Kerche was created in 1988 by Pedro Kraszczuck, Kerche's husband, in Rio de Janeiro. Their objective was to attend to the needs of ballet dancers with products developed by people connected with dance. The products are made using the highest ecologically correct technology for the comfort and health of ballet dancers. Cecilia Kerche pointe shoes are currently produced by So Dança.

Chacott
44-021 21st Street, Ste 302
Long Island City, NY 11101
Phone: 866-MY-FREED
Fax: 718-729-8086
www.freedusa.com
E-mail: info@freedusa.com

The Company was created in 1951 by a Japanese shoe salesman named Makoto Tsuchiya. A famous Japanese ballerina had asked him to make a pair of pointe shoes for her, and after examining her European shoes, he decided to create his own pointe shoe brand and company. Chacott is now one of the largest pointe shoe manufacturers in the world.

Coppelia
Via Orzinuovi, 76
25125 Brescia, Italy
Home: 39-030-35-33-823
Fax: 39-030-35-47-323
www.coppelia.com
E-mail: info@coppelia.com

Freed of London
UK Retail and Mail Order:
94 St. Martins Lane
London, WC2N 4AT
Tel. (0)20 7240 0432
Fax: (0) 20 7240 3061

shop@freed.co.uk
www.freedoflondon.com
UK and Overseas Wholesale
62-64 Well Street
London, E9 7PX
Tel. (0) 20 8510 4700
Fax: (0) 20 8510 4750
UK Email: uksales@freed.co.uk
Export Email: export@freed.co.uk
USA Wholesale & Retail
44-01 21st Street, Long Island City,
New York 11101
Tel: 718 729 7061
Fax: 718 729 8086
info@freedusa.com
www.freedusa.com

Frederick Freed started his toe shoe business in London in 1928, in a small store in St. Martins Lane (near Trafalgar Square), after leaving his job at Gamba's. He started making pointe shoes helped by his wife and an assistant. At the time, he probably did not imagine that his name would be carved in the history of pointe shoes!

Freed produces four to five thousand shoes a week using the inside-out technique, called turn-shoe, and features seven different styles of stock pointe shoes.

Michele Attfield, pointe shoe expert and store manager in St. Martins Lane, has been working with Freed for ever forty years. According to her, "a well-trained foot in a well-fitted shoe is always a pleasure to see. However, the aim of anyone making pointe shoes is that you see the dancer and not the shoe. We must never forget that what we are manufacturing is just a tool of the trade."

Bernard Kohler, a retired former manager at Freed, used to affirm that "of all the pointe shoes on the market, Freed is the kindest to the foot. It is the softest and lightest, with less substance and less weight than other shoes." Kindness, patience, and professionalism are some of Freed's main characteristics, both at the store and at the factory. At the retail store in St. Martins Lane, there is no extra fee to get fitted for pointe shoes; and if you are lucky enough—like I was—you will be fitted by Michele Attfield in person, who is now the store manager, by Sophie or by Beth Chivers, Michele's assistant, who is extremely knowledgeable and very kind.

Ribbons and elastics are supplied free of charge at Freed's, and customers purchasing pointe shoes also receive a free dance magazine of their choice. For custom-made orders, only one extra British pound is added to the shoe price. Michele Attfield is one of the world's most renowned fitters. She explained that, although they are still manufacturing shoes in the old traditional way, Freed's production has evolved to keep up with the dancers' and the choreographers' demands. According to her, after World War II students became bigger. Their technique evolved too, with much higher extensions requiring stronger shanks and different types of vamps.

You can read my interview with Michele in Part VIII of this book. During the few hours we spent together at the store, she shared with me her visions and her secrets about how a pointe shoe should be correctly fitted.

Any dancer visiting the UK should visit at least once Freed's shop and try on some of the newest pointe shoes, like the Classic Pro and the Classic Pro 2.

Freed's cobblers use a traditional technique called turn-shoe making, which was the method used for all shoes until the 1870s. Experienced makers craft 20 to 40 pairs of shoes a day. The store in St. Martins Lane (between Covent Garden and Leicester Square) has barely changed since the time Mr. and Mrs. Freed were alive. The outside has recently been painted in green, and the window displays RAD regulation wear and a basic, white tutu. The inside of the shop is old and traditional and somewhat austere looking. There is a small green velvet couch and two armchairs to help dancers with their fittings. On the walls one can see framed pictures of Margot Fonteyn, Rudolph Nureyev, Tamara Rojo and other famous dancers of the Royal Ballet, with messages of thanks to Mr. Freed and Michele Attfield. In 1987 Freed was bought by Chacott and in 1933 both Companies were purchased by the Japanese firm Onward Kashiyama, a clothing manufacturer, although Freed still operates like they used to in the past.Freed supplies most famous ballet companies throughout the world, like the Royal Danish Ballet, Les Grands Ballets Canadiens, San Francisco Ballet, Pennsylvania Ballet, Carolina Ballet,Les Ballets de Monte Carlo,The Norwegian Ballet, Pacific Northwest Ballet and, of course, London's Royal Ballet.

FUZI INTERNATIONAL
1901 54th Ln SE
Olympia WA 98501
Phone: 888-368-6255
Fax: 360-786-0226
www.fuzi.net
E-mail: info@fuzi.com

This Company was created in 1996 by Xijun Fu and his wife, Fang Li. Born in China, Mr. Fu was a professional dancer originally trained at the Beijing Dance Academy. He continued his career performing with the most prestigious Ballet Companies worldwide.

Besides their famous canvas and leather split-sole flats for both male and female dancers, Fuzi produces a Full Shank and a ¾ Shank Pointe Shoe, a Pre-Pointe Shoe, a Canvas Pointe Shoe, a Split-Sole and a V-Vamp Pointe Shoe.

GAMBA
65 Broadway, Ste 818
New York, NY 1006

Phone: 800-858-5855
Fax: 212-635-0156
E-mail: repettousa@novalys.com

The Italian Jewish Luigi Gamba (1889-1940) is not only the founder of Gamba—the first firm of theatrical and ballet shoes—but he is also the "father" of most shoemakers that came after him. Fredrick Freed, Bob Martin, Capulet's Michael Thoraval, and many other cobblers started learning how to make pointe shoes while working at Gamba's factory.

He came to England at age fourteen, and after working as a waiter, Luigi started his successful ballet shoes business in 1903. By 1912 he started making pointe shoes. Prior to that, all pointe shoes in England had to be imported from Italy and France. Mr. Toscagni, one of Gamba's cobblers, crafted the very first pair of pointe shoes in the United Kingdom. His production was still very small and each of his cobblers could not produce more than two pairs of pointe shoes a day. Over the years Gamba introduced modern machines in his laboratory, including a rotary machine for sewing soles. The production increased to 80 pairs a day. One of Gamba's first customers was the Danish ballerina Adeline Genée. Gamba's traditional shop in London does not exist anymore. It disappeared on November 2005, when Gamba closed and was purchased by Repetto. The store was located in Garrick Street, in the Covent Garden area, and was Britain's oldest ballet shoe supplier. Gamba shoes continue to be made through Repetto and some new styles have just been created.

Stage Pro
This shoe features a longer vamp and a full shank for dancers with strong arches.
Gamba 93
Same as Gamba 97 but with a full shank.
Gamba 97

This shoe is ideal for class, rehearsals or performances. It comes with a ¾ shank, V vamp and wide box. Medium and hard shanks and three choices of width (X, XX, XXX) available

Gaynor Minden
140 W 16th St
New York, NY 10011
Phone: 800-637-9240
Fax: 212-929-4907
www.dancer.com
E-mail: fitters@dancer.com

More and more ballet stars are wearing Gaynor Minden pointe shoes. ABT's principal, Gillian Murphy, has been wearing Gaynor Minden since the age of fifteen and affirms that her shoes provide her with "perfect cushioning for landing." Eliza Minden, founder and president of the company, was a former dancer herself and decided to create a "painless shoe" that would last longer than the traditional ones and cause less pain.

Gaynor Minden pointe shoes are built with no pleats. Instead of a pleated three-piece casing, the shoes are crafted with a separate platform insert, bringing the total to four pieces. This platform insert allows the platform to be totally flat, resulting in a wider balancing surface. Second, it creates a clean demarcation around the edge of the shoe platform, similar to a small darning. This allows the dancer to achieve a better alignment on pointe. Gaynor Minden replaced the old traditional boxes and cardboard shanks with elastomeric materials, which are practically unbreakable and make the shoe totally silent. These new-technology pointe shoes promise to last up to four or five times longer than traditional pointe shoes.

Grishko
241 King Manor Dr, Ste D
King of Prussia, Pa 19406
Phone: 800-474-7454
Fax: 610-239-6441
www.grishko.com
E-mail: info@grishko.com

Grishko is the main supplier of the famous Maryinsky of St. Petersburg and the Bolshoi. Founded by Nikolai Grishko, the main factory is situated not far from the center of Moscow, in a building where about 450 workers produce roughly forty thousand pairs of ballet shoes per month, of which twenty thousand are pointe shoes. The company exports over 80 percent of its production to over fifty-two countries. Grishko's wife, who is a former dancer, had the idea to start the business. Nikolai Grishko guarantees that his shoes are durable and that the entire secret lies in the glue they invented and use to make the box. The Grishko Company today manufactures shoes, costumes, and accessories for ballet and dance.

Grishko makes shoes in five different widths:

X - Very narrow
XX - Narrow
XXX – Medium
XXXX – Wide
XXXXX – Very wide
They also offer five shank options:
SS – Super soft shank
S – Soft shank
M – Medium shank
H – Hard shank
SH – Super hard shank

The newest shoe created by Grishko (at first presented as Limited Edition but now available on line through stores and distributors) is Grishko Miracle, advertised as the lightest shoe on the market. It is a beautiful looking shoe, featuring a box lined in a new spongy fibre making it extremely comfortable to wear. The fitting size and shape of this shoe is exactly the same as the Grishko 2007.

ProFlex

A three-quarter-shank pointe shoe only available in soft-medium-shank strength. Built with a pliable inner sole that helps strengthen the toes, it is considered a good shoe for beginners and professionals.

Harmonie
One Campus Rd
Totowa, NJ 07512
Phone: 800-435-4518
Fax: 800-522-1222
www.harmoniedance.com
E-mail: info@harmoniedance.com

Karl-Heinz Martin
Klassische Balletschuhe
Postafiok 521
H-8601 Siofok, Hungary
Phone: 36-84-887-200
Fax: 36-84-887-201
www.martin-ballettschuhe.com
E-mail: info@martin-ballettschuhe.com

Karl-Heinz Martin stated making ballet shoes in 1964. He is the creator of the pointe shoe Eva, which became one of the most popular on the market and is worn by many principal dancers throughout the world. This shoe is well known for being suitable for ballerinas with strong feet. Michaela Martin, daughter of the founder, took over the factory in 2005 and has since then kept strengthening the reputation of the company.

Other models are Karla and Evita. Arthur Fuchs, or Maker A, has been crafting pointe shoes since age eighteen, following his grandfather's path. He can produce up to forty-three pairs of pointe shoes a day.

Inspire
Inspire Dancewear Limited
Lee Hall
St. Peter's Avenue
Haslingden
Lancs, BB4 6NZ

E-mail: richardswift@futureofdance.com
www.futureofdance.com

Founded by Matthew Wyon, Inspire is the home of the revolutionary Flyte Pointe Shoes.

Designed in 2000 by Dance Scientist Dr. Matthew Wyon, Flyte promises the maximum level of shock absorption and stability. Wyon spent seven years researching in his biomechanics labs in order to create his special shoe: Flyte. This totally innovative shoe, which boasts twenty-eight variations for its inner part, is supposed to last up to five times more the traditional shoe and to move along with the foot. The shank is made of polymer compounds, offering flexibility as well as support. It is the only shoe on the market with a removable outer part, allowing the dancer to replace the satin part when it gets dirty or is worn out.

Merlet
5-7, rue Barthélémy Thimonnier
ZI Nord - BP 1567 87022 Limoges Cedex France
Phone: 0555388778 ou 0555388772
Fax: 0555388779
E-mail: info@merletdance.com

Merlet USA
565 Roma Ct
Naples, Fl 34110
Phone: 800-660-6818
Fax: 800-660-6818
www.merletusa.com
www.merletdance.com/fr
E-mail: info@merletusa.com

The brand Merlet was created in 1973 by Roger James Merlet, who started to design and manufacture pointe shoes. Since 1990, one of Merlet's disciples, Pierre Lassenne, has been continuing the tradition. Merlet's pointe shoes are a blend of tradition and technology, where polycarbonates and resins meet the traditional ingredients. Merlet's pointe shoes are hand-turned by master cobblers and their quality is well known throughout the world.

Prelude

A beginner's shoe providing support and flexibility.

Empreinte

A professional shoe built with traditional materials. It features a wide box and a cardboard shank that molds to the foot.

Dedicace

A shoe that is particularly suitable for wide feet and offers a wide platform and a round vamp.

Premiere

Features a flexible polycarbonate shank and a strong and comfortable box.

Performance

A shoe built with a large and square box, a wide platform and a V-vamp, entirely crafted with traditional materials.

Kaliste

This pointe shoes is entirely made with canvas. A polymer box offers great comfort to the foot.

Pulsion

Shoe built with traditional materials for all levels.

Porselli
6 Piazza Paolo Ferrari
20121 Milan, Italy
Phone: 39-02-8053759
Fax: 39-0206080646
www.porselli.it
E-mail: info@porselli.it

Founded in Milan in 1919 by Eugenio Porselli, this Italian brand of pointe shoes carries with it a lot of tradition. The small store by the Teatro alla Scala is still there, supplying with shoes for the dancers of the ballet company, from students to étoiles like Carla Fracci and Roberto Bolle.

Vanna Porselli explains that they produce shoes for professional dancers, but also for students, for rehearsals, for dancers who wish to develop their instep, for the ones who only need to jump. However, for the little ballerinas of the La Scala Theatre, the decision concerning the type of shoe is totally up to the teacher.

Prima Soft
213 Old York Road
Jenkintown, PA 19046
Phone: 1-800-431-6005
Fax: 215-886-9226

www.prima-soft.com
E-mail: info@prima-soft.com

Prima Soft En l'Air

This pointe shoe is ideal for beginners or dancers with a low to medium arch who wish to have flexibility and ease rolling up and down the pointe. This shoe is described as "feather light," quiet, and very comfortable. Available in X (narrow), XX (medium), XXX (medium wide) and XXXX (wide).

Prima Soft Gala #701

This shoe fits perfectly different types of feet, suitable for beginners as well as for advanced dancers. It features an elastic drawstring and the Prima Soft–exclusive Perfect Placement Toe Box. It encourages dancers to roll through the metatarsal and increases flexibility. It is available in natural or hard graduated shank. Available in the following widths: X, XX, XXX, and XXXX.

Prima Russe tm #702

This is a perfect shoe for dancers with short toes and a medium to wide metatarsal, needing a short vamp. No break-in required, thanks to the graduated roll-through shank, which molds to the foot. Its Perfect Placement Toe Box provides excellent balance.

Prima Soft #PS703 Silhouette tm

Ideal for dancers with strong arches; its special "closed" vamp prevents feet with high arches from "overflowing" out of the shoe. It features a graduated shank that molds to the foot and requires very little break-in. Available in X, XX, and XXX, and regular shank only.

Prima Russe tm Extra Wide #702

Another shoe requiring minimum break-in. This shoe is suitable for the dancer with short toes and a medium to wide metatarsal, requiring a low vamp. The graduated shank easily molds to the foot. Good for dancers with bunions. Available only in XXXX (extra wide) and regular shank.

Prima Soft #PS709 Royal tm

This shoe fits narrow, medium, and wide feet, as well as medium or high arches and features a Russian-style V-vamp. Provides very good foot articulations for dancers with low to medium arches and prevents dancers with high insteps from rolling or knuckling.

Prima Soft #PS710 Volé

Volé is a beautiful shoe featuring the exclusive Prima Soft Graduated Memory shank. This special shank comes back to its original shape anytime the dancer goes from pointe to flat. Perfect for dancers with a tendency to pronate or wing.

Principal by Chan Hon Goh Inc.
2345 Main Street
Vancouver, BC V5T 3C9 Canada
Phone: 604-925-8668
Fax: 604-925-8328
www.principalshoes.com
E-mail: info@principalshoes.com

Repetto
65 Broadway, Ste. 818
New York, NY 10006
Phone: 800-858-5855
Fax: 212-635-0156
www.repetto.fr
E-mail: repettousa@novalys.com

The Repetto stores originally specialized in shoes. Their history dates back to 1947, when Rose Repetto, mother of the world-famous dancer and choreographer Roland Petit, decided to create ballet shoes, in a tiny shop, a few steps from the Paris Opera. She started making shoes for her son Roland and became very popular in the dance world. Dancers from everywhere would travel to her shop to buy her shoes. In 1959 Rose Repetto opened her first store at 22 rue de la Paix in Paris. Since then, the brand Repetto has grown everywhere in France and still continues with the traditional turn-shoe method.

Repetto's pointe shoe factory is located in Saint-Médard- d'Excideuil in the region of Périgord, France.

La Carlotta MS T255

This shoe features a medium box and a flexible sole and is available in different widths and shank strengths.

Russian Pointe
226 S Wabash Ave, 2nd Fl
Chicago, IL 60604
Phone: 866-R-POINTE
Fax: 312-588-4060
www.russianpointe.com
E-mail: info@russianpointe.com

Russian Pointe

This brand offers a selection of six widths and three vamp sizes: short, medium, and long. Shanks are available in Standard, Flexible, and Next Generation.

The Jewels Collection

This collection features lightweight shoes available with or without a drawstring: Almaz, Rubin, Sapfir.

The Polette Collection

These shoes offer extra room inside the box without affecting their elegant appearance, a U-cut vamp, and a drawstring: Polette, Polette 3/4.

Grande

This shoe offers more space around the metatarsal area and is recommended for dancers who want extra room around their toes or use bulky padding, like gel pads.

Classic Collection

Traditional models with V-cut vamp: Brio, Celesta, Dolce, and Entrada.

Sansha
888 8th Ave (at 53rd St.)
New York NY 10019
Phone: 212-246-2138
Fax: 212-246-2138
www.sansha.com
E-mail: franckduval@sansha.com
Or: usa@sansha.com

The creator and designer of Sansha ballet shoes is Franck-Raoul Duval, who was nicknamed "Sansha" during his stay in Russia, where he studied dance. Aware of the dancers' demands for a carefully crafted shoe, he opened a workshop and started, in 1982, producing soft split-sole canvas shoes.

So Dança

So Dança's most popular shoes are the following:

So Dança Nikiya

Suitable for the Greek foot type, promises flexibility and quiet landings.

So Dança Grand Pas

Recommended for the Egyptian foot type, it also offers flexibility and noise reduction.

So Dança F26 Performance

This shoe was designed with the Greek foot in mind, offering flexibility and quietness.

Suffolk
The Suffolk Pointe Shoe Company
Unit 2-3 Churchill Works
Highfield Street Earl Shilton
Leicester, LE9 7HS
United Kingdom
Phone: +44(0) 1455 442767
Fax: + 44(0) 1455 442767
info@suffolkpointe.com

The Suffolk Pointe Shoe Company was founded in 2000 by Mark Suffolk, who boasts twenty years in pointe shoe making and fitting.

Mark Suffolk and his wife Lynn founded the Suffolk Pointe Shoe Company in 2000 after being a pointe shoe maker and a fitter for almost twenty years. In the beginning, Suffolk was making the shoes himself with the help of his wife; now his business has grown into a bigger team of over twenty people and moved to a larger location. His secret paste is a combination of burlap, flour, and dextrin.

Three models of shoes are handcrafted at Suffolk:

Apprentice and Solo

Solo

This is worn by beginners as well as by professionals. It comes in eight widths with three insole types. Many variations are available for company members.

Apprentice

This caters to the more advanced dancer, offering more flexibility, thus still maintaining durability and strength. It is available in eight different widths with the choice of two types of insoles: standard and hard. Just like with Solo, Apprentice can also be customized to the dancer's requirements.

Company Shoe

This is entirely made to cater to each individual dancer's needs.

Captivate

This is a shoe offering a tapered box and a sleek look, though providing space for metatarsals on the inside. Its open U-vamp highlights the dancer's arch.

Ensemble

This is specifically designed for lower-crowned feet and features a wide sole to help with placement.

Instinct

It is a lightweight shoe offering a tapered box with a medium profile and a hammered platform offering stability and quietness.

Suffolk is also the official pointe shoe of the Nashville Ballet.
Widths specification:

N (Narrow)
X N - Fitting between N and X
X
XX N - Fitting between X and XX
XX
XXX N - Fitting between XX and XXX
XXX
XXXX N - Fitting between XXX and XXXX
XXXX

Custom-made orders can include any specification, like different combinations of vamp, side, and heel measurements; cotton or elastic drawstrings; varying box strengths; wider or narrower platform; and higher or lower platform. Suffolk custom-made shoes can offer many combinations of special insoles, including "arch break," which has a built-in "break" at a pre-determined point to conform to a dancer's feet, enabling her to go farther over when on pointe. The "extended heel" can lengthen a shoe by a quarter size (similar to Freed's heel pin), while the "heel reduction" can reduce a shoe's length by a quarter size.

Triunfo
Via Nardones, 107
80132 Napoli, Italy
Tel. +39 (081)404847
Fax: +39 (081) 19362139
E-mail: info@triunfostore.it

These pointe shoes, almost unknown in the United States, are very popular in Italy. Carmine Triunfo started his successful pointe shoe business in 1975. He had to sell his first car in order to buy the machines and the materials he needed to start building his first pair of shoes. Today, more than thirty-five years later, Triunfo is one of the leading brands of ballet shoes on the market, thanks to the quality of its products and the professionalism which is its trademark. Triunfo produces over five thousand pointe shoes a month and distributes his own products in the United States, Japan, England, Germany, France, Austria, and Switzerland.

Here are the different models manufactured:

Triunfo Aurora
Triunfo Effect

Triunfo Europe
Triunfo Pitagora 3/4
Triunfo Technia
Triunfo X-Balance
Triunfo Effect FF
Triunfo Star Soft–Demi-Pointe

The widths available are S, M, and L (Narrow, Medium, and Large), and the shanks can be available in C1 (Soft), C2 (Medium), C3 (Strong), and C4 (Extra Strong). Triunfo offers over one hundred different combinations of shanks, boxes, and widths.

Ushi Nagar
(Custom-made shoes only)
1408 London Road
Norbury SW16 4BZ
London

Ushi Nagar is one of the last "old-style" traditional cobblers. I would describe him as a man with a passion, given his unconditional love for pointe shoes. Trained at Freed's, he has been crafting shoes for over fifty years, and is still in love with the pointe shoes he makes! Nagar does not produce stock shoes and does not have a store or a display. His shoes are not sold at dance stores or through the Internet. Everything is custom-made in his London's laboratory. (See Part II, "Meeting a Pointe Shoe Maker: Ushi Nagar.")

Chapter 2

Finding the Right Shoe for Every Foot

Nowadays we dispose of hundreds of types of shoes. There is a shoe for every foot and for every dancer's requirement. However, the choice range is so wide that sometimes it is hard to know what to buy. Here is a small guide on what shoe could be suitable to your foot or to your needs, but remember, shoes have to be tried on and fitted by an expert!

Here are some shoes according to specifications:

Silent shoes
Bloch Russian Pointe
Bloch Axis S0190L
Capezio Chasse'
Freed Studios Pro
Gaynor Minden
Grishko Miracle
Grishko Pro 2007
Prima Soft En l'Air
Repetto Rushka
Sansha Legende
Harmonie Melody

Three-quarter shank
Bloch Alpha
Capezio Concerto
Freed Studios Pro
Grishko ProFlex
Russian Pointe Polette
Sansha Legende
Sansha Ovation 603
So Dança Clara 31
Triunfo Pitagora 3/4

Soft shank
Bloch SO105 Aspiration
Bloch SO131S Serenade
Chacott Veronese II
Freed Classic Deep Vamp
Freed Studio Opera
Grishko Pro Flex 2007
Hard shank

Easy transition from demi- to full-pointe
Bloch Amélie
Bloch Amélie Soft
Chacott Veronese II
Grishko Elite
Grishko Ulanova I
So Dança Clara 31
Triunfo Aurora
Triunfo X-Balance

Demi-pointe shoes
Bloch RAD Demi-Pointe S0165
Freed Demi Pointe
Gamba Delco Ultra
Grishko Elite Pre-Pointe
Sansha Soft-Toe DP801
Triunfo Pre Pointe Star Soft

High vamp
Capezio Glissé
Gamba Stage Pro
V-shaped Vamp
Chacott Veronese II
Freed Classic Plus
Freed Studios Pro
Grishko Fouette'
Grishko 2007
Grishko Ulanova II
Prima Soft Royale PS709
Prima Soft Silhouette PS703
Sansha Lyrica 404
Square boxes and wide platforms
Bloch Balance ES0150
Bloch B Morph ES0170
Bloch SO131 S Serenade
Bloch Heritage
Bloch SO105 Aspiration
Capezio Sylphide
Capezio Glissé
Capezio Tendu I
Freed Studio II Wider Platform
Grishko Elite
Merlet Dedicace
Merlet Performance
Mirella Advanced MS101A
Prima Soft Volé 710
Russian Pointe Dolce
Russian Pointe Grande
Sansha Etudes
Sansha Recital 202S
Triunfo X-Balance

Padded insole
Russian Pointe Entrada
Sansha Partenaire SAN 303
Shoes ready to go onstage
Freed Classic Pro
Freed New Classic Pro
Gaynor Minden FeatherFlex and Pianissimo
Grishko 2007
Prima Soft Prima Russe
Mark Suffolk Solo Light
Extra room in the block for bunions or bulky toe pads
Bloch's Balance
Bloch Synergy S0100L
Russian Pointe Grande
Shallow Shoes for narrow feet
Bloch Serenade SO131
Bloch Suprima S2132L
Capezio Aerial
Prima Soft Silhouette PS703
Prearched shank
Repetto Willis
Triunfo Effect

Shoes for high arches
Bloch Serenade S0131L
Capezio Sylphide
Freed Classic Wing Block
Freed Classic Plus
Freed Studio II
Freed Studio
Gamba Stage Pro
Grishko Pro 2007
Prima Soft Royale
Prima Soft #PS709 Royal tm
Prima Soft #PS703 Silhouette tm
Russian Pointe Entrada
Sansha Partenaire SAN 303

Shoes for longer second toes
Grishko Vaganova

Lightweight or beginner shoes
Bloch Amelie Soft
Chacott Veronese II
Chacott First Step
Freed Classic Deep Vams (SBTDV)
Freed Studio
Freed Studio Opera
Merlet Prelude
Prima Soft En l'Air
Sansha Debutante D10
So Dança Clara 31
Triunfo Aurora

Narrow heels
Bloch Sonata
Capezio Glissé Pro
Capezio Aria

Chapter 3

Pointe Shoes and Ballet Companies

Ballet companies invest a huge amount of money in pointe shoes to keep their dancers on their toes! Here are some interesting figures.

In 2009, English National Ballet dancers used over 4,992 pairs of pointe shoes! At ENB every company member receives up to ten pairs of shoes per month, with a cost of £100,000 a year. More than 3,600 meters of pink satin ribbon are used by ENB's ballerinas.

In 2009, Oregon Ballet Theatre purchased over 1,500 pairs of pointe shoes, spending more than $120,000. Most dancers at OBT wear Freed custom-made shoes.

At Cincinnati Ballet, every ballerina is allowed only eighty pairs of shoes for the whole season. In 2009 the Company spent $130,000 on shoes.

Edward Villella's Miami City Ballet uses 3,000 pairs of pointe shoes per season, of which 750 pairs are used during Nutcracker performances.

At Atlanta Ballet, female dancers go through over 2,000 pairs of pointe shoes per season, for a price of about $100,000. Young students taking one or two pointe classes a week might use only two pairs of pointe shoes in a whole school year, including the end-of-the-year performance. Dancers with a stronger arch might need three or four pairs, and students in between twelve and fourteen, might outgrow their shoes before they wear them out.

Freed's pointe specialist Michelle Attfield believes that children beginning pointe work and doing ten to fifteen minutes of pointe at the end of class once or twice a week will outgrow their shoes before they wear them out. In her experience fitting students from the Royal Ballet School at White Lodge, she affirms that by the end of the term, most young dancers outgrow their shoes and have to return the second pair provided by the school. Dancing with "dead" pointe shoes can be extremely harmful to the dancer's feet, and shoes should be replaced as soon as they no longer provide proper support to the feet. This does not mean they have to be thrown away. They can still be used in many ways:

- They can be de-shanked and used in class or rehearsal.
- They can be cleaned or dyed and kept as mementos.
- They can be autographed and given away during performances.
- Ribbons can be recycled, washed, ironed, and used for a new pair of shoes.

In the chapter called "How to Make Pointe Shoes Last Longer," you will find a lot of useful information about how to take care of your pointe shoes and prolong their lives.

Chapter 4

32 Famous Ballerinas and Their Pointe Shoes

Svetlana Zakharova The Bolshoi Theatre Grishko (custom-made with extra hard shank and long vamp)	Lucia Lacarra Opera of Munich Bayerisches Staatsballet Principal Dancer Freed
Pollyanna Ribeiro Boston Ballet Principal: Karl-Heinz Martin Klassische Balletschuhe GmbH's Eva	Daria Klimentova English National Ballet Prima Ballerina Grishko Super Flex
Silja Schandorff Royal Danish Ballet Innovation by Bob Martin from London	Svetlana Lunkina The Bolshoi Theatre Principal Grishko Maya I
Melissa Thomas American Ballet Theatre Corps Member Gaynor Minden	Carla Korbes Pacific Northwest Ballet Principal Dancer Innovation by Bob Martin
Alina Cojocaru Royal Ballet Principal Gaynor Minden	Katia Garza Orlando Ballet Company Member Gaynor Minden
Diana Vishneva Kirov Principal Grishko Vaganova	Adiarys Almeida Corella Ballet Principal Dancer Bloch Serenade (special order) Maker Professional
Cecilia Kerche Teatro Municipal de Rio de Janeiro Principal Cecilia Kerche	Laura Bosenberg Cape Town City Ballet (SA) Principal Dancer Gaynor Minden
Gillian Murphy American Ballet Theatre Principal Gaynor Minden	Mia Leimkuhler Oregon Ballet Theatre Freed
Patricia Barker Pacific Northwest Ballet Freed	Courtney Kramer Milwaukee Ballet Capezio

Anne Marie Melendez Ballet Austin Sansha 202S	Ashley Bouder New York City Ballet Principal Freed (custom order) or Mark Suffolk (custom order)
Alessandra Ball North Carolina Dance Theatre Freed	Michele Wiles American Ballet Theatre Principal Bloch Synergy (custom order)
Isadora Loyola de Siqueira American Ballet Theatre II Cecilia Kerche	Aurelie Dupont Paris Opera Étoile Freed (custom-made)
Jill Marlow Cincinnati Ballet Gaynor Minden	Ekaterina Kondaurova Maryinsky Theatre Gaynor Minden
April Giangeruso American Blue Theatre II Capezio Elan	Yuan Yuan Tan San Francisco Ballet Principal Freed (Maltese Maker Cross)
Nadia Iozzo Kansas City Ballet Freed of London, Maker J	Irina Dvorovenko American Ballet Theatre Bloch
Mara Galeazzi Royal Ballet Principal Dancer Innovation by Bob Martin	Kylee Kitchens Pacific Northwest Ballet Freed Forteflex, Maker V
Tempe Ostergren Boston Ballet Freed Wing Block	Jennifer Karlynn Kronenberg Miami City Ballet Principal Freed (custom order)

Chapter 5

Pointe Shoe Master: An Unusual but Fascinating Job!

Keeping dancers on their toes is an important task, especially in a ballet company. You might have never heard about this profession: pointe shoe master or pointe shoe specialist, but nowadays a ballet company's pointe shoe master, or pointe shoe specialist, is an amazingly important person; and only an expert in the matter of dancing shoes is able to fulfill this task properly.

But who is the pointe shoe master, and what is his job in a company?

In large ballet companies, dancers use an incredible amount of pointe and soft shoes, character shoes, and boots due to the innumerable classes, rehearsals, and performances. Companies need to hire an expert who knows exactly how to measure dancers' feet, place orders with the various manufacturers, handle the company's budget, fit and modify shoes, and much more. The pointe shoe master has to cope with all the dancers' demands for shoes and also make sure the shoes fit perfectly and the company members can dance in them without any problem. The so-called Pointe Shoe Room is their kingdom, the place where hundreds of shoes of different brands, sizes, and widths are stored.

My interviews with Michael Clifford, pointe shoe master at Birmingham Royal Ballet in Birmingham, England, and with Julie Heggie, pointe shoe mistress at English National Ballet, are reported below. At London's Royal Ballet, the pointe shoe mistress is Catherine Ladd. Catherine looks after the shoes for the whole company, which includes pointe shoes, "flats" for the boys, and anything necessary for any show within the Royal Opera House.

In the Pointe Shoe Room, every dancer has her own cubbyhole labeled with her name—where her shoes, generally customized and crafted by her own maker—are stored. Each dancer has very specific measures taken of her feet: their width, their length, and their shape. The Pointe Shoe Room is where all the dancers go when they need shoes and where all the shoes are stored. The boys' shoes can be made of leather or canvas, and they range from stock shoes to custom-made leather shoes. Character shoes are also stored in the Pointe Shoe Room, for particular roles, like boots for the czardas or the mazurka in Swan Lake.

Catherine Ladd takes very good care of the dancers' shoes. "They use shoes from the moment they come in," she says, "to the moment they go home!" At present, Ms. Jane Latimer is in charge of the Pointe Shoe Room, replacing Catherine Ladd.

Another pointe shoe specialist is Angel Betancourt, a former dancer himself, who works for New York City Ballet. The walls of his shoe room are lined with bins full of pointe shoes and labeled with the name of the dancer. He claims that the brands they use the most at NYCB are

Freed and Capezio, mainly because they are original turned shoes. He orders shoes in bulk, and the colors vary from pink (the particular shade of pink that Mr. Balanchine liked), white, and sometimes black. All their shoes come custom-made to the specifications of the dancers. Their company has an annual shoe budget of $500,000 for about nine thousand shoes, since some of the main dancers use up to a pair of shoes a day!

Laurent Quéval, a dancer who decided to retire while still young, is the pointe shoe specialist at the Paris Opera. Quéval worked four years for the Company Repetto, where he got most of his knowledge in the field of ballet shoes. According to him, at the Paris Opera men receive two pairs of soft slippers per month, for both classes and rehearsals. In addition to these shoes, they also receive extra ones for performances. The system is the same for women, who also receive pointe shoes. Quéval believes that the glue used to assemble pointe shoes is one of the most important elements.

Julie Heggie is the pointe shoe mistress at English National Ballet in London, and she is in charge of all modifications made on the company's shoes. She also measures dancers' feet in more than twenty-six places. She has been working for twenty-five years at ENB after being a dancer herself, and she reveals that she is the one who does the sewing of all the boys' flat shoes.

At Atlanta Ballet, Kelly Tipton occupies the post of shoe coordinator.

Chapter 6

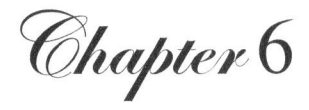

Interviews

Michael Clifford
Pointe Shoe Master, Birmingham Royal Ballet

How did you start getting involved with pointe shoes?

I went to a theater school called Mountview Theatre School, and trained in all aspects of technical theater. After graduating I worked for a while in the West End, then started work for Sadler's Wells Royal Ballet in the men's wardrobe. I used to help the then–shoe supervisor, and after the first year in Birmingham, she left; and I was asked to take over her position.

How would you describe your job as pointe shoe master at BRB?

My job breaks down to roughly three sections:

A. Stock. I am responsible for ordering and maintaining stock for all the dancers. The girls are obviously the main priority. I have the budget control, and I liaise with the shoe companies. I manage the stock control. I do this by issuing the shoes on a monthly basis, and at the end of each month, I do a stock take and send a report to the finance department.
B. I am responsible for new productions. I meet with the designers to discuss their requirements and speak to the choreographers to confirm that what they are wearing on their feet can be danced in! Then do a budget when I have a casting. If there is enough time, I try to make some samples. If not, I go ahead and get the ballet made.
C. Lastly, I am responsible for revivals. This is making sure that any ballet that is revived from our vast repertory looks the same as it would have done if it had been performed fifty years ago. The ballet staff keeps the choreography the same as it was when it was first staged. We call them the heritage ballets.

How does your typical day start?

My typical day depends where we are. If I am in Birmingham, I turn on the computer, make the coffee, and then check my e-mails, as a lot of my suppliers are in different time zones! I usually try to deal with stock issues whilst the dancers are in class. Then I am available directly after class for any dancers who need to either pick up stock or want to talk about anything to do with their stock. When I am on tour, it is slightly different. The main thing is concentrating on the show, so I go around and pick up any performance shoes that need cleaning and do any maintenance on the theatrical shoes, then reset the performance according to the casting. Just out of interest, the girls look after their pointe shoes once taken. Also I am responsible for dying the canvas flats, pointe shoes, and ribbons. I make sure the boys' dyed shoes are clean for the performance. As I'm sure you will be aware, boys will be boys. The girls tell me when they need new dyed pointe shoes. The boys have to be poked with a big stick!

Which is the most popular brand of pointe shoes at BRB?

The most popular brand is Freed.

Are the majority of shoes custom-made?

Out of thirty-five girls, three girls do not use custom-made shoes. They are off the shelf stock measurements.

What do you use to mattify pointe shoes?

The girls use two ways of making their shoes matt:
A. For a heavy matte, they use either aqua color TV white (slightly pink).
B. For a light matte, the girls will use rosin rubbed over the satin with cotton wool. This takes the shine off but leaves a hint of pink.
C. For flesh aqua color OA with 3w, 6w, 5w according to skin color and aqua color ivory.

Do you do any pointe shoe fitting?

I do some fittings as most of our bespoke shoes are made in the UK. I usually have someone in from the company. I can tell if a shoe is too narrow or tight and give advice as to what can be done. In the case of Freed, I can suggest a certain maker. As I have been doing the job for almost twenty years, I have a certain feel . . . I can do emergency quick fixes such as replacing drawstrings and putting suede pieces on the end of the block. If there is a stage cloth, sometimes this acts like sandpaper and shreds the satin and shoes right down to the layers of the block.

What do you do to reduce the noise of brand-new shoes? What if the shoe "squeaks"?

Any girls who wear bespoke shoes made in the turn-shoe method can reduce noise issues by bashing the block on something hard to soften it. Of course this shortens the life of the shoe, but as our girls do not buy their shoes, it is not an issue. If the shoe is squeaking, I tend to put a bit of talcum powder on the inside. As this may be due to the stitching rubbing against the leather outer sole, this can "lubricate."

What are most ballerinas looking for in their shoes?

The girls are looking for comfort but most of all want to have a nice "line" and good instep, and of course, the right size platform for when they are on pointe.

What do you think about the "new technology" pointe shoes like Gaynor Mindens?

We don't have any girls on "new technology" shoes. The ballet staff tends to discourage them. I'm not sure the huge cost and claims about how long they last rings true, with the way we work where we have different requirements for shoes, i.e., dyed, matte, and shiny would be cost effective. It may be better for students who may be looking for length of use versus cost outlay.

How many pairs of shoes a month are given to the company members?

The corps girls can use ten pairs of pointe shoes per calendar month. Soloists can use fifteen pairs a calendar month. If a first artist is doing a lot of corps work and solo work as well, I will allow them to use more, same with soloist girls if they are doing a lot of principal roles. Principals can use as many as they want.

I read that sometimes pointe shoes have to be "sprayed" in the Spray Room. Can you explain the purpose of this operation?

Some pointe shoes are sprayed, and I have a room which was built for the job. It is a booth within a room with daylight-corrected lighting and a very strong extractor with filters, so there are no nasty fumes. I use normal fabric spray in a can.

What is your advice for making pointe shoes last longer?

The girls here use shellac, which they put into the shoes where they want to make it strong, and then leave it to dry somewhere warm. If you go into the girls' dressing rooms on tour, all down the backs of the radiators you will see pointe shoes drying.

How would you prepare a brand-new pair of pointe shoes for a performance?

I leave the preparing of performance shoes to the girls! I make sure they have any dyed pointe shoes well in advance so they have time to do what they need to do.

What type of darning do you think is the best?

Same goes for darning. I have noticed most girls don't darn.

What are ballerinas' most common complaints about their shoes?

Our girls can complain that their shoes do not come quick enough, especially if they have asked for changes. Any orders from Freed that the Royal Ballet companies order can be here with us within three weeks . . . I can get shoes made in less than a week if need be. They don't know how lucky they are! As they are handmade, sometimes there can be some slight variations.

How do you deal with new dancers joining the company? Pointe shoe–wise, I mean.

When a girl is contracted, a form is sent out to them to fill in, which is sent back to me with their pointe shoe requirements. A lot of the time, if they are at the Royal Ballet School or Elmhurst School for Dance, chances are we have used them during the season, so it's not too hard. If they come from another company, I contact the company; and if they have any stock left, I will buy it so there is a smooth changeover.

Can you give your personal advice on how to find the correct pointe shoe and taking care of it?

Try as many pointe shoes as you can. Listen to the person in the shop who is fitting you, and your teacher, when you do settle on a shoe. Buy maybe two or three pairs and rotate them, air them out, and let them dry properly before stuffing them into your bag. They will last longer . . . and not smell!

Julie Heggie
Pointe Shoe Mistress, English National Ballet

Julie Heggie is the "Pointe Shoe Fairy" at London's English National Ballet. The Pointe Shoe Room, where all the shoes are stored—pointe shoes for the girls and flat shoes or boots for the boys—is Julie's kingdom. ENB's main Pointe Shoe Room is located in Kent, outside London, where all the costumes and setting are also stored, ready for tours. In London, at Jay Mews (the Headquarters), ENB has a very small Pointe Shoe Room. There, Julie stores all the shoes the dancers need when in London. Thanks to her work and dedication of twenty-five years, the company dancers do not have to worry about finding the suitable shoe, because this is Julie's task: to keep ballerinas on pointe! Julie made a break in her busy schedule to answer this friendly interview and describe her job as pointe shoe mistress.

How did you start getting involved with pointe shoes?

I was a ballet student working temporarily at the head office when the job came up. I went for the interview, and the rest is history. Since I had danced before and I had worn pointe shoes and knew about them, they gave me the job.

How would you describe your job as pointe shoe master/specialist?

My job is very important. I am the liaison between dancer and maker, the middleman in designs of shoes for new ballets, as I have to ensure that the designer gets the look he/she wants and the choreographer gets the steps that he wants in the shoes. I also manage a vast amount of money tied up in the shoe department budget.

How does your typical day start?

A typical day starts on a train out of London to our shoe storage in Kent. Once I have had my cup of tea, I start up the spray booth and set the heated cabinet going. I mix dye to match the tights the boys will wear and dye their shoes (Nureyev's Romeo has 104 pairs of different-colored shoes in it). I also have to sort out the boots and shoes to ensure that I have a pair for everyone. Other days may see me heading for a meeting with shoemakers, choosing leather to make new boots from. Once a week, I go to the studio in London, where the dancers can talk to me about their shoes.

Which is the most popular brand of pointe shoes in your company?

We buy the shoe the dancer wants, but even now the most popular pointe shoe is Freed's. I also buy from the United States, Russia, France, Australia, and France.

Are the majority of shoes custom-made?

Apart from the American shoes, they are all bespoke made for the individual.

What type of alterations do you generally perform on pointe shoes?

We don't do any alteration inhouse. However, the makers alter the specification for us.

What do you use to mattify pointe shoes?

We use Pan-Cake to powder the shoes down.

Which are the measurements that you take in order to order pointe shoes for a new dancer?

I constantly refit pointe shoes. Foot charts and measurements are taken, and I discuss problems and requirements with the dancer. After injuries and consultation with the physiotherapist, we alter the measurements of the shoe to refit it to the foot after operation or injury. I measure all the joints of the foot, the heel, the ankle all the way up to the leg.

Do you prepare dancers' shoes for the stage?

I expect the individual dancer to prepare her shoes for stage. Banging them on a concrete step works wonders for reducing the noise. Also, a piece of plaster across the pleats of the block is a good solution. The squeak comes from a loose insole, and I frown upon the individual who squeaks onstage.

What are most ballerinas looking for in their shoes?

Every dancer asks something different from their shoe. It is a very personal thing.

What do you think about the "new technology" pointe shoes like Gaynor Mindens?

No comment.

How many pairs of shoes a month are given to a corps de ballet member, a soloist, a prima ballerina, a principal?

All our dancers receive ten pairs per four-week month.

How would you prepare a brand-new pair of pointe shoes for a performance?

I don't do this. The dancers prepare their own shoes.

What type of darning do you think is the best?

Very few dancers darn their shoes these days. They may darn the edge of the platform to even out the bit they stand on pointe on.

What is the type of padding most used among your dancers? Which one do you prefer?

I never wore any padding when I danced. These days there is a massive variety of commercial toecaps, from padded cotton to a type of latex.

What are ballerina's most common complaints about their shoes?

I normally receive endless complaints, usually regarding the shape of the block.

How do you deal with new dancers joining the company? Pointe shoe–wise, I mean.

New dancers are permitted to wear their current shoe unless we consider it totally unsuitable in size or width or strength, then they have to bow to my superior knowledge and change to a shoe I prescribe.

What is your personal advice on how to find the correct pointe shoe and taking care of it?

Very few dancers know what fits well, so I think it is extremely important that they take our advice. The shoes in the company do not last very long, but it is vital to allow pointe shoes to dry out after wear. Re-hardening the block extends the life of shoes as well.

The Magic of Pointe Shoes

Jane Latimer
Pointe Shoe Mistress
The Royal Ballet, London

Jane Latimer is an important figure at London's Royal Ballet: she is in charge of all the dancers' feet and shoes! In this interview, she reveals some of the secrets of her fascinating job.

How did you start getting involved with pointe shoes?

I started here at the Royal Opera House five years ago, but I have a daughter who has danced since the age of five and now dances professionally, so I have been through all stages of ballet footwear development. However, working in ballet footwear is a constant "work in progress and learning curve!"

Where is the Pointe Shoe Room located in the Royal Opera House building?

It is on the fourth floor.

How would you describe your job as pointe shoe master/specialist at the Royal Ballet?

We are responsible for supplying our dancers with footwear from the moment they enter the building—for class, rehearsals, and performances. We fit and supply all character shoes and boots for all productions inhouse and when the company is on tour.

Which is the most popular brand of pointe shoes in your company?

We carry all the major pointe shoe suppliers.

Are the majority of shoes custom-made?

Yes.

What do you use to mattify pointe shoes?

We generally use Pan-Cake.

Which are the measurements that you take to order pointe shoes for a new dancer?

Length, width, insole length, outer sole length, vamp height, back and side heights, strength of shank.

What are most ballerinas looking for in their shoes?

The perfect pointe shoe. Most dancers are always in search of this!

What do you think about the "new technology" pointe shoes like Gaynor Mindens?

They are becoming increasingly popular and are [the company] now customizing for our dancers.

How many pairs of shoes a month are given to a corps de ballet member, a soloist, a prima ballerina, a principal?

This varies enormously depending on the particular repertoire. It can be ten to sixty pairs per month!

Pointe shoes have sometimes to be "sprayed" in the Shoe Spray Room. Does the Royal Ballet Have a Spray Room?

Yes, we have a spray booth in our workroom, here at the Opera House.

What is your advice for making pointe shoes last longer?

Allow the shoes to "dry out" well after wear. Many dancers shellac their shoes in order to prolong their life.

How would you prepare a brand-new pair of pointe shoes for a performance?

Each dancer has her own personal way to prepare a new pair of shoes. She may merely stand on the box, to flatten and soften, or go to quite extreme lengths to remove the insole, so it is loose, cut the insole to a specific length, hammer them, bang them on the floor, or even crush them between a door and the doorframe!

What type of darning do you think is the best?

This is an entirely personal preference. To each individual, whatever works best!

What is the type of padding most used among your dancers? Which one do you prefer?

Some of the dancers wear toe pads, toe separators, or tape.

What are ballerinas' most common complaints about their shoes?

They generally complain about the strength of the shank, the length of vamp, the angle or flatness of platform, and the ability to go over on pointe with ease.

How do you deal with new dancers joining the company?

I check that they are happy with their existing footwear and usually advise a refit and a personally made shoe if they currently wear a stock shoe.

What is your personal advice on how to find the correct pointe shoe and taking care of it?

I recommend that tried and trusted pointe shoe suppliers are used and a proper fitting is undertaken.

Part VII

INTERVIEWS WITH POINTE SHOE MAKERS

Bob Martin
Founder, Innovation Pointe Shoes

This interview was taken in 2010, before Bob Martin's retirement.

How did the Bob Martin shoe factory start? How did you and your wife get involved in the world of ballet and pointe shoes?

Dance Workshop started in 1995. My wife Patricia and I worked for Gamba of London thirty-two years. The factory was bought and sold by many companies over that period of time. We decided to go on our own when it was bought by Repetto.

Your pointe shoes are totally handmade. How many steps does it take to make a pointe shoe? Do you use the "inside-out" technique?

Our shoes are totally handmade. We buy the raw materials and cut everything ourselves. Our shoes are made by the turn-shoe method. They are a Classic Pointe Shoe.

What makes Innovation pointe shoes so unique? What are their main characteristics?

Our shoes are unique because they are made for individual dancers.

How many types of pointe shoes do you make? How many widths and strengths?

We make one type of shoe—Innovation. We have four widths: N, X, XX, XXX.

Is your shank made of cardboard?

The shanks are made from many types of fiberboard depending on the requirement of the customer.

Do you mostly deal with custom orders or with standard orders from dance stores?

All of our shoes are bespoke. The company dancers send me an old shoe of theirs that fits them in the length. I put it on my last to see what size it is. If you wear a 3.5 Freed shoe, for example, then you will be 3 in mine, as our lasts are different. Then I make the shoe and put in the type of insole that the dancer requires. Ninety-five percent of the dancers I make shoes for I have never met. The general public comes to my workshop for fittings. When the shoes are made, we post them to the dancers. You can say that my shoes are 75 percent ballet companies and 25 percent mail order."

Can you name some of the major ballet companies and ballerinas using Innovations?

While I am trading, this remains a secret.

How do you learn to be a cobbler?

We are not cobblers, we are shoemakers. I learned the art of shoemaking at Gamba.

How many cobblers work in your factory? Can you briefly describe a typical day at the factory?

Again, this remains a secret.

What are the most common requests in custom-made shoes? Do you need to see the dancer's feet?

I do not need to see the dancer. They send an old shoe which is a good fit in the length, and I work from there.

When you retire, will the secret of your pointe shoes be lost?

Who knows?

Can you give your personal advice for dancers struggling to find the suitable pointe shoe?

Do not buy any shoe. Make the salesperson listen to what you need, not what they think you should have.

Dawn Terlizzi
Manager Special Make-up
Wholesale Division, Capezio

Your pointe shoes are totally handmade. How many steps does it take to make a pointe shoe? Do you use the inside-out technique? Could you briefly describe some of the stages the shoe goes through before it is ready for the market?

There are five basic steps to make a pointe shoe: cutting, fitting [sewing], lasting, finishing, and packing. Yes, we do use the "turned construction" [inside out] method.

Cutting: All satin is cut by hand using established patterns, or, in the case of a custom pointe shoe, a pattern is made.

Fitting: All pieces of the satin upper are sewn together.

Lasting: The shoes are formed into shape, the pleats are made, and the sole is attached. The pasting is done here also.

Finishing: The shoes are cleaned, inspected, and put in the drying room so that the paste can dry.

What makes your pointe shoes so unique? What are their main characteristics?

Capezio makes all of its pointe shoes, stock and custom. All shoes are handcrafted in the USA. All steps of the process are completed in our factory in New Jersey.

Our paste formula is unique and of a proprietary nature. Our manufacturing process is unique, and again, of a proprietary nature.

Is your shank made of cardboard?

This is proprietary information.

Do you mostly deal with custom orders or with standard orders from dance stores?

We make mostly stock shoes for dance stores.

Can you name some of the major ballet companies using your pointe shoes?

American Ballet Theatre, Joffrey, Nevada Ballet , Les Grands Ballets Canadiens, Metropolitan Opera Ballet, Royal Swedish Ballet, Ballet Austin, Pennsylvania Ballet, Houston Ballet, Boston Ballet, Ballet West, Phantom, Ballet San Jose.

How many cobblers work in your factory? Can you briefly describe a typical day at the factory?

We have just several people working in the pointe shoe factory. The pace is regimented and fast.

What are the main requirements in custom-made pointe shoes?

The following specs can be modified for custom pointe shoes:
Throat shape, vamp length, side height, back height, box strength, wing strength, platform strength, pleat reinforcement, shank strength and length, nail placement, toe shape, and platform shape.

What are the main ingredients of your paste?

This is proprietary information.

How do you learn to be a cobbler?

Most of our cobblers are "born into the trade," meaning that their fathers were cobblers. If this isn't the case, it takes years and years of hard work to become a master cobbler utilizing "on the job training." Most cobblers work their way up the ranks, starting at the bottom and working their way up.

In the case of bespoke shoes, do you need to see the dancer's foot, or you also do it through pictures?

To be properly fit in any pointe shoe, it takes a professional, experienced pointe shoe fitter to work with the dancer's foot and individual needs. We have an expert pointe shoe fitter in our flagship Capezio store in NYC. She is available to visit stores across the USA to instruct shop owners on how to fit a pointe shoe.

Can you give your personal advice for dancers struggling to find the suitable pointe shoe?

Again, the dancer should find an experienced, knowledgeable pointe shoe fitter. These are very hard to find. The dancers should try on several different brands, styles, and sizes, all the while working with an experienced pointe shoe fitter.

Michael Thoraval
Founder, Capulet World Pointe Shoes

Capulet pointe shoes revolutionized a three-hundred-year-old design. The founder of the company explains why their shoes are so different.

How did the Capulet shoe factory start? How did you get involved in the world of ballet and pointe shoes?

Capulet was created in 2003 in London. We all have a Gamba heritage. We were disillusioned by the road taken by Gamba and the constant trouble there, so we decided to start Capulet.

Our main desire was to continue making pointe shoes, but with a difference. That is why we created the D3o, an innovation that has transformed the pointe shoe world.

Are your pointe shoes are totally handmade?

Yes, they are all hand stitched. We do not have a stitching machine.

Do you use the "inside-out" technique for Juliet?

Yes, it is a traditional construction.

Could you briefly describe some of the stages the shoe goes through before it is ready for the market?

We prefer to keep it a secret . . . but the entire outside upper and sole are made traditionally, hand stitched, turned, and finished.

The Magic of Pointe Shoes

What makes Capulet pointe shoes so unique? What are their main characteristics?

There are so many unique points. The D3o itself is a unique material. It is made of intelligent molecules reacting to movement. When not stressed, it is soft, but will react to all movement of the dancer's foot, and protect it by becoming very hard if the dancer stresses her foot during a jump or pointe work.

The toe block is made of hytrel, a polymer with memory. The dancer will not need to break the shoe in, as it will take the shape of the dancer's foot. It also last thirty times longer than a traditional toe block.

The shank is also made of hytrel and will follow the shape of the foot. It is connected to the toe block in a way that will allow going through demi-pointe effortless, but will block when on pointe to support the dancer.

The platform is large, so the shoe is very stable.

We make three types of shanks: soft, medium, and hard. The shoe also offers two shank lengths: three-quarter and full. We offer three different widths: X, XX, XXX.

Which is your "beginner's" shoe?

The D3o soft shank.

Is your shank a cardboard one?

No.

Do you mostly deal with custom orders or with standard orders from dance stores?

We do 50/50.

Can you name some of the major ballet companies and ballerinas using Capulet?

We supply the Royal Ballet, English National Ballet, ABT, and many other companies in Cuba, Mexico, Korea, and Japan.

Can you briefly describe a typical day at the factory?

We start at eight and finish at four.

What is the most common request in custom-made shoes?

High heels.

Do you need to see the dancer's foot or you also accept custom-made orders through pictures and correspondence?

We need to see the foot.

Vanna Porselli
Porselli Pointe Shoes

A friendly interview with Vanna Porselli, the granddaughter of the company's founder, reveals some of the story of the famous traditional Porselli pointe shoes. Eugenio Porselli founded his dance boutique in 1919 in Milan, a town close to the art of ballet where Porselli has always been its symbol. "My grandfather," says Vanna, "used to work for a ballet shoe maker. When the owner of the factory retired, my grandfather took over the business. With huge sacrifices, he carried on the tradition of handmade ballet shoes and gave his name to the company."

Since 1980 a Porselli Prize for Dance (Premio Porselli per la Danza) is awarded every year to a choreographer or dance teacher who is particularly distinguished in his/her work. This prize has been awarded to dancers like Margot Fonteyn, Natalia Makarova, Yvette Chauviree, Martha Graham, Serge Lifar, Maurice Bejart, and Galina Ulanova.

"Today Porselli pointe shoes are still manufactured with selected high-quality materials, and they are proud to be 100 percent made in Italy."

Now Porselli has stores in Paris and London, as well as in the United States and in Japan. It remains the official pointe shoes supplier of the Teatro alla Scala in Milan, as well as the symbol of Italy's love for art and ballet.

Porselli features twenty different styles of stock pointe shoes, in addition to custom-made ones, crafted on the ballerina's own measurements and requirements. The shanks are in leather and come in four different strengths and three widths. Porselli's factory is located in the outskirts of Milan.

Luca Bogarelli
President, Coppelia Pointe Shoes

How did Coppelia start? How did you "enter" the ballet world and the field of pointe shoes?

We started thirty-one years ago with the opening of our first store in Brescia, Italy. Then we opened another store in Bergamo, and finally in Rome. Following this, we founded the DTC, Dance Trading Company, which represents the group Coppelia. DTC produces ballet shoes and dance clothing.

Your ballet shoes are handmade. What are the steps necessary for the crafting of your pointe shoes? Which technique do you use?

Our beginnners' shoes (R-10, R-11, R-12) are machine made, while the special (R14, R-15, R-16 MP) are handmade following the traditional technique.

What are the characteristics of Coppelia pointe shoes? Do you also craft custom-made shoes?

Our pointe shoes are known for the way they mold to the dancer's foot, thanks to their shape and to their vamp—quite high—which holds the foot perfectly. Another characteristic is the flexible shank allowing to execute even demi-pointe work without problems. We do not make bespoke shoes.

How many types of pointe shoes do you produce? How many widths and shanks do you offer?

We manufacture six different types of pointe shoes in two widths, M and W; and we offer three types of shanks.

What type of shank does Coppelia use?

The shank in our beginners' shoes is a typical 2.5 mms. cardboard shank, and for the special shoes, we combine this shank with a 1.8 mms. second shank.

Could you name a few ballet companies and ballerinas wearing Coppelia?

From our store in Rome, we supply the major Italian ballet companies and schools.

How did you learn the technique to make pointe shoes?

We learned from the best international cobblers.

How would you advise dancers who cannot find the right type of shoe?

We leave it up to the teachers, or maîtres de ballet, to give advice to their own students.

Lacy Woodbury
Networking and Marketing, Sansha USA, Inc.

How did your shoe factory start? Can you tell me more about the history of Sansha?

Franck Duval started the company in 1982-1984 by creating the first split-sole canvas ballet shoe, and then opened Sansha in 1984. I know that he was in the town of Sansha, Thailand, when he began his idea for the shoe. He started off with little money, going from ballet company to ballet company, showing them his slipper, which he carried in a briefcase. Franck-Raul Duval was a dancer himself so he has that passion and drive to create shoes he knows dancers can afford, with the comfort and support they look for in a shoe.

Are your pointe shoes totally handmade? How many steps does it take to make a Sansha pointe shoe? Do you use the "inside-out" technique?

We do have select styles that are handmade. Yes, we do use the inside-out technique. After the shape has been formed on the last, the shoe is turned, and the satin is applied and pleated, and the sole is applied. The shoe is then looked over by the maker and sent to quality control, for final testing.

What makes your pointe shoes so unique? What are their main characteristics?

Each shoe is designed with what a dancer's requirements in mind. Not just the shape of the foot, but what a student may need compared to a professional. Each style is designed for a different group of dancers. The students shoes (202, 404, etc.) have a larger, with more of a square shape, platform, for a steady balance. The professional shoes have a flatter box and a rounder platform.

What are the advantages of wearing Sanshas?

There are so many styles to choose from. There is certainly one that fits your foot like a glove.

How many types of pointe shoes do you make? How many widths and strengths?

We make fifteen traditional performance, five decorated, two stage (lace-up and lace-up with tap), three demi-pointe. The DP808 is barre exam standard. We produce five widths in some models; and for the majority of the shoes, we have narrow, medium, wide, and X-wide. Most shanks are medium-hard, and we do have two styles that have a hard shank.

Are your shanks made of cardboard or leather or other?

They are more of a resin and fiberboard mix.

Do you mostly deal with custom orders or with standard orders from dance stores?

For the most part, we deal with stock shoes.

Can you name some of the major ballet companies and ballerinas using your pointe shoes?

San Francisco Ballet, Miami City Ballet, Richmond Ballet, Salt Lake City Ballet, Les Ballet Trockadero, Boston Ballet, and Ballet San Jose. For the dancers, we have Maria Kochetkova (San Francisco Ballet), Emily Bromberg (Ballet San Jose), Keiria Schwartz (Ballet San Jose), Dalay Parrondo (Boston Ballet), and most of the Trockadero Company that goes on pointe. We are the only distributor that has the size range to meet their needs.

Where is your main factory located? How many cobblers work in your factory? Can you briefly describe a typical day at the factory?

Our main factory is based in China. There are at least ten cobblers working at the factory. Our days are really busy. We make so many products, there is always something going on. We produce from tutus to pointe shoes, and from tap shoes to hip-hop. The factory is always on the go.

What are the main requirements in custom-made pointe shoes?

We require a minimum order of at least ten pairs. We need exact measurements and all the details we can get as far as the changes made to the pointe shoe, including current style and size.

How do you learn to be a cobbler?

Our cobblers learn through apprenticeship and study under a current cobbler. It takes dedication and the will to learn.

What are the most common requests in custom-made shoes? Do you need to see the dancer's foot?

One of the main requests is a three-quarter shank or the height of the vamp. These are the most common specifications. We can use a picture or a drawing, but the most important thing is the measurements.

Can you give your personal advice for dancers struggling to find the suitable pointe shoe?

It takes time to know your strengths and weaknesses. Talk to a pointe shoe fitter and salesperson. Tell them everything you can about your foot. And during the fitting, tell them how the shoe feels. That will enable them to help you better.

What is the foot type that best responds to Sansha shoes? Which is your lightest beginner's shoe?

Our 202 would fit the Grecian-type feet while the 101 is for more narrow, long Egyptian-type feet. It really just all depends on the person wearing them. D101 is the lightest shoe we have for beginners, with a flexible shank for barre work. The next one would be the 202 because the platform has great stability.

Marlena Juniman
President, Prima-Soft Pointe Shoes

What is the story of Prima Soft pointe shoes?

Prima Soft revolutionized the dance world in 1992 with the invention of the world's first convertible tights. A design so unique a patent was granted by the United States government patent office (Patent #6,047,571). Prima Soft convertible tights have become one of [the] best-selling, best-fitting tights in the United States and worldwide. In 1996 Prima Soft introduced their pointe shoes, designed with the highest technology available. "Hi tech" does not necessitate using artificial materials. Prima Soft factories are located in Russia and Brazil, and the shoes are designed by me, made to our specifications. They are distributed through the U.S., Canada, and abroad to dancewear stores.

Are your pointe shoes traditionally made?

Prima Soft pointe shoes are made of natural materials, and no plastic, fiberglass, or rubber is used in the shoe construction. Using natural materials allows the shoes to work with, not against, the dancers' feet. The shoes are made on a new, innovative last that allows the dancer's toes to go directly straight down into the toe box, thus preventing the toes from settling into the upper part of the pointe shoe vamp. Toes are correctly placed in the "perfect placement toe box," giving the dancer a connection with the floor. This greatly enhances balance and placement.

What type of shanks do you use?

The shanks of our shoes are made of a combination of materials based on that individual shoe's purpose. The shanks of Prima Soft shoes are graduated, permitting the shoes to mold naturally to the arches, and offers a customized fit from the first wear. In 2005 and 2006, Prima Soft introduced Extension Stretch Ribbon (patent pending) and the Pointe Perfect Toe Pads and the Make It Fit Kit for dancers with two different-size feet in 2008.

Are your shoes crafted with the "inside-out" technique?

We use the "inside out" technique for our shoes. Prima Soft shoes are made by hand and machine depending on the particular shoe.

What makes Prima Soft pointe shoes "different" from the other brands on the market?

Each Prima Soft pointe shoe is decidedly different from each other. Each is made on its own unique last or form, not made on one last and cosmetically changed. This new, innovative last allows the dancer's toes to go directly straight down into the toe box, thus preventing the toes from settling into the upper part of the pointe shoe vamp. Toes are correctly placed in the perfect placement toe box, giving the dancer a connection with the floor. This greatly enhances balance and placement and enables us to fit many different foot shapes and types. Each model has its own characteristics, but each has a perfect placement toe box and graduated shank system.

What is the advantage of wearing Prima Soft?

The advantage of wearing a shoe that has the properties to work with the feet as opposed to "against the foot." This is what we have always strived for.

Do you accept orders for custom-made shoes?

To cut down a heel or vamp is not what we would call "customizing," but modifying. All custom orders must be requested first by a telephone conversation, and then we follow up with an appointment with the dancer to discuss her needs. To customize a shoe specifically, it is best to physically see the dancer's foot.

What is the advice you can give to dancers looking for the right pointe shoe?

If a dancer is struggling with her present pointe shoes and wishes to try Prima Soft shoes, we welcome a "one-on-one" phone consult with her. We also provide her with a questionnaire to answer, and we request photographs of her feet in various positions. We can then make suggestions as to which shoe(s) she could try.

Which Prima-Soft is the most suitable for beginners?

There is no "beginner pointe shoe" per se. A beginner has specific needs, and the shoe she wears should reflect those needs. So a beginner shoe is a shoe that is suitable for that particular beginner. As our shoes are all very different from each other, we feel we are able to fit many different foot types. It is necessary to know your shoes and to know how a dancer is supposed to work in that shoe. That will determine which of the Prima Soft shoes she should try.

Which is your "lightest" shoe?

The lightest Prima Soft shoe is the En l'Air. This shoe is excellent for dancers with a tight ankle and instep, who struggle to get "over the box," need flexibility, and like a quiet and light shoe. It is also a wonderful shoe for the advanced dancer who has a strong foot and does not need a magnitude of support, or is dancing a role that requires a quiet, light feel.

Eliza Minden
President, Gaynor Minden Pointe Shoes

How did the Gaynor Minden factory started?

Our shoes are made at a factory in Lawrence, Massachusetts, that has been making shoes for years. Now they make only Gaynor Mindens, but before that, their specialty was women's satin shoes, especially brides' and bridesmaids' shoes, so they completely understand the importance of immaculate satin fabrics and impeccable stitching. Our website—at www.dancer.com—has information on the company's history.

How did you get involved with ballet?

My mother took me to my first ballet class when I was five, and later to legendary performances by Baryshnikov, Makarova, Kirkland, Fonteyn, and others. They made quite an impression! My own experience of pointe shoes was that at first they were unnecessarily painful and discouraging. It doesn't have to be that way. After graduating from Yale, I worked in the management of dance companies and saw what a terrible burden the expense of pointe shoes is, and what a difference it could make if they lasted longer. I also saw dancers injured from pointe work and wondered if improved shoes could help prevent that. Finally, like so many ballet lovers, I find the noise of pointe shoes clomping onstage extremely distracting—it detracts from a ballerina's performance.

Are your pointe shoes totally handmade? How many steps does it take to make one of your pointe shoes? Do you use the "inside-out" technique?

The internal components—toe box and shank—are machine made by injection molding. Different densities of impact-absorbing foam are cut to exact shapes and then attached to the shank and toe box in critical places. The satin is "combined" to a moisture wicking, silver ion lining, and then cut into uppers, quarters, and platforms (fronts, backs, and tips) in the various sizes and widths. The stitching and lasting are done by hand. We do not need to use the inside-out technique because we don't build our toe boxes out of layers of fabric and glue the way traditional shoes do.

What are the characteristics that make your pointe shoes so unique?

They are the only ones to successfully utilize advanced modern materials to achieve superior durability [confirmed by independent medical research, published in the Journal of Sports and Medicine], as well as greater comfort, impact absorption [also confirmed by independent medical research] and noise reduction. They have also been shown to promote correct, therefore safer, alignment.

How many types of pointe shoes do you craft? How many widths and strengths?

We offer over 2,500 options in total. Five strengths, three box shapes. Narrow heel option. Three widths. Many lengths, also choices of vamp height and heel.

What materials are your shanks made of?

Our shanks are made of thermoplastic elastomerics with "memory" property.

The Magic of Pointe Shoes

Do you mostly deal with custom-made orders or with stock shoes?

We deal with both.

Can you name some of the major ballet companies and ballerinas using your shoes?

Ballet Companies using Gaynor Minden

American Ballet Theatre	English National Ballet
Alberta Ballet (Canada)	Finnish National Ballet
Ballet British Columbia	Greek National Opera Ballet
Ballet de l'Opera de Bordeaux	Het Nationale Ballet (Netherlands)
Ballet de Santiago (Chile)	Hong Kong Ballet
Ballet del Teatro Municipal de Asunción (Paraguay)	Houston Ballet
Ballet du Grand Théâtre de Genève	Hungarian National Ballet
Ballet Estable del Teatro de Colón (Argentina)	Istanbul State Ballet
Ballet Idaho	Kiev Ballet (Ukraine)
Ballet Manila	Konstantin Tachkin's St. Petersburg Ballet Theatre
Ballet Municipal de Lima (Peru)	
Ballet Nacional de Cuba	Kremlin Ballet (Russia)
Ballet Nacional de Guatemala	La Scala Ballet (Italy)
Ballet San Jose	Les Ballets Grandiva
Bayerisches Staatsballett (Germany)	Les Ballets de Monte Carlo (Monaco)
Béjart Ballet Lausanne	Les Ballets Trockadero de Monte Carlo
Bolshoi Ballet (Moscow)	Lithuanian National Ballet
Bolshoi Ballet Theatre of Belarus	Macedonian National Ballet
Boris Eifman Ballet	Maryinsky (Kirov) Ballet Company
Boston Ballet	Metropolitan Opera Ballet (New York)
Cape Town City Ballet (South Africa)	Miami City Ballet
Cincinnati Ballet	National Ballet of Canada
Companhia Nacional de Bailado (Portugal)	Nevada Ballet Theatre
Compañia Nacional de Danza (Mexico)	New Jersey Ballet
Corella Ballet de Castillon y León	New York Theatre Ballet
Dance Theatre of Harlem	Novosibirsk Ballet Theatre
Den Norske Opera Ballett	Opera Nationala din Bucuresti
Dortmund Ballet	Royal Swedish Ballet
Estonian National Ballet	Royal Winnipeg Ballet

Scapino Ballet Rotterdam	Tulsa Ballet
State Ballet Theatre of Kazan (Russia)	Victor Ullate Ballet (Spain)
Suzanne Farrell Ballet	Washington Ballet
The Royal Ballet (England)	West Australian Ballet

Ballerinas

Gillian Murphy	Alina Somova
Maria Riccetto	Ekaterina Kondaurova
Yevghenia Obraztsova	Ekaterina Osmolkina
Kristi Boone	Nadia Gonchar and many other at the Maryinsky Ballet
Zhong-Jing Fang	
Veronika Part of American Ballet Theatre	Erica Cornejo of Boston Ballet
Alina Cojocaru	Ekaterina Shipulina of the Bolshoi Ballet
Zenaida Yanowsky	Aria Alekzander of Houston Ballet
Vanessa Palmer	Deanna Seay of Miami City Ballet
Francesca Filpi of the Royal Ballet	

What are the most common requests in custom-made shoes? Do you need to see the dancer's foot, or it is enough to see a picture of the foot?

It is hard to answer the first question because there are so many different types of feet. Certainly, we have a range of our most popular sizes, and because you select from six size variables when fitting Gaynor Mindens, each stock pair is a virtual custom fit. It is ideal to fit Gaynor Mindens in person. However, we do have an excellent online fitting system that allows dancers to submit foot tracings, photos, and general information about themselves. With these combined details, our fitters are able to suggest an initial Gaynor Minden fit within a relatively small margin of error.

Can you give your personal advice to dancers struggling to find the right shoe?

Essential in a pointe shoe selection of any brand is a good fitting. A dancer needs to place herself in capable, skilled hands when selecting a pointe shoe, with fitters who are familiar with dancers' needs, foot types, and fitting options. Education is important as well, so a dancer should thoroughly research whatever pointe shoe she wishes to try to better understand her options with that brand. And open communication with the dancer's teacher is also helpful. Teachers have the best lens on a dancer's individual needs and should always check a dancer's pointe shoe fit before she sews and wears her shoes.

Where should dancers interested in having custom-made Gaynors send their orders?

All the information you need is on the Gaynor Minden website. Click "Pointe Shoes" and "Let Us Fit You" for all the details. Pictures of the foot are certainly helpful, but foot tracings and other comparative information is even more important—age, height, weight, pointe work level, arch height, preferences, previous pointe shoe brands, cushioning you want to wear when dancing on pointe, etc.

Jean Teplitsky
Teplov Pointe Shoes
34 Sergeant Street, Somerset West, Western Cape
South Africa 7130
Phone: 021 851 4331
Fax: 021 851 5263
E-mail: www.teplov.co.za

Teplov Ballet Shoes, the first professional ballet shoe manufacturer in South Africa, opened its doors back in 1979.

How did your shoe factory start? Can you tell me more about the history of Teplov?

Teplov was started by two international ballet stars—namely, Diana Teplitsky (formerly Cawley) and her husband, Georges Teplitsky—who were both dancing for the state opera ballet in Munich, Germany. When Georges was forced to give up his professional career because of an arthritic hip, this was both physically and emotionally painful, as he had worked his entire life to come to this point in his career, having danced the lead in all the famous ballets around the world. Georges retired from the stage in his late twenties. At that time, all the ballet shoes were custom-made inhouse by a master craftsman. When he offered Georges to teach him his craft, he promptly accepted. On returning to South Africa, Diana's home country, Georges started a small atelier in Bree Street in Cape town (the first ballet shoe maker in the southern hemisphere) whilst Diana carried on [with] her professional career with Capab Ballet, now Cape Town City Ballet. The production started with one pair a day, all hand cut and made, except for the use of a sewing machine brought back from Germany, to stitch the uppers!

Are your pointe shoes totally hand-made? In how many steps are your pointe shoes crafted? Do you use the "inside-out" technique?

We do not use the turn shoe technique. Our shoes are completely handmade in several steps: cutting of the uppers and lining, upper lining lamination, shank construction, prelisting, block construction, final lasting, block setting in a warmer area for several days.

What makes your pointe shoes so unique? What are their main characteristics?

One of our defining characteristics is our ability to custom-fit shoes for clients, from last alterations to vamp height, and shank alterations.

What are the advantages of wearing Teplov?

Their solid classical construction, suited mostly for beginners and amateurs.

How many types of pointe shoes do you make? How many widths and strengths?

We have two types, namely, Delco's (softer block) and the Points. They come in five different widths and several back strengths.

What type of shanks do you offer? Which is your softest shoe, the most suitable for beginners?

We offer full backs [shanks] and three-quarter backs (for stronger more arched feet). These come in soft, medium, hard, and double hard. In the case of beginners, all depends on their foot type, usually medium back.

Do you mostly deal with custom orders or with standard orders from dance stores?

We deal with both, but the bulk of our shoes go to shops.

Can you name some of the major ballet companies using your pointe shoes?

Cape Town City Ballet and the State Ballet Theatre.

Where is your main factory located? How many cobblers work in your factory?

Our factory is located in Somerset West [Cape Town]. We have ten cobblers working for us, and most of them have been here for almost twenty-five years! We have a great work ambiance!

What are the main ingredients of your paste?

This is a trade secret!

What are the most common requests in custom-made shoes? Do you need to see the dancer's foot?

The most common requests are back alterations and vamp heights, and we prefer to see the dancer's foot!

Can you give your personal advice for dancers struggling to find the suitable pointe shoe?

Very few shoemakers have actually danced themselves. This makes it difficult sometimes for the dancer to get what they need.

Which is the foot type that best responds to Teplov pointe shoes?

We can cater for most foot types.

Which is your lightest beginner's shoe?

This would usually be our soft back.

Part VIII

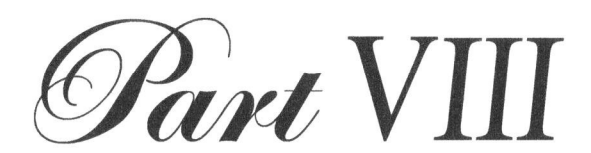

INTERVIEWS WITH POINTE SHOE FITTERS AND SPECIALISTS

Michele Attfield
Managing Director and Pointe Shoe Expert
Freed of London

Michele has worked at Freeds for over forty-five years and was honored by the Queen last year with an MBE for her services to the industry. Her expertise is requested by many international and UK companies and schools to fit, as well as to organize talks and lectures to students and professionals. She was appointed director of Freed in 1996 and is also a lifetime member of the Royal Academy of Dance.

This interview took place at Freed's retail shop in St. Martins Lane, London. Michele is a fine lady with a sharp sense of humor and an immense knowledge in the fitting of pointe shoes.

Michele, how did you start getting involved in pointe shoes?

When I was a girl, I danced. I was ten when I was first fitted by Mrs. Freed. I had very high insteps right from the beginning. I got a particular scholarship, and the teachers invited me to be fitted by Mrs. Freed, and since then I'd always come to Freed to fit my shoes. When I stopped dancing, I started performing in the theater, and then I started teaching and working here at Freed part-time. So for about four years, I worked here and taught. Then when my teaching job was finished, Mrs. Freed asked me to start working here all the time. So I stopped working and started working full-time at Freed's. I was then twenty-eight years old and stopped only when I had my babies. Even when my babies were small, I continued to do the fitting for the ballet companies. I've fitted the Royal Ballet, English National Ballet, Birmingham Royal Ballet, the UK ballet companies with continuity during that time. I had the chance to meet lots of dancers. I got to help some, which is great for me. When I go to companies abroad to do fitting, I get to watch rehearsals or classes, which you know, if you're interested in dancing, is really good.

What are the steps to follow to help find the suitable shoe?

When I start fitting, I look at people's feet, and then I look at the rest of their body. You can't just fit the feet, particularly when they're beginners, but you really can't just fit only their feet at any time because you have to have a look at where the weight distribution is. When you're first fitting particularly, you're looking at very young children that are in prepuberty. The pelvic girdle is undeveloped, and you have to have a very light shoe because they cannot get the instep over if their hip is only that wide.

From that point of view, we always start with a light shoe. It's something that's peculiar to the schools of ballet that are famous for footwork, this idea to start young people in a light shoe. So in the UK and in the USA, we do that. It's no secret that since the '60s our companies are famous for the terre à terre footwork, the ability to use the feet. In some other countries, they have the opposite approach, and they think that you should start with a shoe that is like a piece of scaffolding to hold you up, but the feet this way never get any stronger. So I always start with a very light insole for beginners. Obviously you also have to look at the child's weight, and you can't guarantee how a twelve-year-old child will develop.

So we have to take practicality into account. By the same token, if you're fitting a very small child, she is going to outgrow her shoes anyway, so the issue of whether they have longevity, whether they are strong or weak doesn't really matter.

What do you do if they are beginners but the arch is really pronounced?

Generally, in most dancers' feet, people with high arches have intrinsically weak feet. People with high insteps have very lazy metatarsals, and the theory that we use to fit pointe shoes is, the part of your foot that does all the work, that part that supports you on pointe, the part that enables you to develop your pointe work is the metatarsal or the cou-de-pied, and that's the part of the foot that we look at all the time. The argument of where the toes are long, short, is actually quite irrelevant. I need to see if the student is actually able to use her metatarsals.

So quite often, you find that girls that have that exceptional high instep find pointe work really difficult, because they have weak metatarsals. We send them away from here to do metatarsal exercises, to try and get on a three-quarter pointe, generally to do lots of things like that to develop that part.

So if you line up a group of children and make them all point their toes really hard, what you are looking at is the metatarsals. Insteps are irrelevant, pretty, very pretty, and not intrinsically strong. The part of your foot that's working is your metatarsal, that's the part that does all the work.

The series of pointe work is so easy, so logical, there's no magic, no smoking mirrors. The most important thing is to have flexibility in the ankle, in the demi-pointe and demi-plié.

What do you suggest when the heel of the shoe slips off?

One of the biggest reasons the shoe comes off of the heel is because they're narrow. Again, a lot of the excess fabric, bagginess of the heel when you're on pointe, when you demi-plié is not evident, and it means that you're not using your metatarsals. If you're not using them, your foot just slides into the shoe.

If the metatarsal is working, then you stay in the shoe. If it's not working, then you slip into the shoe.

At Freed we move our soles back. Bloch shoes have much longer soles, so they'll cut a poke on everybody.

What do you do when the second toe is longer than the first?

It makes no difference because you are not fitting the toes, you are fitting the metatarsals. So when you point your toes, the longer one curves with the other toes, and you are wearing toe pads anyway.

What do you think about toe pads?

I don't mind thin ones, but most toe pads are too padded underneath, and you can't feel the floor. Also, students leave them in the shoes, and they become like a nest of bacteria where they put their feet back in every time. It's not hygienic, and it stinks.

Does Freed make a shoe "ready for the stage"?

If you are looking for a shoe ready to go onstage, the nearest choice is the Classic Pro. So if you are doing Swan Lake, you need one pair of shoes quite broken in for the white act, and one pair of shoes not broken at all to do black act.

What shoe do you prefer for beginners?

If the beginner is very lightweight, I would like to go with a light shoe. If she is not very lightweight, I am not going to go with a light shoe because she's going to kill it in the first class.

Which is the best way to sew ribbons?

The ribbons are very intense. They should be sewn very low down and slightly angled, and they should pull the sole against your foot, not the upper.

What do you think about elastics?

I don't think you should need elastics to hold your shoe on. I'm quite happy with professionals to use elastics to make themselves feel more secure, but to be frank, if I go to the ballet and I can see too much elastic, then I think it looks ugly. We don't mind the lightweight elastic, be we don't like the thick ones.

How do you think pointe training should start?

The first two or three months, students should only work at the barre, doing rises, relevés, and échappés. By the end of the first two months, they should be doing relevés on one foot and from two to one.

Do you think having custom-made shoes is important?

Most professional dancers have custom-made shoes because they want something specific and they want continuity. They prefer custom-made shoes because they get twenty or thirty at a time and they want them to be identical. And because they can do what they want with the shoe—I want this up, that down—they can do anything. Freed shoes are durable. It depends what shoes you have, to be honest. I mean, obviously, Freed shoes are all hand lasted, and they only use natural ingredients, which are biodegradable. There is no plastic, there are no polymers, everything is natural; and also, the other thing, which is very important with children,

Freed shoes are never stronger than your foot. Nowadays, there are shoes made of plastic. One of the problems we had in the UK is that these shoes are very expensive—they cost £70, and ours cost £35; and because they are plastic, they win. The foot doesn't win, the shoe will win.

From that point of view, one of the things that make Freed's shoes successful is just that. Obviously, how long they last depends on how you wear them and how you look after them, and how much work you do. It's always a misnomer what people would say when they are talking of pointe shoes and know nothing about it. How long will they last? I understand that some ballerinas wear two pairs in a performance. Yes, but they wear the same two pairs in five other performances as well, so it's difficult, and again it depends. You get one dancer who wants her pointe shoes really hard or she can't dance on them, and you have someone else who wants them really soft, or she can't dance on them.

Obviously, if you ask for a strong block, it will last longer. If you stump on them, and put them in a doorframe, they will go quickly.

What do you advise to do in order to break in Freed shoes?

I don't. For a beginner, I would say don't. I am so tired of people having teachers and seniors bending them when they're cold and snapping them, so I would say that all Freed shoes have what we call the spring. In fact, it's because of the way the block substance is layered, and the way they are baked in the oven. There is air in the shoe, so there is always a small movement. They are never completely rigid. When the foot gets hot, the air expands and acts as a shock absorber, which helps to reduce stress injuries and makes the shoe more flexible. When you're warmed up and you're dancing, you think, Oh, they feel really fine. But if you put them on when you're cold, you say, "I can't do this." That's what does that. When you take your shoes off, take your toe pads out, stuff your shoes with paper, and put them somewhere to dry, and they will last longer. If you put your toe pads back and your shoes in your bag, next time you take your shoes out, they are still wet; and they are not going to last too long. Children will give the shoe to some kid in their class who will snap their shoes, and then their mothers will come, saying, "The insole is broken." We will repair them. We are lucky we have a factory, but it's a problem.

Exercise: Just in a natural position, quarter-pointe, half-pointe, and three-quarter pointe and come down. So tell kids to start to learn that when they do not have a lot of body weight. It's a very good idea because it makes them use their metatarsals; and also, if you're teaching it, it lets you know how strong they're going to be on pointe before you put them in pointe shoes. So without turning out, quite naturally, just comfortably go up till the three-quarter pointe and then half-pointe. Try and get the center of the metatarsal off the ground without curling your toes, and then go back down. When you get to the half-pointe, just take the center of the metatarsal off the ground. This is an exercise that I learnt when I was a RAD scholar, when I was ten. It gives you a heads-up on how their feet work.

Zoe Cleland
Pointe Shoe Fitter, Capezio

How does a typical fitting start at Capezio's?

Our typical fitting starts by measuring both feet on a Brannock device. It is important to assess many different qualities of the dancer's foot in the very beginning. By measuring the foot, you will immediately know which is the longer or narrower foot and which foot is the smaller or the wider. Also look at the length of the toes, as well as the placement and flexibility of the dancer's arch. Then discuss with the dancer about which padding she prefers, so you can adjust the size accordingly. Finally, ask the dancer what technique she is studying, so you can complement her style of dance.

What are the basic steps you follow to help a beginner find the suitable shoe?

Typically, I start first-time pointe dancers with a basic beginner shoe, which is the softest, lowest-vamp shoe (and most similar to a demi-pointe shoe). This way I can assess their needs. If they have weak arches or strong arches, if they are tense in the ankles, or need something to hold them back. Also look at the amount of support or glue they need to achieve proper technique and alignment.

How long does a fitting generally last?

It lasts about forty-five minutes.

How short do you think nails should be trimmed?

I believe the nails should definitely be trimmed to be flush with the dancer's toe. Also make sure the corners of the toenail are not digging into the cuticles. Any extra pressure points on the toe will cause bruising or infection in the toenails.

Are Capezio shoes built inside out?

Yes.

How many types of pointe shoes does Capezio produce?

Capezio manufactures twelve different styles, most of which can be found in a normal shank and an ES shank. We also manufacture four different styles of pointe shoes for Special Make-Ups.

Can you name a particularly popular shoe for beginners?

Tendu II.

Do you advise soft shanks or hard ones for beginners?

Softer is better. However, it is not that black-and-white. Ideally, I look at where the dancer is bending the shank when she is up on pointe. If it is bending around the metatarsal of the foot, then she possibly needs more support from her shoe.

What about in the case of a strong arch and instep?

Strong arches and insteps will learn to articulate better in softer shanks. I have also found that higher crowns will help give big arches room for articulation, as well as allowing the shoe to hug the foot better when on pointe, and ultimately make the shoe last longer because there is less pressure on the shank. Sometimes a three-quarter shank may help in this case. The three-quarter shank allows the dancer to get proper support from the metatarsal area without compromising the durability and life of the shoe. With strong arches, the dancer often needs less support from the shank, but because of the increased demand they are putting on the shank, as well as desired flexibility, the three-quarter shank allows for the arch to work without putting strain on the top quarter of the shank. However, if the foot is strong and flexible, they may need a longer vamp to hold them back.

What do you suggest in case of very low arches?

I prefer to put dancers with low arches in shoes with shorter vamps so it's easier for them to get over the box, and they don't have to fight with the shoe for proper alignment from the whole body.

What do you advise for students with a longer second toe, in order to reduce the pain?

Lower crown and/or tapered boxes to reduce the pressure on the toes. Inside the shoe, I recommend a little more padding, either gel toe pads or lamb's wool.

What if the first toe is longer than the second?

Same thing as longer second toe.

What type of accessories would you recommend, if any?

Besides lamb's wool or gel toe pads, I would recommend toe spacers to help create greater lateral support.

I often notice that students have problems with the heel of the shoe. Heels are often too high compared to the dancer's heel. Are there any "low-heel" pointe shoes you advise, or any "trick" to conceal the bagginess of the shoe?

Capezio has two awesome shoes for this problem. The Glissé Pro has a shortened heel for dancers looking to show off their arches. Capezio also makes a shoe called the Aria, which has a heel seam cut down three-eighth of an inch shorter than most heel seams. The shortened heel seam cuts out the excess bagginess. We also provide this service with our Special Make-Up pointe shoes. With an SMU, we can shorten heels to any specified length for this problem. Also, for a heel that is too baggy, Capezio creates a split last for dancers with narrower heels, such as an A heel width but a C box width.

How do you think a beginner's shoe should fit?

The shoes should feel snug but should not pinch. A dancer is not supposed to feel like the foot can move around inside the shoe, but rather, the shoe and the foot should move as one. The longest toe should feel the platform without feeling curled. Students should feel like they can move their foot freely without restriction, be in charge of the shoe and not let the shoe do the work for them or pull them off pointe. There should be no space between the top of the foot and the crown of the shoe. When on pointe, there should be no more than a quarter of an inch of excess fabric at the heel. The shank should bend slightly to their arch. If there is no bend in the shank, the shoe is too hard; and if it bends too low, the shank is too soft.

Do you think students should use toepads and if yes what type do you think is the best?

Bunheads Ouch Pouches in combination with lamb's wool or toe tape, if needed. The less stuff in the shoe, the better, especially in the first six months. I like the dancers to feel the floor and their toes. They need to feel a little pain so they can adjust their technique and shoes accordingly.

What type of shoe would you advise for professionals wishing a shoe "ready to go onstage," offering the maximum flexibility thus still supporting?

I would suggest a shoe with a three-quarter shank.

What type of shank, block, and vamp do you recommend for beginners?

Soft shank, wide platform, and short vamp. Soft shank so they can develop their own strength, wide platform to assist in balance while ankle strength is being developed. Short vamps so they can have easy roll-through to gain foot articulation.

How do you think students should break in their new Capezio pointe shoes?

If they are beginners, they should break the shoe in with their feet to gain strength and help mold the shoe to the foot.

Are there any special steps to follow?

If the dancer is more experienced, she already knows what kind of arch she has and where she needs support. For Capezio pointe shoes, I do recommend a little breaking-in. However, I also recommend different types of breaking-in, depending on the shoe and the dancer's feet. Also, each shoe has its own special attributes (as does each foot).

My general advice for breaking-in is,

1. Flatten the box a little by placing the palm of your hand on the crown of the box, and gently press down to soften the glue and flatten the crown from being high and round to a little more flat and a little bit more reflective of your foot's crown height. This also makes the shoe a little bit wider.
2. Take your thumb and index finger and gently work the glue in the wings to soften it a little. This will decrease the pressure on your metatarsal bunion area.
3. Put your thumbs on the top of the shank near the heel, and put the heel of the shank on the floor, and roll the shank at the three-quarter into a small arc so the shank follows the natural arch of the foot better and the shoe becomes more supportive.
4. Lastly, if rolling through demi-pointe is difficult because of the glue in the box or the stiffness of the shank behind the ball of the foot, I recommend, once the ribbons and elastic are sewn on, to run across the floor with the shoes on, in demi, just a little.

If you do any of these techniques too much, you will kill the shoe and its support. I recommend making subtle, gentle changes to the shoe and then trying it on after each step before doing more.

Are you against elastics?

No, I am not.

Which is the most suitable spot for elastics according to you?

It varies depending on the foot and the dancer's needs.

How do you solve the problem of the heel slipping down or looking too baggy?

For a heel that is slipping down, this depends entirely on the dancer's foot. Sometimes the shank is too hard and snaps the shoe off the foot during roll-through, so I suggest a more flexible shank. Sometimes they may need a higher heel seam. Most often I try to fit the dancer in an alternative shoe, because the shoe is just not fitting their foot correctly. Some quick fixes are sewing the elastic close together behind the heel or sticking rosin on the inside of the heel, so it's less slippery. Alternatively, Capezio can cut down or lengthen the heel seam.

Do you have special guidelines for the students for sewing their ribbons?

Folding down the heel of the shoe and placing the back edge of the ribbons at the crease. Also sewing the ribbons deeply into the shoe at a slight angle forward that also runs parallel to the crease creates tension to keep the ribbons tight during repeated transitioning from flat to on pointe.

How do you think ribbons should be tied?

They should be tied into the divot behind the anklebone.

What is the correct way to sew elastics?

It depends on the dancer, but if possible, as far down inside the shoe, as close to the shank as possible. This helps the shoe hug the foot better as it breaks in.

Most dancers think that Capezio shoes are only good for narrow feet. Is it true, and if yes, to what extent?

Historically, yes. However, times have changed, and we have a range of shoes for almost every kind of foot. Especially in our newer shoes, we tend to have squarer boxes these days.

Is there a particular exercise you teach your dancers in order to improve their arch?

Tendu correctly, never letting your toes leave the floor and extending through the front of the leg to pointe. Avoid scrunching the heel and Achilles tendons. Also, Thera-Band exercises help.

When do you think a dancer has to choose custom-made shoes instead of the ones already on the market?

After they have danced in them and wish for just one or two small differences. Also at a professional level, dancers' needs become extremely specific, and we can address those needs without all the unnecessary stuff.

Do you think Capezio shoes are durable, and what do you advise to make them last longer?

I think they are durable. Capezio shoes are amazing for this reason. They are durable without compromising the articulation and line of the foot. To make pointe shoes last longer, I recommend drying them out completely before wearing them again.

What is your personal advice for beginners' pointe?

Communicate all your concerns with fitters and teachers. That way you can understand your feet, technique, and shoes better for yourself. Honesty and patience is the best way to achieve a perfect fit from your pointe shoes. Don't worry about the fitter's feelings or time spent. They are just a bridge between you and your ultimate feet on pointe.

Mary Carpenter
Professional Fitter, Freed USA

Mary Carpenter trained at the College-Conservatory of Music, the official school for the Cincinnati Ballet Company. She went to Butler University and continued her training at David Howard Dance Center in NYC on scholarship. She danced professionally with the Metropolitan Opera, Lexington Ballet, Ohio Dance Theatre, Charleston Ballet, Maryland Ballet, Festival Ballet of New Jersey, Granite State Ballet, and many others. She has worked as a professional pointe shoe fitter for Repetto USA, Gaynor Minden, Capezio, Freed of London and USA and been interviewed for many magazines on fitting tips. Mary is also the featured instructor in two of RizBiz's ballet videos "Budding Ballerinas" and "From Tights to Tutus." She also works for Roper Records and has directed nine classroom music CDs as well as starred and directed "The Magical World of Ballet" DVD for teaching young students. Mary is on faculty at Steps on Broadway, NYC; Barnard College, and the New School university.

Mary shared some of her wisdom and experience during this very interesting interview.

How do you assess the ability of a student to start pointe work? What is, according to you, the age range for going on pointe?

This is a tough question in America. There is no standardization for dance training in this country. You have to be certified to do someone's hair or nails, but no certification is required to be a dance teacher. I am working on my certification for Pilates mat training right now. Why do I have to certify in that, but I don't have to do anything to teach ballet and pointe? This is why there are so many problems with bad ballet technique and the pointe work you sometimes see that makes you cringe.

When I fit someone for the first time here in NYC and parents ask that question, I usually answer this way: If you are not going to a very serious training conservatory (ABT's JKO school or Ballet Academy East, to name a few), then you have to be taking ballet continuously for three years in a row, three times a week, and be at least twelve years old. That includes studying over the summer!

Having stated that, I have seen amazing kids in very fine schools go en pointe at age ten, and they are nurtured and not overworked, and the studios get amazing results. Some of the schools that come to mind are Seiskaya (Valia Seiskaya, St. James, Long Island) and Central Pennsylvania Youth Ballet—one of the most fertile training grounds in this country. SAB waits until they are twelve usually. I personally have rejected customers when the child is aged eight or nine. I've gotten a lot of angry parents, a lot of tears, and I have had to play the bad guy. I really cannot endorse anything under age ten. The feet are so undeveloped, as well as the muscle tone. Many kids still have their round "baby" bellies under age ten.

Do you advise soft or hard shanks for beginners?

Another good question—there are two schools of thought on this. One is to get the first-time pointe dancer into something soft so they can "get over" easily and develop strength on their own. The idea is that they develop strength on their own and don't rely on the shoe. The second philosophy is that if you put the student in something hard, they have to work against it and work hard to get en pointe, and they will develop the strength from the hard work and the resistance of the shoe. Both of these ideas are useful. As a professional fitter, I am there to make the teacher happy and work my fitting into their personal philosophy. I know all the teachers around NYC and all the major schools, so I try to fit to what they want. As a teacher and someone who dances en pointe, I think pointe work is a privilege, not a right. I don't think everyone is suited to go en pointe, and to be honest, many, many dancers are put en pointe too soon, in my opinion. It is so backwards—get the shoes and then the technique will come and you will be able to get over. That is the wrong idea. The dancer has to display a technical level that shows they are worthy of getting those shoes. Pointe work is an extension of good technique—you have to have good technique first. The shoes aren't magic! As David Howard always says, "It's called pointe work, not pointe easy!"

I do fit the individual dancer according to their needs. I assess their training, technique, level, foot shape, and body type. All of those factors go into what type of shoe they need and the strength and box shape. Any good fitter should be doing that for their customer. In the broadest terms, low arches want soft shanks, high arches want harder shanks. Weak feet should be strengthened first and then get the shoes later. Cross-training with things like a stretchy band and Pilates is very important.

What do you advise for students with a longer second toe, to reduce the pain? What if the first toe is longer than the second?

This is hard to answer in writing. When I fit dancers in NYC, I always try to make sure that there is good alignment with their bones. Hips, knees, ankles should line up correctly with the metatarsals en pointe. The same goes for the phalanges. If you don't have even toes, there are all kinds of constructive things you can do to help out.

I often notice that students have problems with the heel of the shoe. Heels are generally too high compared to the dancer's heel, and they give that "baggy" look. Are there any "low-heel" pointe shoes you advise or any "trick" to conceal the bagginess of the shoe?

Many dancers have a diminishing heel, or a triangular appearance, to their foot. There is nothing they can do about that from an anatomical standpoint. You can improve the appearance by getting a slim-cut heel, [getting] a lower-profile shoe, stitching the ribbon and elastic differently, and, if you can afford it, getting a custom order with cut-down sides.

Custom orders are not practical until the dancer has finished growing. The first thing I would do is check the fit of the shoes. Many American dancers wear their shoes too wide, and they are swimming in the shoe. They get a shoe that is too short, and then go wider to compensate.

How do you think a beginner's shoe should fit?

I have worked for Repetto, USA; Gaynor Minden; Capezio Ballet Makers, and currently I work for Freed of London/USA. I have also fit Bloch, Grishko, Cecilia Kerche, Principal, Fuzi, Chacott, Gamba, and Sansha. In addition to that, I am familiar with Suffolk, Prima Soft, Eva Martins, Solos, Russian Pointe. I am what they call an "across-the-board" fitter. I could never say that one type of shoe was the only shoe for this or that. That would be a disservice to my customers. I try to give very honest advice about what type of shoe will go well on what foot. I do like Freed pointe shoes for professionals. I have worn them since I was seventeen!

Do you think your students should use toe pads?

This is the age-old debate. Most every dancer needs some kind of padding, even if it is a small amount. I do like the Bunheads products. They are made with a non-silicon polymer gel, and they have mineral oil in them. They are also washable and reusable.

What type of shank, block, and vamp do you advise for beginners?

Whatever fits the best!

How do you teach students to break their new pointe shoes in?

"Some brands require a lot of work; some require no work before entering class. When I fit a dancer in NYC I give them the "courtesy crunch." I flatten out the box for them a bit; also I like to curve the shank under their arch so it hugs. Water works if the wings are too stiff."

Do you hold a special "introductory" pointe class before the start of pointe work?

"Everybody should. I used to make my firsttimers sew their own shoes the first class, and then we would learn to tie them, etc.
This is where I love the European method of training, where they use a "demi-soft" shoe. I think it is a great idea, kind of like training wheels on a bicycle.

How do you teach your students to sew their ribbons? How do you want them to be tied?

The most basic method for first-timers is to fold the back half of the shoe down and make a diagonal mark with a pen. Follow the pen line and stitch the ribbons all the way down on the diagonal by the shank. Then put the elastic behind the ribbon, not in front of it. You can follow the same diagonal line with the elastic.

How do you like the elastics to be sewn?

It is a science experiment, and you are the scientist. You have to try different things to see what works.

Could you give a sample of a first class on pointe?

Learn to put the shoes on, tie the shoes, and go to the barre. Learn how to stand correctly at the barre without using it like it is a crutch. Slow elevés and some relevés on two feet. Learn how to properly store the pointe shoes in between wearing.

Can you describe two barre and two center exercises suitable for the first two to three months on pointe?

Échappés are always good. Elevés are always good. No relevés on one leg for a while.

Is there a particular exercise you teach your dancers in order to improve their arch?

Yes! They are called tendus! Also working on a very high demi-pointe in technique class is mandatory.

What is your personal advice for beginner's pointe?

Congratulations and good luck. Don't panic, and work hard!

Judy Weiss
Fitter, Grishko's Pointe Shoes

Judy Weiss is a veteran in the fitting of pointe shoes. Her career, which she started as a dancer, gave her even better knowledge about the requirements of a dancer. She is a master pointe shoe fitter at Grishko in New York and has been fitting pointe shoes for over thirty years. Judy created a shoe for Capezio called Prelude.

How did Grishko start? Can you tell me more about the history of Grishko?

Pointe shoes are no longer made within the theaters. Grishko started pointe shoe production in 1989. They are made in accordance with all traditions of the nineteenth century. The secrets of pointe shoe making were passed by word of mouth. Each maker added something new to the technology.

How did you start fitting pointe shoes?

I danced for twenty years and started fitting and selling pointe shoes when I decided to stop.

Are Grishko shoes totally handmade? Do you use the "inside-out" technique?

Yes, the shoes are all made by hand. The pattern, the way the uppers are cut, the binding and the drawstring sewn to the upper, and the box made of layers of different materials, built inside out then the sole sewn on. The shank is then added, and the shoes are set to dry. This is what I remember after visiting our factory in Moscow. It is not totally accurate.

What makes your pointe shoes so unique? What are their main characteristics?

They are beautiful on the foot and lengthen the line of the leg. The foot becomes an extension of the leg. The shoes with the V throat give the foot a lovely Russian look.

How many types of pointe shoes do you make? How many widths and strengths?

We have eleven different models, five widths and sizes starting at 1 and go up to 8.5 in some models. We make three different shank strengths. Some are full shanks and some are three-quarter.

Are your shanks made of cardboard or leather or other?

They are made of some kind of fiberboard.

Do you mostly deal with custom orders or with standard orders from dance stores?

Both.

Can you name some of the major ballet companies and ballerinas using your pointe shoes?

Bolshoi, Maryinsky, Diana Vishneva.

Where is your main factory located? How many cobblers work in your factory?

The one factory is in Moscow and has three hundred people working for it. Pointe shoes, ballet slippers, tutus, dancewear, and active wear are all made in separate areas within this factory.

What are the main requirements in custom-made pointe shoes?

We can do anything. Lower or higher vamps, sides and heels are most common.

What are the main ingredients of your paste?

I can't reveal.

What are the most common requests in custom-made shoes? Can you fit through pictures and correspondence?

I have and will "fit" shoes with correspondence and pictures. The order can be sent to me at our NYC store. A picture is not enough. I need pointe shoe size and style to begin with. If [the dancer is] not wearing Grishko, it is difficult to find the right size or style unless the shoes are tried on.

Can you give your personal advice for dancers struggling to find the suitable pointe shoe?

Go to a retail store where there is somebody who really knows how to fit shoes. Do not buy something because it is the only size or style shoe they have at that moment.

What is the foot type that best responds to Grishko shoes?

There is a style for dancers of all levels, from beginners to professionals.

Esther Juon
Professional Pointe Shoe Fitter, ABBO
Author, Pointe Shoe Secrets
Linda Reid-Lobatto
Professional Pointe Shoe Fitter
www.pointeshoefitting.co.uk

How do you assess the ability of a student to start pointe work? What is, according to your experience, the suitable age to start pointe work?

I think the student should be answering "yes" to all of the following questions:

- Have you started your periods or had your second growth spurt?
- Have you had permission from your teacher?
- Are you taking at least two to three classes a week, every week, and studied for a minimum of four years?
- Do you have sufficient strength to do the following:
- Hold your turnout while dancing
- Hold your heel forward toward the big toe when you point your toes with no sickling
- Hold a passé balance on demi-pointe without any wobbling
- Be able to point your foot without curling your toes

The above points should be taken into consideration before pointe shoes are fitted. If we feel a dancer is not ready for pointe shoes, we encourage the fitting of demi-pointe/soft-blocked shoes. A dancer coming to me for a fitting is advised that we may not fit the shoes if we feel she is not ready or physically developed enough. We do not like to fit a dancer before the age of twelve years, but we are also aware that some dancers are in full-time dance school from an early age. If pointe shoes are fitted early, we highly recommend that they are taken off pointe when a growth spurt starts. To dance en pointe during a growth spurt can cause many serious problems.

Do you advise soft shanks or hard ones for beginners? How do you fit students with strong or weak arches?

We both have no hard-and-fast rules on what shank we would fit a beginner in. We would normally start dancers in a medium shank. In my experience, I have found that the softer the shank, the more core stability a dancer requires. A medium-shanked shoe is supportive both for the arch and ankle. We both have no rules or regulations for different-strength arches. A high arch usually is a weak arch, where a flatter foot has a stronger arch. Every dancer is an individual and must be fitted as such.

What do you advise for students with a longer second toe to reduce the pain? What if the first toe is longer than the second?

We both often fit dancers with a longer second toe, but it will depend on how the length differs to how it is dealt with. Normally we try and use the Grishko Vaganova shoe. This has a longer-tapered box. Pop a little toe sock on the tip of that toe and fit the shoe to the length of that longer toe. It is then a good idea to fill in the space between the big toe and the platform of the shoe. You can purchase a small silicone disc that sticks to the bottom of the platform, where the big toe would sit. It will normally fill that space. The most important issue is that the longer toe is straight and that the foot does not slide down the shoe at all. A well-fitted shoe that holds the metatarsal heads securely is most important here. The principles of fitting with a longer first toe are exactly the same as [with a] longer second toe.

How do you solve the issue of "baggy heels"? Are there any "low-heel" pointe shoes you advise or any "trick" to conceal the bagginess of the shoe?

If a shoe is fitted too long or too wide, the heelpiece will automatically bag. It is most important here that the shape of the shoe is the correct style for the dancer. There are shoes that are designed for a narrow heel.

If the shoe is fitted correctly, the dancer is held in the shoe, and no slippage occurs. This usually points to a good, correct fit. If even with a good fit the heel slips, then I would either use a heel grip that can be bought in any good shoe shop, or ask the dancer to apply rosin to the heel of her tights. We would never ever fit a shoe with a pinch of satin to spare.

Do you have a special brand of shoes you prefer for your students? How do you think a beginner's shoe should fit?

We both will only ever fit Grishko Pointe shoes. We dislike the Gaynor Minden shoe, but if a pointe shoe is correctly fitted where the foot is held, and there is no slipping of the foot down the shoe, then all pointe shoes can be used. We use the same principles of fitting for every dancer we fit, whether they are beginner or advanced. The importance with a beginner is that you take your time to explain how to stand correctly when [on] en pointe and how the shoe should feel.

Do you think students should use toe pads?

We never fit using toe pads as we have found that this changes the correct shoe sizing as width and length need to be increased to fit in the ouch pouch.

What type of shank, block, and vamp do you prefer for beginners?

We have no hard-and-fast rules for a beginner's shoe. The shoe we would use will depend on the foot shape and what gives the dancer's foot the maximum support.

How do you teach students to break their new pointe shoes in?

To break in a pair of shoes, we would strongly recommend that the dancer does pony trots at the barre. We like to use the barre to prepare pointe shoes. We find that very few dancers are prepared to put in the amount of time to prepare pointe shoes ready to work in. This means that many dancers are dancing in an unbroken shoe. This makes pointe work much more difficult.

An introduction to pointe work day is always highly recommended before pointe work commences, and we both participate in these one-day courses at dance schools.

Do you have special guidelines for the students for sewing their ribbons? How do you want them to be tied?

We recommend that the ribbon is sewn in one continuous strip rather than cut into two pieces, and that the ribbons are tied using the inside ribbon first. Also to make sure that the ribbon is not knotted so it sits on the anklebone.

How do you want the elastics to be sewn?

Hopefully, if a pointe shoe is well fitted, then elastics do not need to be used.

What barre exercises do you advise for the first two to three months on pointe? Can you describe two barre and two center exercises?

The first three months of going en pointe should only consist of only basic barre work. No centre work as the feet are just not stable enough.
Feet in parallel, step up onto pointe and roll down through the shoe.
Two exercises we give all dancers we fit are 1) the metatarsal lift and 2) Kissing Toes from Eric Franklin.

We also recommend the use of a Thera-Band and wobble board, as these help to strengthen the feet. Our personal advice for a new dancer about to go en pointe is the wearing of soft blocks/demi-pointe shoes for six months to a year leading up to pointe work.

Make sure you get a well-fitted pair of pointe shoes from an experienced fitter. Do not buy the first pair of shoes you are fitted with. There are many different shoes on the market and many different styles. Look at your foot shape and the shape of the shoe, see if they match. If they are completely different shapes, then ask to see more. Take your time. They are your feet, and you have to dance in them.

Part IX

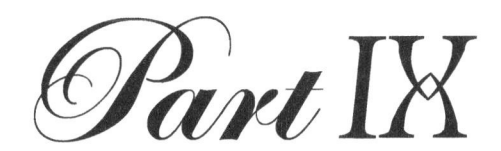

BALLET AND POINTE-RELATED INJURIES

HOW TO PREVENT THEM AND TREAT THEM

Chapter 1

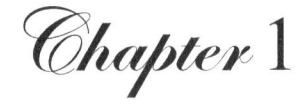

Common Problems

Before we approach any of the problems related to the practice of ballet and pointe work, I would like to say that most of these issues are related to poor training and incorrect technique.

Overturning feet, rolling in, tension in the shoulder, jumping without putting the heels completely on the floor, going on pointe too soon, or dancing without warming up properly . . . the list could go on forever. All of these factors contribute to future injuries and malformations of the foot, spine, and legs.

Dancing on a hard or non-sprung floor can cause or accelerate injuries such as tendonitis, small fractures, plantar fasciitis, shin splints, and sesamoiditis.

Stephen F. Conti, MD, and Yue Shuen Wong, MD, in their article "Foot and Ankle Injuries in the Dancer," affirm that "dancers subject their bodies to the same stresses that athletes do. The difference is that dancers have an additional artistic component to consider." They also claim that the majority of dancers' injuries affect the lower extremities. They reveal that according to most studies, it has been proven that 60 percent to 80 percent of injuries in dancers involve the foot, knee, and ankle. They also believe that the dancer's physique can affect the rate of injury. "The slim dancer with good turnout and joint mobility is less likely to be injured than one who is heavier and with poor flexibility." Fatigue injuries are also among the most common, especially for professional dancers who dance and rehearse full-time all week. Margaret Papoutsis is a well-known osteopath and nutritional therapist in England. She has been a consultant for many ballet companies like the Royal Danish Ballet, London Festival Ballet, and English National Ballet. She believes that the most important function of a teacher is to recognize that a structural problem exists, and to refer the dancer to a suitable therapist in order to obtain a correct diagnosis and appropriate treatment. The role of the teacher is of the maximum importance. It is up to her/him to detect tendencies like hyperextension, bow-leggedness, flat or hypermobile feet and work with them accordingly.

I am going to analyze some of the most common injuries occurring in the ballet field.

Chapter 2

Different Types of Injuries

Ballet and pointe-related injuries can be of different kinds:

- Sprains
- Strains
- Fractures
- Hairline fracture
- Bruises
- Metatarsalgia
- Plantar fasciitis

Ankle Sprain

Ankle sprain is the most common severe injury in dancers. In her book Preventing Dance Injuries, Ruth Solomon states that "perhaps the most important reason of ankle sprains is inadequate rehabilitation of previous ankle sprains, since these injuries are often taken too lightly." She also believes that poor technique could be one of the main causes for this type of injuries, especially in landing from jumps with the foot supinated.

Solomon believes that certain steps, like entrechats six, are more at risk than others. Also, she stresses the importance for dancers to know their limits and when it is time to stop rehearsing. Late-afternoon or evening rehearsals are more prone to cause injuries since the body is already tired. Ankle sprains generally involve the lateral ligaments and are caused by forced inversion of the foot when landing from a jump or coming down from pointe. Dr. Mark A. Caselli, DPM, suggests that we could divide ankle sprains in three different degrees, according to their severity.

Grade I ankle sprain involve stretching or partial tearing of the fibers of the muscles. This type of sprain can be treated with taping or Aircast. Icing, rest, and elevation have to be observed by the patient until the swelling persists.

Grade II sprains involve a total tear of the anterior talofibular ligament with different degrees of damage to the calcanealfibular ligament. Swelling is generally present, and as soon as it decreases, serial taping or an Aircast can be used.

Grade III ankle sprains involve complete or almost-complete tear of both the calcanealfibular and the anterior talofibular ligament. Immobilization is generally the only cure, but each case might be slightly different and require different treatments.

Dr. Caselli stresses the importance of physical therapy, regardless of the degree of the sprain, before being back to regular exercise.

Binding Sprained Ankles

You will need to be taught how to do it by a doctor or a physical therapist. It is important to know this, as dancers are often confronted with this type of injuries.

Use ankle-support bandages or premade ankle supports when you have a problem, but do not overuse because this will cause the ankle to become dependent on these, and therefore weak.

Stress Fractures

Dr. Lisa M. Schoene, a podiatrist specializing in sports medicine, stresses that dancers typically experience stress fractures of the second or third metatarsal. Continuous jumping and landing may be the cause of this injury. A hard floor with little or no shock absorption can also lead to stress fractures in the foot. Dr. Lori Weisenfeld, a New York–based sports podiatrist, affirms that most dancers' injuries occur between 4:00 and 6:00 PM. She believes that at that time, after a whole day spent dancing and practicing, the mind is tired and physical control has decreased. "I have never seen a ballet dancer whose feet were not abused," she said in a recent interview.

It is sometimes hard to determine the existence of a stress fracture. Plain radiographs may not show the evidence of fracture, and a bone scan may be the best way to confirm the diagnosis.

Bruised Toenails

Bruised toenails are generally due to improperly fitted pointe shoes, nails left too long, or knuckling of the toes while on pointe. The nail becomes dark, which means there is some bleeding underneath, and starts to appear thick and "elevated." If you have a bruised toenail or a blister, wear a Jelly Toe for padding.

There are a few things you can do to try and rescue the nail and prevent it from falling:

1. If you see any bruising, apply an ice bag for ten minutes and repeat three times a day.
2. Show the nail to your dance teacher and refrain from dancing on pointe for a least a week.
3. Apply micro foam tape over the end of the nail in order to compress it and keep it intact.
4. Clip the nail short, but not under the soft tissue under the nail.
5. Consult your doctor if the symptoms worsen.
6. Have your pointe shoes checked by a fitter or by your teacher. Maybe they are too short, and your toes are curling under.

Sometimes dancers can deal with a partially torn nail by avoiding pointe for a few days and by taping the loose nail down with a Band-Aid (only the non-sticky part should be in contact with the nail) until a new nail plate forms underneath, which can take up to three months.

Metatarsalgia and Plantar Fasciitis

Metatarsalgia is a term that indicates a painful condition in the metatarsal area of the foot (commonly called the ball of the foot). Metatarsalgia (ball–of-foot pain) is often situated under the second, third, and fourth metatarsal heads, or near the big toe. You could also experience numbness in your toes and sharp pain with a burning sensation. This foot condition is very common, and it causes one or more of the metatarsal heads to become inflamed, usually due to excessive pressure over long periods of time. The main causes usually are the following:

- Improperly fitted shoes. Tight shoes with thin soles and high heels should be avoided.
- Pointe shoes too narrow in the box.
- Jumping on hard floors.
- Standing for too many hours, like in the case of ballet teachers.

Pain can be relieved by resting and icing, using a metatarsal pad or gel metatarsal cushions and metatarsal bandages. These pads relieve some of the pressure in the ball of the foot. In order to prevent this condition before it appears, you can use shock-absorbing insoles or arch supports.

Plantar fasciitis is an inflammation of the longitudinal arch caused by excessive stretching of the plantar fascia—a broad band of fibrous tissue running along the bottom surface of the foot, attaching at the bottom of the heel bone and extending to the forefoot. When the plantar fascia is excessively stretched, this can cause plantar fasciitis, which can also lead to other issues like heel pain, arch pain, and heel spurs. You will experience pain at the bottom of the foot, often near the base of the heel or near the inside of the foot, where the heel and the arch meet. Overpronation (flat feet) is the major cause for plantar fasciitis. The pain is often acute either first thing in the morning or after a long rest, because while you're resting, the plantar fascia contracts back to its original shape. As the day progresses and the plantar fascia continues to be stretched, the pain often disappears.

Treatment and Prevention

One of the best treatments for plantar fasciitis is basically rest and reduced or no activity to keep the inflammation under control. When the cause is overpronation (flat feet), an orthotic with rear foot posting and longitudinal arch support is an efficient device to reduce the overpronation, and allow the condition to improve and heal. If you have high arches, which can also be a reason for plantar fasciitis, cushion the heel, absorb shock and wear suitable footwear that will accommodate the foot.

Icing is an excellent treatment to reduce the pain. If you do not have an ice pack handy, Dr. Jonathan Cluett, MD, suggests freezing some twelve- or sixteen-ounce plastic water bottles and then rolling them under your foot for ten to fifteen minutes.

Other popular treatments include stretching exercises, anti-inflammatory medications, shoe inserts, plantar fasciitis night splints, wearing shoes with a cushioned heel to absorb shock, and elevating the heel with the use of a heel cradle or heel cup. Heel cradles and heel cups provide extra comfort, cushion the heel, and reduce the amount of shock during everyday activities.

Every time your foot strikes the ground, the plantar fascia is stretched. You can reduce the strain and stress on the plantar fascia by following these simple instructions:

- Avoid running on hard or uneven ground.
- Lose any excess weight.
- Wear shoes and orthotics that support your arch to prevent overstretching of the plantar fascia.

Achillis Tendonitis

In a dancer's career, Achilles tendonitis is a frequent, most dreaded condition.

Why is it called Achilles tendonitis? In a few words, we could describe it as an irritation or inflammation of the tendon at the back of the heel. But why is it called Achilles tendonitis?

In order to explain this, we have to go back to the ancient Greek mythology. The legend says that Achilles was a half-divine Greek hero and the greatest warrior of the Trojan War. He was the son of a sea nymph called Thetis, one of the fifty Nereids, and of Peleus, of Thessaly, king of the Myrmidons. Thetis tried to immortalize the little Achilles by dipping him into the waters of the river Styx. Thetis held her son by the heel while dipping him into the waters, so all of his body became invulnerable except for his heel. However, during the Trojan War, Paris shot a poisoned arrow into Achille's heel, causing his death. Following this legend, the tendon connecting the heel to the calf was named Achilles tendon.

This unpleasant condition starts with pain that comes and goes at the back of the heel. When you get up in the morning, you find it hard and painful to walk barefoot, and the pain slowly decreases as you warm up with other movements. In class you might experience discomfort, or even pain, when rising on the demi-pointe or even doing a demi-plié, a battement tendu or rolling through jumps. These are warning signs telling you that you have the first symptoms of Achilles tendonitis.

Michelle Arnot, in her book Foot Notes, compares the Achillis tendon to a piece of rope that can wear out after being used repeatedly. She affirms that some experienced dancers manage to diminish the pain by warming up that area with a moist heat pack, then to massage it with a mild cream (liniment). The next step is wrapping the foot in plastic and a woolen sock. After class, the dancer can apply ice or cold water for about twenty minutes. Wearing higher heels might give a feeling of decreased pain, but this will also keep the muscles tighter.

According to Dr. William Heinz, MD. and Doctor Michael J. Mullin, ATC, PTA, Achilles tendonitis is more often due to:

1. Rolling in or out when on pointe
2. Incorrect tendu or relevé technique
3. Forced pointe
4. Tight calf muscles
5. Increased pronation
6. Not putting down the heels when landing from a jump

7. Incorrect placement of pointe shoe ribbons or elastics

When the Achilles tendon feels strained or inflamed you can use one of these treatments:

- Ice application
  In case of swelling, apply ice or an ice pack for at least ten minutes, three times a day.
- Moist heat
  If no swelling is present, apply moist heat and gently massage the calf muscles manually.
- Massage
  A massage using a tennis ball is usually very helpful. Sit on the floor and place a tennis ball right under the calf muscle. Lift your hips up with your hands. Using your heels as a pivot, roll the tennis ball along the calf muscle for one minute and repeat three times a day.
- Stretch and contraction exercise
  Sit on the floor keeping your back straight and perform the following exercise 5 times keeping your knee straight. Repeat 5 times with your knee bent. Put a towel around your foot and pull your foot towards you with the towel while relaxing the tendon at the front of your ankle. Maintain this position for 5 seconds and repeat the whole exercise 5 times. Repeat 5 times with the knee bent. Perform three times a day.
- Functional and strengthening exercises
  1. Heel lifts
     Execute a small rise (just lift your heels from the floor) on both feet and roll down slowly on one foot. (Use 3 counts to go up and 3 counts to come down). Repeat at least 20 times alternating legs. You should feel a contraction in the calf muscle when rolling down.
  2. Arch strengthening
     Stand on demi pointe on one foot with the other foot off the floor and to the side. Try to balance with only one finger on the barre or against the wall. You should feel the muscle in the back of the hip of the supporting leg. Hold the position for 30 seconds and repeat 5 to 10 times.

Ingrown Toenails, Blisters and Bunions

When a toenail is ingrown, the nail curves downward and grows into the skin, creating redness, irritation, swelling and pain. Ingrown toenails are generally caused by improper nail trimming. Cutting nails too short and wearing shoes that are too tight or too short are among the main causes. It could also be the result of a trauma, like stubbing your toe or having something heavy fall on your toe. Wearing tight and pointed shoes can also be one of the causes for ingrown nails, and sometimes even ballet tights—or regular hosiery—constricting the toes. What happens when the nail is ingrown is that the side edge of the toenail grows into the soft tissue of the skin, causing severe irritation and sometimes also infection. This condition generally affects the big toe, but it can also appear on the smaller ones. Proper trimming of the nails can prevent this painful condition. Always trim your toenails straight across with a slight rounding on each end. Do not round the nail to the point where it pokes (digs) into the skin on either side of the nail bed. If you have an ingrown toenail, you should try and soak your foot in 110°F water two or three times a day. Then apply a thin piece of cotton under the edge of the nail. This procedure will lift the nail slightly from its bed, providing relief from pain. If the pain continues, you should see a podiatrist.

Dr. Elizabeth H. Roberts, DPM, suggests that the only home treatment for a noninfected ingrown nail is to insert a few strands of cotton between the nail and the skin using an orange stick from a manicuring kit. In case of infection, Roberts believes you should soak your foot in warm water for ten minutes a day for at least three times a day until you go to a podiatrist.

Surgery to correct an ingrown toe-nail is a very simple in-office procedure. The surgeon will numb the toe and remove a small border of nail or, in worst situations, the whole nail.

Blisters

Blisters are a dancer's nightmare! At some point, we all deal with painful blisters, especially if the shoes are new, ill-fitted, or if we are switching to a new brand. Pointe beginners are especially concerned since their feet are still tender, but the good news is that with time and practice, the skin gradually hardens and blisters stop appearing. Alessandra Ball of North Carolina Dance Theatre affirms that taping and a little cushion helps with absorbing some of the pressure. The most important thing is preventing the blister, because once it appears, you have to deal with it. I will give some advice on how to prevent having blisters, what causes them, and how to take care of them and avoid infection when you have them. Also, how to dance if you have to, with blisters!

First, don't panic! As I already mentioned above, usually with time feet become stronger, and the skin in your toes hardens, so you will get less and less blisters.

Rubbing your toes every day with surgical alcohol will make the skin gradually tougher, and in the long run, you will stop getting blisters.

But let's analyze which are the causes and how to try and prevent them.

1. Too much friction
   Blisters are often caused by ill-fitted shoes and by friction onto the skin. If your shoe is too long or the box is not fitting right, your foot will slide inside and rub against the shoe, resulting in a blister.
2. Too much moisture
   Be sure you give your shoes and your toe pads enough time to dry in between classes. Let your paddings dry separately from your shoes, which might take up to forty-eight hours to dry. If you take pointe more than twice a week, you should have two pairs of shoes and toe pads.
3. Not enough strength and control in the toes.
   Always be sure that when you go on pointe your toes are lengthened and not curled. If your toes are bent, the knuckles will rub against the shoe and cause blisters.

The feeling is like a "hot spot"; I always advise my students to take their shoes off if they feel they are developing a blister. The spot will look very red and feel sore, and gradually the skin will become thinner and thinner, eventually break and form a blister. Blisters take a few days to heal; this is why you don't want to have one the day before a performance. How can you prevent this from happening?

1. Make sure your shoes are the right size and there is no sliding of the foot inside the shoe.
2. Gently smash the box with your hands so the sides will be softer.
3. Protect the spot where you are generally likely to have a blister with moleskin, New Skin, a new product called Blister Block, or with surgical tape. I do not advise Band-Aids, as they never stay up long; medical tape in rolls is preferable.

Thalia Mara, in her book On Your Toes, suggests using New Skin on the blister, in order to cover it with a protective layer until the skin grows back again. She also advises dancers to put a dab of boric-acid ointment on the blister, after using Mercurochrome on it, then cover it with a waterproof bandage. In my personal experience, New Skin is good, but not once the skin has already broken. The contact between New Skin and the raw skin can be very painful, so I would refrain from using this type of product once you already have an open blister. If you are prone to getting blisters, try to avoid wearing your pointe shoes without tights, since there is much more friction directly on the skin which would cause more frequent blisters.

Bunions

What we commonly call bunion is in reality a deformity of the big-toe joint. According to William Heinz, MD, bunions, otherwise called Hallux valgus, result from a loosening and collapse of ligaments in the arch. He affirms that the tendency to develop bunions is largely inherited, but says that wearing shoes with arch support can prevent this development. He believes that rolling in is also one of the main causes, since when you roll in, you put a lot of pressure on your first metatarsal.

Make sure your everyday shoes are wide and comfortable in the front and not tight and narrow.

In my experience as a ballet teacher, I noticed that overturning is one of the major causes for bunions. When the dancer overturns, the foot tends to collapse forward (rolling in), thus putting a lot of pressure on the first metatarsal. In the long run, it will result in bunions and weakening of the ankles.

I have seen students at the age of fourteen with big and inflamed bunions due to incorrect training and forced turnout.

Some schools require a 180-degree turnout when standing in first position. Students who do not have that amount of turnout just force themselves in a position that causes a large amount or rolling in.

When dancers with bunions choose pointe shoes, they need more room around their big-toe joint to avoid painful pressure on the bunion, and therefore will have to opt for shoes with a wider box.

Dancers with this problem can get some relief by using Bunheads Bunion Buster (see in "Pointe Accessories" for description) or should tape the metatarsal area with good sports tape.

Bunion cushions are excellent to protect and isolate the bunion from the shoe and reduce friction. Pedifix Visco Gel Bunion Guard is an amazing product made of soft gel enriched with vitamin E and mineral oil. It absorbs most of the pressure and soothes the pain. It is available in one size that fits in most shoes and gives immediate relief.

Lisa Howell, a physical therapist based in Sydney, Australia, and author of The Perfect Pointe Book, claims that it is "preferable to tape under the head of the first metatarsal before drawing the tape up and over the knuckle, de-rotating the first metatarsal. The tape is then wrapped around the big toe."

This helps align the toe more correctly in the shoe. A tape can also be employed to keep the head of the first metatarsal in closer to the second, to minimize the sideways drift. She also suggests creating custom-designed pads by cutting pieces out of a simple foam rubber shoe inner sole, available from any drugstore or supermarket. Cut a circle larger than the inflamed area, and then remove the center portion so that there is no pressure on it. Put the padding onto the foot to keep it in place using thin hypoallergenic white tape so that it does not move around when you're dancing.

Dr. Lowell Scott Weil, a podiatric surgeon specializing in dance-related problems, recommends wearing boxy street shoes, giving the toes enough room, instead of high-heeled, tight, and pointy ones. It has been proven that women are much more predisposed than men to get bunions; 90 percent of people affected by bunions are women, due to the type of shoes they wear. His advice is to wear a bunion splint at night and to avoid pointe work before the feet have acquired the necessary strength. Chinese medicine recommends treating the bunion internally with homeopathic silica, to reduce the inflammation and restore the body's balance. Also, drinking chamomile tea and then using the tea bag for external relief by placing it on the bunion can lessen the swelling.

Since bunions generally cause the big toe to collapse toward the smaller toes, spacers can also help maintain proper alignment, prevent friction, and provide relief from pressure.

At the end of the day, if your bunions hurt and look red and inflamed, apply an ice pack to reduce the swelling and inflammation.

In very severe cases, bunions have to be surgically removed, but this is not advised for dancers.

Hammertoes and Overlapping Toes

Hammertoe is a deformity of one or both joints of the second, third, fourth, or fifth toe that causes it to be permanently bent, looking like a hammer. The base of the toe points upward while the end of it points down. Some people are structurally or genetically prone to developing this type of deformity. Highly arched feet are more inclined to develop hammertoes, due to the positioning of the ligaments. Wearing shoes that are too short or too tight can also be a cause for hammertoes. This problem can be corrected by using shoes with larger boxes or by using splints or tape. Padding can be helpful in providing relief from some of the pressure. Surgery can also be an option, but not advisable for dancers.

Overlapping Toes

Overlapping toes are substantially a form of hammertoes and can cause friction and irritation. Dr. Suzanne Belyea, DPM, CPed, believes that overlapping toes are one of the most common causes of pain in the forefoot for people of all ages. She also claims that inflammation and soreness are the most common symptoms.

Nowadays toe spacers are one of the best solutions for toes that overlap, along with comfortable shoes with more room in the toes area.

Overpronation (Flat Feet), Shin Splints, and Sore Feet

Flat feet, more commonly called fallen arches, can be a problem in pointe work; but this does not mean that dancers with flat feet should give up dancing on pointe. I have met many dancers who had flat feet and through hard work managed to develop a decent arch and a brilliant career. It all depends on the type of flat feet.

According to dance physiotherapist Lisa Howell, there are two types of flat feet.

- Anatomically or genetically flat feet
- Flat feet with very mobile ligaments and poor muscular support

Dancers with genetically flat feet have better chances of achieving satisfactory pointe work, although feet won't have the desired look required by many ballet companies. Flat feet and very mobile ligaments could be too weak and prevent the dancer from progressing in pointe technique. Only a medical professional will be able to assess the real nature of a flat foot and advise accordingly.

Shin Splints

The most common symptom of shin splints is pain along the shinbone, or tibia—the large bone situated in the front of the lower leg.

According to world-acclaimed ballet master David Howard, shin splints happen because of the tightness at the top of the bone. Howard believes the main causes for shin splints can be either of the following:

- Hard floors
- Walking too much
- Bad posture

David Howard also stresses the importance of making sure the pain is not due to the beginning of a hairline fracture or a more serious problem with the tibia.

According to UK osteopath Margaret Papoutsis (anatomy and physiology consultant for the Royal Ballet School Teacher Training Course), there can be many other causes for pain in the shin, ranging from periosteal irritation to osteoid osteoma.

Sore Feet

This is not a syndrome or a disease, but who is the dancer who never experienced sore, swollen, aching feet? After a full day of rehearsals or after a pointe class, all dancers feel like their feet need a break!

One of the best things is soaking your feet in warm (not boiling!) water with two tablespoons of Epsom salts for about ten minutes in order to obtain immediate relief.

If you do not have Epsom salts, baking soda is an excellent substitute. It leaves your feet immediately rested and refreshed.

Corns and Calluses

Both of them can be very painful conditions, but there are ways to manage the pain, and sometimes even to avoid their formation.

We should also take into consideration that dancers do need their calluses because they provide protection when using pointe shoes. Calluses need to be treated only if they get infected or if they cause serious pain. "Corns and calluses are a necessity for ballet dancers and should not necessarily be seen as a pathologic condition," says Professor Stephen F. Conti, chief of the Division of Foot and Ankle Surgery at the University of Pittsburgh, Pennsylvania.

According to Elizabeth H. Roberts, DPM, corns and calluses, if observed under a microscope, are "identical cellular structures. The callus develops in flat planes while the corn is shaped like a cone with the tip penetrating into the tissue. This is why a corn is so painful on direct pressure."

Corns and calluses are caused by friction or pressure, usually caused by the wrong type of shoe or standing for long periods. Soft corns are more present between toes, mostly caused by one toe rubbing against another.

Use moleskin to protect and isolate your calluses, and preferably, insert gauze in between the moleskin and the callus itself. Let your callus breathe during the night in order to avoid the formation of excessive moisture. Do not shave or scrape your calluses and avoid over-the-counter corn removers containing acids. If you have a corn, you can protect it and isolate it by wrapping it in lamb's wool or using a band-aid like Band-Aid Spots. Do not use band-aids that wrap around the toe, which cause constriction and even more pain. Wear comfortable walking shoes that offer sufficient room in the box and avoid tapered and high-heeled footwear.

Chapter 3

Treating Minor Injuries

Some minor problems can be treated at home, as long as done properly. Any severe injury or strong pain lasting more than forty-eight hours should be checked by a physician or an orthopedist.

Here is a list of over-the-counter remedies commonly used by dancers:

Ace Bandage (or Athletic Tape) Ankle Supports

Epsom Salts

It is just the generic name for magnesium sulfate originally obtained at first by distilling the waters in a town called Epsom, in Surrey, Great Britain. Use half of the Epsom salts in two parts of warm (not hot) water. Soak for ten to fifteen minutes when feet feel tired or sore. If you have blisters, it makes them dry out and heal faster.

Analgesic Cream

There are many brands available on the market. I am just going to list a few. Most of them are made exactly the same way and use the same "ingredients," so just read at the back and see the percentage of each component used. When I danced in France, most dancers were "addicted" to Laodal, a miracle product that was unfortunately withdrawn from the market. It was a kind of white, milk-looking liquid that could heal muscle sprains and strains in two to four days! Besides that, it would immediately warm up your muscles as if you had worked an hour at the barre, act as an anti-inflammatory, and provide immediate relief from pain! I don't think anything like Laodal exists on the market; however, I have compiled a list of recommended creams and gels that will prepare your muscles before class or "repair" them when they feel sore.

Biofreeze

Biofreeze is a deep-penetrating gel and provides an immediate cooling sensation to the area applied, which decreases pain and increases blood flow. The increased circulation to the injured tissues promotes healing and relaxation of stiff, sore muscles. The effect of Biofreeze lasts for several hours. It is used to provide relief from arthritis, sore muscles and joints, back pain, as well as minor strains and sprains.

Tiger Balm

This is the best product of this kind on the market, at least according to my opinion. Used for centuries, Tiger Balm is a general analgesic, pain-reducing rub. It is a unique formulation of herbal ingredients derived from ancient Chinese sources, and it became famous in more than one hundred countries. It provides effective relief from most symptoms of muscle strains and sprains. It smells like menthol and is really effective. It contains camphor, menthol, cajuput oil, mint, and clove. These essential oils contained in the balm help dilate the peripheral blood vessels, thus helping the blood move closer to the skin's surface and increase the circulation. By raising the skin's temperature, the balm creates a local analgesic effect, which reduces pain and soreness. It is also available in patches.

Bengay

This cream provides temporary relief from minor aches and pains of muscles and joints associated with simple backache, arthritis, strains, bruises, and sprains. It contains three pain-relieving ingredients: camphor, menthol, methyl salicylate.

Aspercreme

This analgesic rub is an odor-free, salicylate cream that provides temporary relief from minor muscle aches and pains. It penetrates quickly and deeply into painful areas, relieving pain without aspirin and without burning.

Glucosamine

Glucosamine is a gel widely associated with joint health and is now available in a dermatologically tested clear topical formulation. Non-sticky and non-greasy, Glucosamine is easy to apply.

Neosporin

An antibiotic ointment used to prevent and heal minor infections and accelerating the healing of wounds. Also known as the triple antibiotic ointment, it contains three different types of antibiotic: bacitracin, neomycin, and polymyxin B.

Nurofen

A topical analgesic and anti-inflammatory gel that provides relief from pain and inflammation in conditions such as backache, muscular pains, sprains, strains, etc. It contains 5 percent ibuprofen.

Mentholatum Ibuprofen Gel

A topical analgesic and anti-inflammatory ibuprofen gel to relieve pain and inflammation. Optimal for conditions such as muscular pains, sprains, strains, etc., and contains 5 percent ibuprofen.

Deep Freeze Cold Gel

Deep Freeze Cold Gel is a fast-acting pain-relieving cold gel very popular among dancers. Its cooling, penetrating action goes deep down to relieve the aches and pains of overworked muscles, tendons, and joints.

Deep Heat Rub

A warming muscle rub for relief from muscle aches and pains. It contains eucalyptus oil, which is proven to reduce muscle pain.

Radian B Ibuprofen Gel

An anti-inflammatory ibuprofen gel that relieves pain and inflammation from backache, muscular pains, sprains, strains, and sports injuries.

A general rule for all these creams: wash your hands thoroughly immediately after use and do not touch your eyes. Gently rub the cream onto the skin to prevent redness and itching. Softly massage the cream until it penetrates into the skin. Do not apply any of these creams on scrapes or cuts.

Antiperspirant

To avoid sweaty feet, you can apply an antiperspirant before you dance. Washing the feet before, during, and after dancing will also reduce the need for using an antiperspirant. It should not be used all the time, though, as overuse can itself cause pore blockage. Change your tights often and always wash them as soon as you get home. There are many brands of antiperspirant deodorants available over the counter in all countries. Read the label first, to make sure that you get what you need. Absorbent solutions, such as Drysol, containing aluminum chloride will help to decrease sweating when used on a regular basis. In the old days, simple cornstarch was the answer to sweaty feet.

Antibiotic Cream

Antibiotic creams can reduce bacteria presence. This means that such a cream can help reduce the incidence of bad-smelling feet. It should only be prescribed by a podiatrist or doctor. Antibiotic creams are sometimes used in the treatment of and for recovery from badly calloused heels.

Betadine

It is very popular and one of the oldest topical antiseptics used to fight local infections. Betadine solution contains povidone-iodine, which is excellent for fighting against viral, bacterial, or fungal infections. It does not sting.

Blister Block

Apply whenever you feel you are going to get a blister. Rub it on the sore spot; it works wonders.

Analgesics and anti-inflammatory drugs can do more harm than good sometimes. It is well known that dancers like to self-diagnose when it comes to health issues and use a lot of over-the-counter medicines like ibuprofen (Advil, Tylenol, etc.). These drugs should never be taken simply to keep dancing in class or in a performance. Do not dance if you are injured. Give your body time to get better, and eventually, see a doctor. These medicines can cause damage to the liver and stomach lining and can have long-term side effects.

Chapter 4

Little Accessories to Make Life Easier

This generation of dancers is so blessed by having technology working with them side by side. So many accessories have been created to help them feel comfortable on pointe and to relieve their pain; it's just a matter of combining the right shoe with the right accessories, and pointe work could become totally painless!

When I was a student, we had none of these accessories, and even toe pads did not exist! We had to use cotton or paper instead. I think nowadays dancers are really lucky compared to the dancers of the past.

Here is a list of the most useful accessories, what they offer, and how to use them:
- Super Spacer and Pinky Pad by Bunheads Inc.
  www.bunheads.com
  Super Spacer is a larger version of Bunhead's Spacers and is an excellent solution for dancers with long toes. Placed in between the big toe and the second toe, it aligns the big toe joint and correct bunions.
  Pinky Pads are excellent for relieving pain and pressure from small corns or blisters on the pinky toes. Made of soft polymer gel, they can also be used on the smaller toes.
- *Gel Tip Max by Bloch*
  www.blochworld.com
  It reduces pressure and bruising on dancers with a long first toe.
- Space Enhancers by Bloch
- Extension Stretch Ribbon by Prima Soft
- Lamb's Wool by Capezio/Ballet Makers
- Corn cushions (non-medicated)
  They provide relief from pain and pressure due to corns. They cushion and protect.
- Nylon Ribbon by Prima Soft
- Toe Wrap by Gaynor Minden
  www.gaynorminden.com
- Mesh Elastic by Chacott
- Pointe Shoe Ruffer by Freed of London
  Available at www.dancedistributors.com
- Soft Pointe Pro Gel Toe Pads by Leo's Dancewear
- Jet Glue Pointe Shoe Hardener
  The perfect solution to re-harden and give some extra life to your old pointe shoes. Apply this powerful glue (always use gloves) to the inside and the outside of the

box, on either side of the shank inside and outside, under the shank and to the pleats and seams. Let it dry completely in a well-ventilated space before wearing the shoe.
- Rock Rosin
- Lacquer Sizing Pointe Shoe Hardener
This spray acts against the sweat that makes your shoes softer by creating a barrier between your foot and the shoe, to prevent and delay softening of the box. Just spray it into the shoe block and let it dry before you wear your shoes.
- Pointe Shoe Vamp Elastic by Gaynor Minden
This elastic is perfect for giving extra support in the vamp area for dancers who go too far over the shoe or for high arches that "pop out of the shoe." This elastic (three inches wide by fifteen inches long) can be sewn in the throat of the pointe shoe or crisscrossed.
- Heel Grippers
They are a wonderful solution for heels of pointe shoes slipping down, or to fill that little extra space at the back of the shoe. You can find them at any grocery store or drugstore, and they are a lifesaver for dancers with short heels or dancers in between sizes. These self-sticking heel grip pads fit inside the heel area of the shoe to fill extra space and prevent heel slippage while adding comfort to the heel area.
- Gaynor Minden's pointe shoe heel grippers are perfect for dancers with narrow heels.
- Softpointe Gel Toe Pads by Leo's Dancewear
- Moleskin
Very cheap and found in every pharmacy, drugstore, or grocery store, moleskin is every dancer's forever friend. Its general purpose is to cushion and isolate. It is sold in a pack that generally contains several sheets of approximately three inches by four inches. It looks like a beige soft felt on one side with a self-sticking layer on the back side. You can cut it into the shape and size you want, according to your needs.
What can you do with Moleskin? Here are some ideas:
   * Stick it to the tip of your pointe shoe to avoid slipping (Always remove the excess of frayed satin first.)
   * Place it under your heel for more cushioning.
   * Stick it inside your platform if you don't want to use toe pads.
   * Use to protect and cushion calluses underneath your metatarsals.
- Stitch Kit by Bunheads
This small container provides dancers with one hundred yards of waxed pink/salmon thread plus two big-eyed needles and written instructions. The best solution for sewing ribbons and elastics. Makes sewing really easy and fast, and the thread is practically unbreakable! Available in three colors: professional pink, white, or black. A must for every dancer! I personally could not do without it!

- Pointe Shoe Shank Tacks by Bunheads
  Each container has fifty tacks to reinforce soft or broken shanks. Good for dancers with strong insteps.
- Knot Keepers by Bunheads
  These invisible adhesive strips help keep ribbons securely tucked in place. There are twenty-four in a package and will give your shoes a more professional look.
- Gellows (Reversible Toe Pads)
- Pointe Shoe Full Sock Liner by Gaynor Minden
  These pink insoles are very useful for reducing excess material on the heel and side of the shoe. Ideal for dancers with narrow feet.
- Jelly Tips by Bunheads
- Jelly Toes by Bunheads
- Bunion Buster by Bunheads
  An elastic fabric tube with a gel coating on the inside, created to protect the big toe and bunion area. It helps to relieve some of the pressure on the big-toe joint.
- The Big Tip
- Clear Stretch Tips
- Toe Spacers by Bunheads
- Cushy Cuts by Bunheads
- SoftSpacers by Danz Tech
  www.danztech.com
  SoftSpacer pads are ideal for relieving pressure from your toes. These newly created pads are made from a material called Gelastic, which is a soft and hypoallergenic gel. Made with pharmaceutical-grade mineral oil, they help soothe and protect your feet. They are really thin and do not take up much space in the pointe shoes. They are excellent for easing discomfort caused by soft corns in between toes. Each one has a different purpose:
    * Wedgies go between the big toe and the second toe to reduce pressure and improve alignment in case of bunions.
    * Tweenies go between the toes to relieve sore spots and to prevent toes from overlapping and fractioning. All the pads are trimmable and can also be washed, powdered, and reused. Each kit includes four short spacer pads, two long spacer pads, and two wedge pads.
- Toe Savers Skinny Dips by Danz Tech
  These toe pads are extremely soft, cool, and stretchy. You feel like touching them over and over—they are as smooth as silk! They are also very lightweight and thin and not bulky at all when placed in the shoe; you hardly know you are wearing them! They are also indicated for dancers with bunions or wide feet. You can trim them and also wear them upside down. The inside is made of stretchy cotton, and the outside is the super-

soft gel. Their hypoallergenic components provide relief from pressure and sore toes. They come in two sizes (small/medium and medium/large) and in four colors.

My advice: Trimming the bottom part will allow you to have a better feeling of contact with the floor and will also take up less space in the shoe!

- Pliers

  A small pair of pliers always comes in handy to ballerinas when they wish to remove the tack from the shank of their pointe shoes.

- Scissors

  A good pair of scissors is a must in a ballerina's dance bag. Dancers use them to cut pieces of tape, trim their ribbons or drawstring, cut thread, and for many more usages!

- One Exacto or Stanley knife.

  Invaluable tool, always in a ballerina's dance bag, especially employed before performances! Use the Exacto knife to three-quarter the shank, remove the satin from the platform, make cuts on the outer sole for more flexibility or to roughen the top layer of it, and to perform other types of "surgery" to the shoe! Many ballerinas, like Tamara Oughtred, first Soloist at Birmingham Royal Ballet, shave their soles with a Stanley knife, before wearing them on stage.

- Your small pharmacy kit to carry around during class and performances:

  * Band aids of different shapes
  * Toe tape
  * Blister Stop: this stick is wonderful to prevent blisters!!! Rub onto the affected area as soon as you feel your skin getting sensitive.
  * Icy Hot or Tiger Balm or any other brand of rubbing cream
  * A knee brace
  * An ankle brace
  * Ibuprofen or Tylenol
  * A pair of scissors
  * New Skin
  * Neosporin
  * Moleskin

Chapter 5

Interviews with Health Specialists

Doctor Frank Sinkoe, DPM

Doctor Sinkoe has been practicing podiatry in Atlanta, Georgia, for twenty-one years. He worked in dance medicine for six years and is currently the podiatrist for the Atlanta Ballet and for local dance schools. Dr. Sinkoe started having an interest in dancers when his daughter started to dance.

Dr. Sinkoe, what are the reasons why a child should not be on pointe before age eleven to twelve? In your experience, what could be the negative effects?

I consider going on pointe to be a process. Dancing on pointe obviously requires core strength and proprioceptive agility on one foot. Regarding the foot, students should first develop intrinsic muscle strength within their foot, isolating the muscle groups, with exercises such as tendus against resistance and doming exercises. In girls, bone maturity and growth plate closure usually occurs at age twelve to thirteen. However, the growth plates of the ankle may close later. Prior to this, the bones are fairly "elastic" and thus can become deformed with injury or increased stress. Parents are reasonably concerned that their daughters may develop bunions when getting into pointe shoes and on pointe. In my opinion, increased stress to the first MPJ (metacarpophalangeal joint), and thus development of deformities such as bunions, occur when the foot chronically "rolls in." I find that they are able to stand in first and second positions effectively turned out. However, when they land from jumps, etc., they are frequently rolled in.

I therefore emphasize exercises to improve turnout at the hip. This will help them to learn to engage their turnout muscles. I have them use a physiotherapy ball and perform core exercises with the foot in parallel and turned-out position. I use this exercise to treat a number of foot pathologies, which are caused by rolling in of the foot—that is, first MPJ pain and flexor hallucis tendonitis. My answer to your question is this: bunions and first MPJ pathology can result from rolling in due to poor turnout. In a skeletally immature dancer, this occurs more readily. In addition, lack of strength of the foot may cause the dancer to "go over" on pointe, and thus cause posterior impingement of the ankle. Lack of strength causes the dancer to "sit back" on pointe, which may cause Achilles tendon strain.

How would you treat the first symptoms of Achilles tendonitis? When ice is required and when heat is required? Which is best? In what case could the Achilles tendon "snap" and require surgery?

Achilles tendonopathy is the result of overuse in a dancer with tight gastrocnemius, soleus, and/or hamstring muscle. I particularly see Achilles tendonopathy in the young dancer during their growth stage. The bones are growing longer, but the muscles/tendons are still short. The Achilles tendon should be stretched with the knee straight and bent due to the two muscles involved (gastrocnemius and soleus). Apply ice during the initial stage of tendonitis, and always if swelling is present.

Ice should be applied for 10 minutes within an ice bag. When the tendonitis resolves, heat can be applied for a few minutes prior to stretching. I also have the dancer roll their calf on a tennis ball to stretch the muscle, and treat trigger points after the acute stage. The Achilles tendon will usually not rupture in a young person. As we age, the blood supply to the Achilles tendon diminishes and, therefore, [it] is susceptible to rupture when the foot is forcibly dorsiflexed, like when landing from a jump.

Can you suggest a few exercises to prevent injury?

Stretch the Achilles tendon passively with a towel with the knee straight for 30 seconds, and knee bent for 30 seconds by 5 repetitions. The gastrocnemius-soleus / Achilles tendon complex crosses the knee, ankle, and subtalar joint. I have the dancers perform relevés on an ankle disc and single-leg exercises on a half foam roller. I am therefore treating the Achilles tendon in the sagittal and frontal planes. Most injuries occur when the muscle is eccentrically strained. I therefore emphasize exercises to eccentrically strengthen the hamstrings and posterior calf muscles.

Do you think hyperextension can be corrected with proper training? Should hyperextended students be encouraged to keep their heels together in first position?

This is not my area of expertise. I am a podiatrist and not a dance teacher or dancer. However, I have read two articles which encourage the students to focus on proper alignment: "The Hips" in June 2010 Dance Magazine and "The Freedom of Movement" in December 2008 Pointe Magazine.

Students often complain of having pain under their arch when they point in a battement tendu. What could be the cause?

Overuse of the posterior tibial and peroneal muscles [stirrup muscles] may be the cause, particularly if their insertion sites are at the site where the shank bends. I encourage the dancer to work the foot intrinsic muscles using doming-type exercises and tendu against resistance with a Thera-Band. This will teach them to use the toes to bend the foot.

Another common complaint of students aged eight to fourteen is pain around the kneecap. What are the possible causes?

I do not treat knees. However, it sounds like Osgood-Schlatter's disease. I believe tight quadriceps will aggravate this condition.

Can you describe an effective way of taping bunions? How do you treat them when they are inflamed?

Bunions are the result of increased stress on the first MPJ in a child who may have a foot structure, metatarsal adductus, which makes them prone to bunions. As I stated in question 1, increased stress may be caused by rolling in of the foot. I therefore will have the dancer improve her turnout with external hip strengthening. I will have her treat the inflamed bunion with ice application for 10 minutes at least three times a day. Rather than taping a bunion, I have the dancer apply a foam or silicone padding within the first webspace, to better align the first MPJ and hallux.

Calluses underneath the metatarsal area are common in dancers due to the amount of hours standing and the friction caused by the shoe. What would you do to reduce soreness and inflammation? Would you place a pad underneath the affected area or place a pad in the shoe in the corresponding spot?

Dancers find that calluses toughen the feet. I do tell them that painful calluses and corns should be treated. I will shave the callus to a comfortable level. I have placed padding on the foot and the shoe. I leave it up to the dancer to see what works the best.

Which exercises would you suggest for stretching and improving the look of the arch?

I have the dancer strengthen the foot intrinsic with doming exercises, what I call toe push-ups, and tendu against resistance with a Thera-Band. I explain to them that there are several joints in the foot. The hinge joints are the ones best capable of providing them with the best arch. I therefore have them focus on these joints when performing the exercises. I tell them to never perform stretching exercises with their feet under a couch or other such subject. Over-stretching and straining these dorsal ligaments can be harmful. The best method of stretching the foot is via engaging the intrinsic foot muscles.

Ginette Hamel, BSc(PT)
Diploma in Sports Physiotherapy
Certified Mat Stott Pilates Instructor

Mrs. Ginette Hamel is a physiotherapist with more than twenty-five years of experience. She has treated dancers, actors, and musicians of all types in the clinic, backstage, and on movie sets. For the past twelve years, she has been one of the few physiotherapists worldwide working almost exclusively with ballet dancers. Presently, she is the consultant physiotherapist at the National Ballet of Canada and at the Artists' Health Centre.

Among her clients are performers from the National Ballet of Canada, the National Ballet School, the Toronto Symphony, the Canadian Opera Company, the Canadian Brass, and the stage shows from the area.

Mrs. Hamel has also worked with the Royal Winnipeg Ballet and in ballet schools in Stuttgart and Copenhagen; and she has presented at international dance medicine conferences. She designed and produced two exercise conditioning DVDs—Stability with Mobility—volume 1, Exercise Program for Dancers, and volume 2, Exercise Program to Promote Freedom of Movement for Musicians.

Mrs. Hamel, what are the reasons why a child should not be put on pointe before ages eleven to twelve? What could be the negative effects according to your experience?

Before the age of eleven or twelve, a child's growth plates are not fully closed, and the bones might be more vulnerable to trauma. It has been my experience that if children go on pointe too early, they have weak muscles around their ankles, making them more vulnerable to ankle sprain. Also, because their muscles are weaker, they have more chances of getting tendonitis in the lower legs from overuse.

How would you treat the first symptoms of Achilles tendonitis? Would you advice icing the part or applying a moist heat pack? In what case could the Achilles tendon "snap" and require surgery? Can you suggest a few exercises to prevent injury?

If the first symptom of Achilles tendonitis is swelling, I would use ice at least 2 or 3 times per day for the first 48 hours on the onset of the symptoms. After 48 hours, if the pain persists, I like the effect of contrast bath. I tell my clients to put their foot in hot water for 3 minutes, and then in ice water for 1 minute. They should repeat the process 4 times, finishing with the cold. I find that Achilles tendonitis is associated with poor pointing technique. Often the dancers use the plantar flexing muscles the wrong way. They start using the foot muscles too early, and do not get a relaxation of the tendon at the end of the movement. I developed an exercise that helps to do this:

- Pointe flexed with elastic band from Stability with Mobility volume 1, Exercise Program for Dancers.
- The next three exercises are done with an elastic band. They will help you to warm up and strengthen your calves and some key muscles in your feet. In dance, these muscles assist you in being stronger on relevé or on pointe. You will also get a stretch as you strengthen.
  - * Exercise number 1
    Starting position: Start by sitting in an upright position. You can bend one leg at the knee if you have problems sitting with both legs straight. Place an elastic

band under the calf of the straight leg, coming up under the foot and toward the front of your shin.

Movement: Point against the elastic band while keeping your toes pointing up. Flex or return your foot back to the initial position. Keep your toes towards you throughout the whole exercise. Repeat 10 times on each foot.

* Exercise number 2

   Starting position: Start in the same position as the previous exercise, sitting with one leg bent and one leg straight. Again, place an elastic band under the calf of the straight leg, coming up under the foot and toward the front of your shin.

   Movement: Point the foot against the elastic. It is important to begin the pointing movement from the heel and then point your toes at the end of the movement. Keep your toes pointing straight. This will engage the muscles on the bottom and inside of your foot. Moving in this manner will also allow the Achilles tendon to relax into the heel. The movement is now the flexing of the toes against the resistance of the elastic band. Do not move at the heel. Repeat 10 times on each foot.

* Exercise number 3

   The next exercise is a combination of the previous two.

   Starting position: Sitting with one leg bent and the other straight, place an elastic band under the calf of the straight leg, coming up under the foot and toward the front of your shin.

   Movement: Point your foot against the resistance of the elastic band while keeping your toes flexed (pointing toward you) and then at the end of the movement, point your toes. Make sure that you point from the heel and then point from the toes at the end of the movement. Hold the position for 3, 2, 1 and bring your toes up towards you and then flex the foot towards you, returning to the starting position. Repeat 10 times.

An Achilles tendon tear is usually associated with fatigue of the muscle and tendon, and the tear usually occurs in the landing or the start of a jump or a sudden start.

Here is a way to stretch the Achilles tendon stretch from the DVD Stability with Mobility volume 1, Exercise Program for Dancers.

Calf Stretch

1. Starting position: Place a one-foot-long half foam roll against the wall, flat side up. The angle of the roll depends upon your flexibility. Stand with one foot on a half roll, flat side up, and your heel on the floor.
2. Movement: Lean forward toward the wall by bending your elbows. Hold for 3 to 4 long breaths (15 to 30 seconds). Repeat on the other side.
3. Now bend your knee. Repeat the stretch. Hold for 3 or 4 breaths (15 to 30 seconds). Repeat on the other side.

Do you think hyperextension can be corrected with proper training? Do you think students should be encouraged to keep their heels together? How would you make them understand the concept of not overstretching their knees but to use the muscles in their thighs?

Hyperextension of the knee is related to overall looseness of the ligament in the individual. Hyperextension of the knee is usually associated with beautifully pointed feet. I believe that dancers need to learn to work with their hyperextension. They need to learn how to pull their kneecaps up by using their quadriceps muscles (with emphasis on the VMO [vastus medialis oblique], the muscle on the inside of their quad) and keep their weight toward the front of their feet so that they do not lock their knee back or bring their weight on their heels. They will only be able to do this if they are allowed to keep a space between their heels. When they stand on one leg, their leg needs to be kept in a lengthened position, and they have to use their hyperextension. If they do not, their leg will be slightly bent when they stand on one leg, and this will decrease their stability.

Students often complain of having pain under their arch when they point in a battement tendu. What could be the cause?

I think that students get pain in their arch during pointe in battements tendus because they overuse the foot muscles that are weak and they are cramping.

Another common complaint among students aged eight to fourteen is pain around the kneecap. What are the possible causes? Would you advise rest or just wearing a knee brace and icing the part several times a day?

Pain around the kneecap is usually associated with tightness in the quadriceps muscles and weakness of the vastus medialis obliquus [or oblique] muscle, the muscle on the lower inside of the thigh. That muscle helps to pull the kneecap straight up. Usually, I would recommend rest from jumping and see if it helps. I would start an exercise program to strengthen the VMO. If the pain does not go away, I would recommend full rest for 48 hours and see if that works. I do not use bracing because I find bracing too restrictive, but I do use Leukotape (a rigid strapping tape) or Kinesio Tape to bring the kneecap where it needs to be and stimulate the activation of the proper muscles. I do believe that icing 2 or 3 times per day helps, mostly if there is swelling.

Can you describe an effective way of taping bunions? How would you treat a child with enlarged and inflamed bunions?

I find that bunions are often associated with pronation (flattening) of the feet. I often use the tape for the treatment of extensor hallucis tendonitis illustrated in Dance Technique and Injury Prevention by Justin Howse and Shirley Hancock (p. 116) but I use Kinesio Tape or Elastoplast half-inch tape. I also use a Leukotape taping, where I start by putting two pieces of Hypafix tape going first around the arch area from the top of the foot, toward the outside of the foot, going under the foot toward the middle of the foot coming up and finishing at the top. After applying the under tape, I apply Leukotape, leaving one-half inch at the top of the white tape. I close the tape in standing position and plié to make sure that the taping is not too tight. I would advise the child to use icing and tell him or her to avoid relevé for a few days until the inflammation has decreased.

Students sometimes complain about their hips "popping." What is the cause, and how dangerous can it be? What should a ballet teacher advise in this case?

Popping of the hip can be painful or bring pain relief; rarely in my experience is it dangerous. If the pain happens during développé, it is often due to weakness of the psoas and that muscle needs to be strengthened. The popping can be due to snapping of a muscle over another one or snapping of a muscle over a bone. If the pain or snapping is on the outside of the hip, the snapping is due to the iliotibial band going over the greater trochanter. In that case, the tensor facia lata and the ilio-tibial band need to be stretched. If the pain persists, the movement that is painful needs to be avoided, and ice needs to be used.

Calluses underneath the metatarsal area are common in dancers due to the amount of hours standing and the friction caused by the shoe. What would you do to reduce soreness and inflammation? Would you place a pad underneath the affected area or place a pad in the shoe in the corresponding spot?

I would place the padding directly on the skin and secure it with Hypafix tape. That way you minimize friction that would happen if the pad moved on the skin.

Which exercises would you suggest for stretching the arch and improving the look of it?

I believe that the plantar flexion exercises given in question number 2 help the shape of the foot and the arch.

What are the symptoms of "fallen arches"? Should dancers stop activity for a while if this happens? What are the symptoms, and what is the therapy recommended?

Arches do not fall all of a sudden. It usually happens overtime and often during a growth spurt of the feet. It is due to laxity of the ligaments around the joints of the foot. If the pain happens suddenly, it is due to inflammation so the arch needs to rest. The child can use ice and should get orthotics for his/her everyday shoes and be taped for dancing.

What are the symptoms and treatments for shin splints?

The symptoms for shin splints are pain on the inside or outside of the shin associated to jumping or running. If the diagnosis is not made early, the pain can also be there during walking or even at rest. A differential diagnosis has to be made. Shin splints pain can be due to tendonitis of the tibialis posterior or the tibialis anterior. It can be due to periostitis of the tibia, stress fracture of the tibia or fibula, or due to compartment syndrome.

Treatment will depend on the diagnosis, but the first thing to do is avoid the activity that hurts. To relieve the pain, you can try ice bath or contrast bath. Stretching and self-massage of the lower leg can help to relieve tightness in the area. Also, if the shin splints pain is due to the tibialis tendon, that muscle needs rest, and that can be achieved with taping of the arch or of the tibialis tendon.

Margaret Papoutsis, Osteopath
The Margaret Papoutsis Practice
London

Doctor Papoutsis, what is your opinion on hyperextended legs?

This problem can be corrected with a combination of therapeutic exercises and expert corrective teaching. I find that the main difficulty to overcome is the lack of motivation in the dancer themselves, particularly if previous teachers have encouraged/ordered them to "pull up their thighs" or "fully straighten their knees." Changing such habits is difficult and physically hard work, so many dancers tend to revert to old habits when tired or bored. If the dancer has naturally lax ligaments in her knees, she may well need to rely on correct muscle usage to maintain stability for her whole career; so the sooner the corrections start, the better. As my approach is necessarily holistic, rather than orthopaedic, each dancer will have a different therapeutic protocol, even though they may be suffering from similar injuries.

My emphasis is always on etiology and prevention—however well a bunion is strapped, it is no help to the dancer if they have weak "turn-out" muscles, for example.

My own opinion is that the most vital function of teachers is to recognize that a structural problem exists, and to refer the dancer to a suitable therapist in order to obtain a correct diagnosis and appropriate treatment. It is impossible, for instance, to give an opinion on "shin splints" without actually seeing the dancer involved. There are many causes of pain in the shin, ranging from periosteal irritation to osteoid osteoma. Similarly, "fallen arches," "popping hips," etc., are not accurate orthopaedic expressions.

Teachers always give the best service to their pupils when their own diagnostic skills are directed towards the mechanical and technical problems, which are at the root of virtually all injuries—and these, of course, vary from dancer to dancer.

Dr. Simon Costain
The Gait & Posture Centre Ltd.
Flat 6, Harmont House
20 Harley Street
London W1G 9PH
Tel. 020-7636-4465
www.gaitandposture.net

Dr. Costain is the owner and founder of the Gait & Posture Centre Ltd. based in London. With over thirty years of experience in the field of podiatry, Costain was the GB Olympic team podiatrist, has coauthored a CD-ROM of Sports Injuries of the Foot and Ankle and published various papers and lectured nationally and internationally on the subject.

Dr. Costain, what are the reasons why a child should not be put on pointe before age eleven to twelve? What could be the negative effects according to your experience?

I believe that a child should not be put on pointe before the age of eleven to twelve because of the risks of foot complications, especially the toe joints; and the structure of the foot could be compromised because the foot is simply not strong enough before that age.

How would you treat the first symptoms of Achilles tendonitis? Would you advice icing the part or applying a moist heat pack? Which is best? In what case could the Achilles tendon "snap" and require surgery? Can you suggest a few exercises to prevent injury?

I would treat the first symptoms of Achilles tendinosis (it is no longer referred to as tendonitis in the medical literature), with eccentric stretching gently at first and increasing the ballistic nature of it according to the literature currently available on Achilles tendinosis. I am not an advocate of the use of heat or cold on Achilles tendinosis but would use taping as I see very little evidence in the literature of the Achilles tendon "snapping" following a patient suffering with Achilles tendinosis.

Do you think hyperextension can be corrected with proper training? Students standing in first position with a big gap between their feet, should they be encouraged to keep their heels together or not?
They sometimes cannot understand the concept of not overstretching their knee but to use the muscles in their thighs. How would you help them?

The stretch block system and eccentric stretching remains the treatment of choice. I do think hyperextension can be corrected with proper training, and I think that the student standing in first position with a big gap between their feet should be encouraged to increase the external hip rotation strength and perform good Pilates exercise routines to ensure that they can eventually keep their heels together and do not hyperextend their knees. I think that a student will understand not overstretching their knees and to use the muscles in their thighs, providing it is explained carefully to them in an anatomical and physiological sense.

Students often complain of having pain under their arch when they point in a battement tendu. What could be the cause?

Arch pain is generally caused by foot weakness, and so exercise to enhance the intrinsic and extrinsic muscle strength of the feet most of the time will solve the problems. Avoiding walking barefoot or in too flat a shoe will also make sense out of dance hours, as would the use of some temporary orthoses.

Another common complaint of students aged eight to fourteen is pain around the kneecap. What are the possible causes? Would you advise rest or just wearing a knee brace and icing the part several times a day?

Kneecap pain is caused by poor muscle control of the vastus medialis and other quadriceps muscle groups around the knee, for this is also linked with the poor biomechanics of the feet and internal and external hip rotators. I would not advise rest or wearing any form of knee brace, or icing, unless it is particularly severe; but I would address the functional cause of the problem and try to correct that with exercise.

Can you describe an effective way of taping bunions? How would you treat a child with enlarged and inflamed bunions?

The best way of treating any form of bunion problem is to identify the cause of the bunions, and this, generally speaking, is caused by poor rear foot function and the podiatrist needs to identify what precisely is causing the bunions. Taping bunions is relatively ineffective, but using low dye antipronation taping to the subtalar and midtarsal complexes works extremely well with bunion problems.

Students sometimes complain about their hips "popping." What is the cause, and how dangerous can it be? What should a ballet teacher advise in this case?

The phenomena of "hip-popping" often relates to hypermobility and poor muscle control around the hip and pelvis and a sensible strengthening and stretching programme needs to be designed for the dancer by the physiotherapist.

Calluses underneath the metatarsal area are common in dancers due to the number of hours of standing and the friction caused by the shoe. What would you do to reduce soreness and inflammation? Would you place a pad underneath the affected area or place a pad in the shoe in the corresponding spot?

Calluses underneath the metatarsal area are common in dancers, but this is not caused by the shoe. Calluses and corns are caused by poor foot function and not bad shoes. Someone needs to examine the patient's foot function using a gait analysis system, and it needs to be a podiatrist experienced in this field.

Which exercises would you suggest for stretching and improving the arch?

Arch stretching and strengthening is linked with calf muscle stretching with a stretch block or squats are very useful for stretching the arch. Strengthening is important, as is proprioceptive rehabilitation for the arch, and this is performed using the modified Rhomberg exercise, amongst others.

The modified Rhomberg exercise is in essence a balancing exercise to enhance "proprioception or position sensing." It involves nothing more than "standing on one leg with your eyes shut" . . . a minute a time for up to 5 minutes a day on both legs morning and night.

What are the symptoms of "fallen arches"? Should dancers stop activity for a while if this happens? What are the symptoms, and what is the therapy recommended?

Arches do not "fall," but they begin to function in an abnormal manner, which makes them look as if they are falling. Aching can occur in the feet and lower legs, and some serious strengthening routines with the intrinsic and extrinsic musculature of the feet is important, as is addressing the correct type of footwear and avoiding too flat a shoe at all costs. Some orthoses can be of great help in strengthening the arches of dancer's feet. It is a myth that properly designed orthotics can weaken feet for they will strengthen feet rather than weaken them.

What are the symptoms and treatments for shin splints?

Shin splints is a passé term. It is now referred to as medial tibial border stress syndrome and pain in the lower legs is usually the symptom, but there are a myriad of causes for shin pain, and this needs thorough podiatric and physiotherapy assessment. A universal stretch, though, is the calf muscle stretch, which should be used for all symptoms in the lower limb. Dancers should be aware of how to do this.

We encase our feet in leather coffins most of the day and totally restrict their movement, unlike our hands, which are constantly being exercised as we carry out our normal, everyday tasks. No wonder they feel mistreated—they are!

Part X

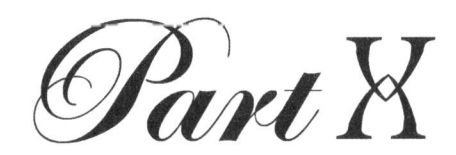

PRESTIGIOUS SCHOOLS AROUND THE WORLD AND INTERVIEWS WITH PROFESSIONAL STUDENTS

The Royal Ballet School
Upper School: 46, Floral Street
Covent Garden, London WC2E, 9DA, UK
Tel: +44(0)20 7836 8899
Lower School: White, Lodge,
Richmond Park, Surrey TW10 5HR, UK
Tel: +44 (0)20 8392 8496
E-mail: enquiries@royalballetschool.co.uk
www.royal-ballet-school.org.uk

In 1926, a young dancer of vision and determination opened a ballet studio in London. From a handful of pupils, modest premises and limited financial resources, she would build up for Great Britain the world-famous Royal Ballet School, the Royal Ballet and the Birmingham Royal Ballet.

This message, written on a commemorative plaque, welcomes visitors at the entrance of the Royal Ballet School in Floral Street. The Royal Ballet School is one of the world's most renowned institutions for classical ballet training. Its Royal Charter connects it with the Royal Ballet companies and assures its commitment to perfection in training.

The school was founded in 1926, when Dame Ninette de Valois (1898-2001) opened her Academy of Choreographic Art. Born in Ireland on June 6, 1898, Ninette de Valois—whose real name was Edris Stannus—had been trained by Edouard Espinosa, Enrico Cecchetti, and Nicolas Legat. She became a leading dancer with the Diaghilev Ballet and the Royal Opera House. In 1931, the dancers trained by de Valois formed the Vic-Wells (the future Sadler's Wells) Ballet and School. In 1947 Sadler's Wells Ballet School was established and moved to the Royal Opera House, Covent Garden. White Lodge, a neo-Classical Palladian building that used to serve as a Royal Hunting Lodge, developed into the home of the Royal Ballet Lower School in 1955, becoming residential and offering its pupils ballet training as well as general education. It is located in the center of London's Richmond Park, and the White Lodge Museum occupies a crescent wing of the building. In October 1956, the school was granted Royal Charter, and along with the companies, they were renamed the Royal Ballet School, the Royal Ballet and the Sadler's Wells Royal Ballet (renamed Birmingham Royal Ballet after its move there in 1990). Since March 27, 2003, the Upper School is located on Floral Street, Covent Garden, right behind the Royal Opera House. The studios are connected to the Royal Ballet by an aerial award-winning bridge called Bridge of Aspiration. It was Ninette de Valois's dream to connect the school to the company, and this bridge fulfilled her wish.

It is the policy of the Royal Ballet School not only to produce dancers of excellence, but also dedicated, balanced, well-mannered thinking individuals who will be an asset to any community and in any environment, not only a joy to watch but a pleasure to know.

—Gailene Stock, AM, Royal Ballet School Director

Royal Academy of Dance
36 Battersea Square
London SW 11 3RA, UK
Tel: +44 (0)20 7326 8000
www.rad.org.uk
info@rad.og.uk

 The Royal Academy of Dance is one of the largest and most influential dance education and training organizations in the world. With over 14,500 members and branches in over eighty-two countries, the RAD strives for excellence in ballet and trains well-prepared and inspiring teachers. Over 190,172 children take RAD exams every year, from Pre-Primary Level to Solo Seal.

 The Royal Academy of Dance offers a unique range of internationally recognized dance teaching qualifications, like degrees and diplomas, university-validated or validated by the RAD as a chartered body.

 The academy was founded in 1920 by a group of eminent dancers like Tamara Karsavina, Adeline Genée, Lucia Cormani, Edouard Espinosa, and Phyllis Bedells, with the aim of improving dance teaching levels in Britain. It was first known as the Association of Teachers of Operatic Dancing in Great Britain.

 In 1935 it was granted a Royal Charter and was renamed the Royal Academy of Dancing. The RAD started to expand and moved its headquarters to the present location in Battersea. A children's syllabus was created by its former president, Dame Margot Fonteyn. Following her retirement and death in 1991, Dame Antoinette Sibley, DBE, was appointed as the new president. Lynn Wallis, former Royal Ballet dancer and ballet mistress, is today the RAD's Artistic Director.

 The Academy's patron is Her Majesty Queen Elizabeth II.

Paris Opera
(Ecole de Danse de l'Opéra National de Paris)
20, Allée de la Danse
9200 Nanterre, France

 In 2013 the ballet school of the Paris Opera (Ecole de Danse de L'Opéra de Paris) will celebrate its three hundredth year. It is the world's oldest school and, as Director Elisabeth Platel explains, its mission is the same as the one given by King Louis XIV: "to train ballet dancers and provide dancers with professional training." The school, created by Jean-Baptiste Lully and Pierre Beauchamp in 1672, survived three centuries and obtained a reputation of superiority and perfection as the oldest school in the West. In 1987 the school moved from the Palais Garnier in a newer building in Nanterre.

 The school accepts students from age eight to age eighteen who attend regular school classes from 8:00 a.m. to until noon and dance classes during the afternoon. Children are admitted to the school between ages eight and thirteen. Pupils between eight and eleven will go through a six-month course starting in January and ending in June, which will decide their admission to the school. Children aged eleven to thirteen will follow a course from September to June. The youngest dancers are called petits rats, which mean "little mice." About four hundred children audition every year, hoping for admission. Candidates go through very meticulous medical controls; they are checked for size and weight, have to pass two selections, different trial periods according to their age, and a final exam. Only twenty children will be chosen to join the school, whose tuition is free. The selection will continue throughout the eight years of school, through yearly examinations, performances, and the omnipresent risk of injuries. The selection is one of the hardest: by the final years, there will only be four or five students left.

The training at the Paris Opéra School is structured over a period of six years. Alongside ballet students will follow classes in contemporary and character dance, jazz, folklore, mime, anatomy, and history of ballet. The classes, called divisions, are divided into six girls' and six boys' levels. Beginners in the sixth division work on placement, posture, and ballet basics. At the end of each year, students are examined to determine whether they will move to the next division or stay in the same. Students of the first division (which is the most advanced) take part in the entrance competition to join the Paris Opera Ballet School or leave the school and join other companies.

Academie de Danse Princesse Grace de Monaco
5, Avenue de la Costa
98000 Monaco (France)
Tel: +377 93307040
E-mail: danse.princesse.grace@monaco.mc
http://academiedansemonaco.com

This prestigious school operates under the presidency of Her Royal Highness the Princess of Hanover.

Started in 1952 as the School of Classical Danse (Ecole de Danse Classique de Monte-Carlo) by the late Marika Besobrasova, it became the Princesse Grace Academy of Danse in 1975, when Princesse Grace and Prince Rainier III of Monaco moved the school to Casa Mia, now its permanent home. Russian-born Madame Besobrasova worked with Mikhail Fokine with Les Ballets de Monte-Carlo and started teaching in 1939. She continued her mission and taught class every day up to the age of ninety-one. Luca Masala undertook the direction of the academy after Marika Besobrasova.

Casa Mia is a beautiful Mediterranean-style building surrounded by trees and flowers. This mansion was purchased by the French government with the aim of opening a professional ballet school. At the academy, the subjects taught span from classical ballet to contemporary and character dance, music education, as well as regular French school education.

The Royal Swedish Ballet School
(Kungliga Svenska Balettskolan)
PO Box 17 516
118 91 Stockholm, Sweden
Tel. +46-(0)8-508 33 510
E-mail: info@kunligasvenskabalettskolan.se
www.kunligasvenskabalettskolan.nu

This old and prestigious school traces its origins back to 1773, when King Gustav III founded the Swedish Ballet and Opera. It is considered the third oldest in Europe, celebrating thirty years since its opening in 1981. Students are trained in classical ballet as well as in modern and contemporary dance. The Royal Swedish Ballet School offers Junior School and Upper Secondary School. The Junior School offers locations in Stockholm, Gothenburg, Malmö, and Pitea; and its aim is to prepare pupils both artistically and technically to be accepted in the Upper Secondary School's professional course for dancers. Classical ballet is the main part of the education, but children also study jazz, contemporary, character, as well as acrobatics and improvisation. The professional course for dancers offers complete professional education in dance, combined with the study of theoretical subjects. Students from Sweden and all other Scandinavian countries are accepted. Entrance to the Upper Secondary School is only by audition.

Royal Danish Ballet School
Auguste Bournonville's Crossing 2-8
1055 Copenhagen K
E-mail: lehj@kglteater.dk
www.kgballetskole.dk
Tel: +45 (33)696701

Considered one of the oldest ballet schools in the world, Det Kongelige Teaters Balletskole was established around 1770. Auguste Bournonville, who was trained by Auguste Vestris at the Paris Opera, was appointed ballet master in Copenhagen in 1836 and remained there until 1875.

After Bournonville's death, his repertoire was revived by Harald Lander, who was appointed ballet master in 1932.

At the Royal Danish Ballet School, they do not just teach correct technique, but they work on developing real artists of the stage.

"Bournonville is about beauty and love," says Lis Jeppesen, former soloist with Royal Danish Ballet and now a professor at the Royal Theatre. Bournonville, in fact, did not like anything showing "technique." He just wanted to show beauty and love and tell a story that people would remember afterward for the rest of their lives.

Since their younger-age children are used in productions as an integral part of the company, especially in works from the Bournonville repertoire. The ballet school at the Royal Theatre includes approximately sixty to seventy pupils from age six to sixteen, and the school is particularly well known for developing strong male dancers, also a part of Bournonville's legacy. Being a dancer himself, he raised the position of the male dancer—who in his days was only confined to the role of supporting the ballerina—to a role of equal importance.

All children at the school receive daily ballet tuition and a comprehensive education at the Reading School. All tuition is free of charge and the school is government funded. Anne Marie Vessel Schlüter was in charge of the school for about eighteen years and then was followed by Niels Balle, who has taught there since 1992 and was also trained at the Royal Theatre Ballet School. In 2003 he was appointed deputy head of the School of Ballet and became director in 2006. In 1996 a branch of the school was established in Holstebrö with Theresa Jarvis as the director, a former principal with the company. Students have the opportunity to perform with the Peter Schaufuss Ballet, which is based in the same town.

Another branch was opened in 2002 in Odense, directed by former soloist Henriette Muus, with around twenty students. These branches make it possible for more students coming from other parts of the country to attend classes at the Royal Theatre School.

Every spring, generally around March, there is an audition held at the three Royal Theatre Ballet School's locations. Students are admitted between ages six and eleven. They prefer students with no prior dance training, and the assessment focuses on charisma as well as physical and rhythmic skills. The children who are selected take part in a training period of two to four weeks, at the end of which the school decides which child they want to offer admission to the ballet school.

Students are taught every morning one and a half hours of classical ballet from Monday to Friday, and from the third grade on, they have classes also on Saturday. Bournonville steps are incorporated into the ballet classes, and from the seventh year, the students take two full Bournonville classes a week. The curriculum also includes music, stage makeup, pointe work for the girls and gym for the boys, as well as contemporary dance and drama. Students are divided into training teams by age and level.

All ballet school's ballet teachers have a background as professional dancers. Virtually everyone has been a former pupil of the school or has danced in the Royal Ballet.

The ballet school is affiliated with the local school systems; it has its own physiotherapist, sports psychologist, and a specialist who follows the children's development closely in all three departments. The Royal Ballet also works with a dietician who regularly teaches and mentors in nutrition and healthy eating. The academic classes are held within the theater complex, and the school has a parent board, meeting several times a year to discuss all aspects of the children's development. Ballet exams are held every spring, and the different dance teams show their skills in front of a jury composed of the principals of the ballet school and company, ballet school teachers, and an examiner.

Once students—aged more or less sixteen—reach the ninth academic year, they can be recruited as apprentices, or aspirants, for the Royal Ballet for a period of two years. Applicants follow ballet training with the adult dancers and take part in performances. The students follow a so-called pre-aspirantår, where they both follow candidates' training and receive instruction in subjects closely related to their impending time as dancers.

The Royal Theatre Ballet School has existed on Kongens Nytorv since 1771 and has trained generations of dancers for the Royal Ballet.

School of American Ballet
70, Lincoln Center Plaza, New York, NY
10023-6592
Phone: 212-769-6600

The School of American Ballet was founded by Lincoln Kirstein and George Balanchine in 1934. Kirstein was a famous American impresario, writer, and dance authority, whose dream was to establish an American school of ballet, and a ballet company that would be as famous as the ones existing in Europe. When he met George Balanchine, at the time working in Europe, he convinced him to come to the United States and help him realize his dream. The School of American Ballet opened its doors in January 1934, at 637 Madison Avenue, New York City, with only thirty-two students enrolled.

The school's early faculty included prestigious teachers like the Russian Pierre Vladimiroff (who had partnered with Anna Pavlova in many occasions), Muriel Stuart, and Dorothie Littlefield. The syllabus for the children's division classes was established by Antonina Tumkovsky and Hélène Dudin and is still in use today. In 1956 the school moves to a larger location on Broadway at Eighty-second Street, in Manhattan; and in 1964 Balanchine adds to the faculty ballerina Alexandra Danilova, former star of the Ballets Russes de Monte Carlo, and Stanley Williams of the Royal Danish Ballet.

The school starts producing very talented dancers like Merrill Ashley, Suzanne Farrell, Gelsey Kirkland, and Robert Weiss. In 1969 SAB moves again, this time at the Juilliard School's new Lincoln Center Headquarters, closer to New York City Ballet's new location at the New York State Theater. After Balanchine's death in 1983, Peter Martins becomes chairman of faculty and co-ballet master with Jerome Robbins. In 1991 the school makes its final move into the newly built headquarters in Lincoln Center's Samuel B. and David Rose Building, including a residence hall able to host up to sixty-five students.

In order to increase male dancers' enrolment, Peter Martins creates a tuition-free boys' program and the faculty includes former dancers like Jack Soto, Darci Kistler, and Katrina Killian. Today SAB is considered the most prestigious professional ballet institution in the United States, still training its students following Balanchine's teaching principles. Admission to the school is by audition only, and students from six to eighteen years old are accepted. In

SAB's children's division, girls and boys study separately, except for pupils in Preparatory A1 level. The School of American Ballet has trained some of the best dancers in the United States, who joined the New York City Ballet or other established Ballet companies.

La Scala Ballet School
(Scuola di Ballo del Teatro alla Scala)
Via Campo Lodigiano 2
20122 Milano
Tel. +39 (02) 92882100
E-mail: audizioni.ballo@accademialascala.it
www.accademialascala.org

The ballet school of La Scala in Milan was founded back in 1813 by Benedetto Ricci and was originally known as the Imperial Royal Academy. Famous dancers like Carlo Blasis, Caterina Beretta, Olga Preobrajenska, and Enrico Cecchetti have been directors of this prestigious school. Today the school is directed by Anna Maria Prina, who was a pupil of the school and a soloist in the company. Frédéric Olivieri has been the head of the dance department since 2003.

The ballet school program lasts eight years, and the technique is based on many styles: Italian, French, Russian, and Balanchine.

Bolshoi Ballet Academy
2nd Frunzenskaya Str, 5
Moscow 119146
Russian Federation
Phone: 007-(095)242 86 12
www.balletacademy.ru
E-mail: balletacademy@yandex.ru

One of the most prestigious ballet schools in the whole world. It is known today as the Moscow State Academy of Choreography and was founded in 1773. Their curriculum, based on the Vaganova technique, includes classical ballet, pointe, repertoire, pas de deux, jazz, character, and historical dance. Admission to the school for children from nine to eighteen is strictly through audition, and many of the students sleep in the school dormitories. The Bolshoi Ballet Academy offers twenty large studios with special dance floors, a study area, a physiotherapy room, showers, and changing rooms with lockers. The academy is directed by Marina Leonova and former Kirov ballerina Altynai Asylmuratova, who is the artistic director.

Vaganova Academy
2, Rossi Street
St. Petersburg
191011 Russia
E-mail: academy@vaganova.ru

The school was founded on May 4th, 1738 in Saint Petersburg, by order of the Empress Anna Ioannovna. From the Vaganova Academy legendary dancers like Vaslav Nijinsky, Anna Pavlova and Tamara Karsavina have graduated and each year new talented dancers leave the school to join the Maryinsky Ballet Company, formerly called Kirov. The school takes its name from the famous ballet pedagogue Agrippina Vaganova, who laid the foundations of the Vaganova technique and the Russian school.

Since 1999, the school has been directed by former prima ballerina Altynai Asylmouratova.

Miami City Ballet School
2200 Liberty Avenue
Miami Beach, Fl 33139
Phone(305)929-7007
E-mail: school@miamicityballet.org

Miami City Ballet School was founded in January 1993 by Edward and Linda Villella and is one of the most renowned ballet schools in the United States and throughout the world. Edward Villella trained with the American School of Ballet in New York and later joined New York City Ballet as an artist. The aim of the school is to educate dancers according to Villella's style and principles and incorporate them into the ballet company.

Linda Villella, Director of the School, declares that by developing contacts with different teachers around the world, the school has become a world-wide known entity in the field of ballet. The school's Principal is ballet master Alexander Carter.

Miami City Ballet accepts students throughout the year from age 3 to age 19. The school offers a Winter Program that goes from September to mid-June and a Summer Program from the end of June through the end of July. Classes are held in a modern and fully equipped 63,000 square-foot building, located right in the heart of Miami Beach. Every other month parents are invited to come and observe class and monitor the high quality of the teaching and the students' progression. The school offers a Children Division and a Pre-Professional Division, as well as a Jazz Division. The Children Division includes Mommy and Me Music and Movement Class, Creative Movemment, Ballet Preparatory I and Ballet Preparatory II. The Pre-Professional Division aims to prepare students for a professional career. The Curriculum focuses on ballet technique and includes Pointe Work for girls, Variations, Partnering classes, Jazz and also Character. All lessons are accompanied by a pianist and are taught by world-renwned teachers of Miami City Balet School's Faculty.

English National Ballet School
Carlyle Building, Hortensia Road
London SW10 0QS, England
E-mail: info@enbschool.org.uk
www.enbschool.rg.uk

The English National Ballet School (ENBS) was founded in 1988 and celebrates its glorious twenty-third year as one of the best ballet schools in the world.

It was founded by Dame Alicia Markova and Sir Anton Dolin and was originally based at Markova House, in the borough of South Kensington. The school is now located at Carlyle Building, Hortensia Road, in the heart of the Royal Borough of Kensington and Chelsea. Here is the school's mission:

To be a centre of excellence for young dancer development, providing intense ballet training in preparation for students to enter a professional career.

ENBS provides training for students aged sixteen to nineteen years old, as a preparation for a professional career, working toward the National Diploma in Professional Dance. Over 35 percent of the graduates join the English National Ballet or other distinguished ballet companies. ENBS curriculum includes choreography, Benesh movement notation, dance and voice, dance on film, dance through time, professional employment skills, music, and singing. The school works continuously in raising money for scholarships in order to help talented students who lack financial means reach their goals. The school works under the direction of Wayne Eagling, who is also the director of the Ballet Company, and Verena Cornwall, BA (Hons) PG Diploma.

Interviews with Twenty-two Professional Students

- Jemma Babayeva – School of Canadian Ballet Theatre
- Portia Van De Braam – Arts Educational School (Tring Park, England)
- Merrit Howard – The Rock School for Dance Education, (Philadelphia, Pennsylvania)
- Nicole Ciapponi – Pacific Northwest Ballet School
- Lilit Hogtanian – Academie de Danse Princesse Grace de Monaco (France)
- Emma Layne – Central School of Ballet (London, England)
- Emily Smith – Australia Trainee, Vienna State Opera Ballet School
- Rebecca Croan - Bolshoi Ballet Academy (Moscow)
- Nicola Wills-Jones – Queensland Ballet Professional
- Sarah Elizabeth Johnson – The Ballet Conservatory (Lewisville, Texas)
- Aimee Higgs – Royal Ballet School
- Ilka Felsen – Duke University (Durham, North Carolina)
- Tiara Watts – Prudence Bowen Atelier (Mudgeeraba, Queensland, Australia)
- Brooke Newman – Prudence Bowen Atelier (Mudgeeraba, Queensland, Australia)
- Katie Chachich – University of Maryland (Baltimore County)

- Katie Partridge
- Heidi Landford – Prudence Bowen Atelier (Mudgeeraba, Queensland, Australia)
- Kirsten Wicklund – Washington Ballet Studio Company
- Liana Vasconcelos- Youth Ballet Company of Rio de Janeiro (Brazil)
- Sarah Lamkin - Prudence Bowen Atelier (Mudgeeraba, Queensland, Australia)
- Myriam Ernest - Professional Division Student, Pacific Northwest Ballet
- Josephine Cheung – Bolshoi Ballet Academy (Moscow)

Jemma Babayeva
Student, Grade 11
School of Canadian Ballet Theatre

Jemma was ten years old when she started pointe. She wears Grishko Maya I, size 5 1/2, width XXX H.

Her feet are highly arched with very long and bendable toes. In order to soften her pointe shoes, she breaks the toe box with a hammer, just enough to soften the block and widen it, but she never breaks the arch part of the shoe. As far as how many pairs of shoes she uses in a month, she says it depends on her schedule. If she has lots of rehearsals and performances, she uses up to five to six pairs per month. During school days, when she only has pointe, variations, and pas de deux classes, she uses only one pair of shoes a week. She does not Pan-Cake her shoes for performances very often, but whenever she has to, she uses powder. Here is her technique to sew in elastics and ribbons:

First she divides the 5/8" elastic into two equal halves and then sews it in a semicircle from the back of the shoe where the seam meets on either side. Then she takes the ribbon and cuts it into four equal lengths, and she burns the top of the ribbon lightly against a flame to prevent it from fraying. In order to find the correct place for the ribbons, she folds over the back of the shoe to the sock liner. After that she places the ribbon at about a thirty-five-degree angle running toward the top of the shoe so that they lie flat against her ankles when she ties them.

Jemma strengthens her feet with Thera-Bands before every class. She does not use any trick to make her arch look better, but she says she always tries to point her feet a little bit more, and this makes them look better onstage. She also suggests stretching the knees to the max to achieve the perfect look. Her toe pads are Bunheads Pro Pad.

Jemma always works a little bit on the floor before class to avoid injuries. She executes some turn-out exercises, like "the frog," while lying on her stomach, some splits, and some abs workout. At the barre she performs several warm-up tendus with demi-plié to "warm-up the thighs and tendons of the leg." She has tried different types and brands of shoes but Grishko Maya I is the one that works the best for her. Asked what she does if she gets a blister before a show, she answered that she uses toe tape. "It works well, and the pain goes away!" She also likes Second Skin even if it's more expensive. Her advice to dancers: "You should always work doing your best. Ballet is a hard profession, but if you believe in yourself and always work hard no matter what, you'll make your dream come true!"

Portia Van De Braam
Arts Educational School
Tring Park, England

Portia is nineteen years old. She trained from the age of eleven at the Royal Ballet School, White Lodge, and then moved on to broaden her theatrical horizons to the Arts Educational School, Tring Park. Portia started pointe at eleven at the Royal Ballet School. Her feet are wide, high arched, and quite strong.

How old were you when you started pointe?

I was eleven, but I didn't do a lot at that tender age of course!

What pointe shoes do you use?

I used to have to use Freed at White Lodge, which, don't get me wrong, are great shoes for many, but they didn't really suit my highly arched feet as they'd soften or break easily. Now I use the perfect shoe for a high arch, which is Sansha Lyrica. I'm a size 9 (that's an American size). I'm a 6.5 with toe pads, wide fitting. I think most of the shanks on Sanshas are high. Somehow they always spring back to life in the sole and last for ages . . . they just need shellac-ing in the ends!

What type of foot do you have?

High arched, and quite strong.

How do you soften your pointe shoes?

By firstly standing on the tops and sides too. Give them a little bending of the sole, then I just wear them around the house, so they mold well to my feet. Another way is to just use them in class.

How do you make your pointe shoes less noisy?

My fabulous Sanshas don't actually make noise! Another thing they are brilliant for is that they are sort of padded right underneath the hard-toed part, and don't really need any noise banged out of them. They're great, I'm telling you!

How many pairs do you generally use weekly or monthly?

Before, I'd go through maybe one or two pairs each fortnight, but now I have had the one pair of Sanshas for over a month.

Do you Pan-Cake shoes for shows? What do you use?

Yes, I do Pan-Cake them, unless otherwise told. I use calamine lotion.

How do you sew your elastics and ribbons?

I sew the elastic from the right at the back of the heel, so that they are almost touching, as my shoes tend to slip off the backs. The ribbons are sewn on just in front of the crease when I fold the heel over.

Is there any exercise you practice to strengthen your instep?

Clingy-band exercises: Using the clingy/Thera–Band round under your foot, just point and flex, altering the tension in the band as required. Also, metatarsal exercises are great for strong feet articulation, especially in pointe shoes: lay foot flat on the ground and draw up the toes, but without rounding or crunching them underneath you. You can do this exercise on a towel or tissue and try to draw the end of the towel or tissue closer.

Do you use any tricks to make your arch look better?

No, fortunately I don't need to! But I am against arch enhancers.

Can you suggest a warm-up exercise at the barre or in the center?

Just good old-fashioned rising and lowering, slowly and going right through the feet. Then relevés.

Do you always use the same brand and type of shoes, or do you change?

No more will I change from my lovely Sanshas!

What do you do when you get a blister before a show?

Just grin and bear it! I have found in the past that it hurts more when I strap them up, as it gives less room in the shoe and therefore squeezes it even more. Just add lots of antiseptic cream to keep it from getting infected, and I wear toe pads, which helps enormously. Another thing is that I find, and I'm sure many others will agree, that somehow you don't feel the pain when you're actually performing, although just before you go on, the pain is unbearable and you think you won't make it. It's a thing that just is . . . It's the magic of performing!

Any advice you would give to beginners?

Take it slowly, and don't get too excited as you may end up with an injury.

Do you use any padding in your shoes?

I use Bunheads toe pads. They have this gel inside that really protects. However, I will either alter them or get a new pair, as I think it's not important and unnecessary to have the gel padding underneath the foot . . . you don't get blisters there, and it makes dancing in pointe shoes harder to balance, and one can't feel the floor so well. But I know that toe pads with just material underneath are available, so that's OK!

Portia, do you have any personal suggestions?

Another good exercise to stretch the arches and improve them is, rise up in a wide first position holding on to the barre. Then bend your knees and just "go over" on pointe, without retracting the foot as you would usually do for jumping en pointe. No more suggestions, really. Pointe work is wonderful (if you don't have blisters!). It is like dancing to the max, stretching right through and up high on your toes!

Merrit Howard
The Rock School for Dance Education (Philadelphia)
Professional Division

Merrit wears Bloch European Balance Size 5.5 XXX with a medium shank. She has also tried Russian Pointe, Freed, and Grishko; but she is happy with Bloch at the moment. Her foot is wide, with a narrow heel. Her favorite toe pads are Pillows for Pointe by Gellows. She crisscrosses her elastics and ties her ribbons on in the traditional manner, and she softens the shoes by bending the arch and stepping on the vamp. She uses an average of three pairs of shoes per month, and if she gets a blister, she opens an Advil Liqui-Gel and spreads the gel on the blister and after tapes it with toe tape. The only alteration she makes to the shoe is scraping the bottom with scissors and cutting off the satin on the tip. Merrit doesn't usually Pan-Cake the shoes for performances, but if she is asked to do so, she uses calamine lotion or Pan-Cake makeup.

Nicole Ciapponi
Pacific Northwest Ballet School
Professional Division Program
Winner of the Silver Medal
Adeline Genée Competition 2008
Top 12 at Youth America Grand Prix 2009

Nicole started pointe at ten. She uses Suffolk's Solos or Apprentice, size 4 1/2 XXX or 4 XXXX, according to what she can get. She likes this brand at the moment, but she might switch to Freed in the future.

She has a Giselle foot, all the toes of the same length, very square and very wide. Nicole does not soften her pointe shoes. "I like them hard," she says. "I eventually add more glue to make them harder." She goes through one or two pairs of shoes a week, depending on what she is doing. If she has Nutcracker or end-of-the-year show rehearsals, she uses up to three to four pairs.

In order to protect her toes, she uses the end of socks. "The toe part of the sock," she specifies. She also likes lamb's wool or tape.

She doesn't Pan-Cake her shoes because "it leaves marks all over the floor." Nicole crosses her elastics and attaches the ribbons to the front end of the elastics, then she sews around where the drawstring is on the shoe. In order to strengthen her feet, she practices about thirty-two quick relevés. Nicole does not use any trick to make her arch look better. "I just make sure I sew my ribbons to pull my shoe up, so my arch can show more." If she gets a blister before a performance, she sprays on New Skin—"which burns, but it's very helpful." Then she puts a bandage on it. Her advice for beginners is to make sure they get fitted by an experienced fitter, and then have the teacher check the shoes before sewing them.

Lilit Hogtanian
Académie de Danse Classique Princesse Grace
Monaco, France

Lilit started pointe at age ten and uses Russian Pointe, model D, width 3, vamp 2, with a medium-hard shank. She sometimes also wears Grishkos, and now she is looking for another type of shoe "with a slimmer look, and less bulky!"

Lilit has narrow feet with wide toes. She doesn't soften her shoes but lets them mold to her foot by using them in class. Her shoes can last from two weeks to a month, depending on how much she is dancing. Lilit protects her feet using a toe pad and a half sock to prevent blisters from sweating. She does not Pan-Cake her shoes for performances. "I Like the color and shine of Russian Pointes," she says. Lilit hand-sews her elastics and ribbons using Bunheads Stitch Kit. Before class she does a lot of pointe and flex exercises to prepare her feet.

She suggests an interesting warm-up exercise at the barre: "Three relevés without plié and two slow with plié in first position 8 times, then on one leg, 4 times each leg." If Lilit gets a blister before a show, she ends up forgetting about it! She advises young students to work hard and always accept feedback. "Pay attention to all the details of how you work your feet to prevent bad habits, and also listen to what your teacher says."

Emma Layne
Central School of Ballet, Fifth Year
London, England

Emma started pointe work at about twelve. She wears Bloch Sonata 4C (at the moment), and her feet are "small and quite shallow." To soften new shoes, she lightly stands on the blocks to flatten them slightly, then puts some water on the top of the block near the drawstring to soften that area for demi-pointe. The she sits down, puts the shoes on her feet, and pushes over onto demi-pointe, holding the back of the shoes on her heels. Still remaining seated, she pushes over onto pointe and bends the backs slightly. She then walks around in them for a while so they begin to mold to her feet.

Once she has sewn the ribbons on, she executes a few basic rises and relevés. She uses a few new pairs of shoes each term, but as she says, "I like to save all my pointe shoes, and after hardening them using Klear [floor polish], I often can then wear my old shoes again for repertoire classes."

She uses calamine lotion to make her shoes matte. "I dampen a makeup sponge and apply the calamine lotion lightly using the sponge." Emma likes to sew her ribbons on an angle so that there is no bulging around the satin. She sometimes sews elastics just behind the ribbons to keep the heel of the shoe on while dancing, but only if necessary.

She pads her toes with Happy Toes gel pads. "The padding covers the top of the toes but does not cover the ball of the foot, which I prefer so that I can feel the floor more when I am dancing."

She strengthens her feet by pointing and flexing using a Thera-Band for resistance. To enhance her arch, she just bends the back of the shoe a little. If Emma gets a blister before a performance (although she says she is quite lucky because she does not generally suffer from blisters), she uses Germolene New Skin, which protects the blister, and uses Gaynor Minden gel patches, placing them on one side of the blister to relieve the pressure.

"Satin can be slippery," says Emma. "To reduce the risk of slipping, you can darn the platform, but I find that scoring the platform with a Stanley knife, or cutting away the platform satin completely with the knife, is just as effective.

Her advice to young dancers:

1. Build up strength at the barre first.
2. Work through the feet.
3. Don't wear pointe shoes that are too hard—you must be able to stand fully on the platform.

She also suggests using several pairs of pointe shoes at the same time. For example, a hard pair for pas de deux, a comfortable yet supportive pair of pointes for pointe class, and a softer pair for variations. "Be prepared to try different pointe shoes," she says, "as you go through your training. Your feet will change. They will become stronger, and they will also widen."

Emma likes to keep the old shoes once they are broken or have become too soft. She tears out the backs and makes them into soft blocks!

Emily Smith
Royal Ballet School
Vienna State Opera Ballet School

Emily is from Australia; she grew up in the small rural town of Gordonvale, just outside of Cairns, Far North Queensland. She started ballet when she was eight years old, doing just one class a week along with jazz. When Emily was twelve, her love for ballet grew stronger, and in 2004 she successfully auditioned for the Interstate Junior Program with the Australian Ballet, which she was a part of for three years. In 2008, at the age of sixteen, Emily left home and moved to Sydney to study full-time ballet at Tanya Pearson Classical Coaching Academy.

During her time with Tanya Pearson, she competed in many prestigious competitions, both nationally and internationally. She was a semi-finalist in the Sydney McDonald's Performing Arts challenge for two consecutive years, a finalist in the Society of Dance Arts, and she was selected to compete in the Finals of the Youth American Grand Prix in New York in 2009. It was at this competition that Emily was offered a full scholarship to the Vienna State Opera Ballet School and the Royal Ballet summer school. Emily finished all of her RAD exams with distinction, and it was upon completion of her final exam that she qualified for the Genée International Competition in Singapore, also in 2009, where she was one of twelve finalists. It was a very busy year for her, and at the age of seventeen, she successfully auditioned for the Prix de Lausanne held in Switzerland in 2010. Here Emily was offered her third year (graduate year) at the Royal Ballet School in London. In September Emily moved to Vienna to commence her one year placement at the Vienna State Opera Ballet School, but has since returned in preparation for beginning her final year of training at the Royal Ballet School commencing in September. In this interview Emily shares her "little secrets" and good advice.

What pointe shoes do you use?

"I currently wear Serenade BLOCH. I am a 3C. I need them because they have quite a hard full sole shank and the vamp is reasonably high."

What type of foot do you have?

I have an Egyptian foot, where my big toes are the biggest and the other toes taper accordingly. I have a very high arch, which is difficult to hold back on. I always need to dance in a shoe that has a hard shank.

Do you wear any type of padding?

Yes, I wear a Pro Pad. It has padding on the top but not the bottom. They are very thin, but just enough to take the discomfort away.

How do you like to sew your ribbons and elastics?

I sew my ribbons farther forward than most. I attach them near the arch to help the shoe mold to the shape of my foot. Otherwise, I get a huge gap between my arch and the shoe. I then sew the elastics on right at the back of my heel to keep it from coming off. I use really thick elastic.

What technique do you use to break in your shoes?

I sometimes bend the sole about three quarters the way up the shoe where my arch would sit so that I get a straight line up until my arch and then it bends. So almost like a ninety-degree angle. But I cannot do too much to a shoe, if I want them to last a couple of weeks. I always just do slow rises and tendus in them.

How do you protect your toes from blisters?

I'm pretty lucky with blisters—they are never really a problem for me. But if I do happen to get them (mainly when the weather is hot), I put a piece of Second Skin on it, with a piece of white tape on it, to hold it in place, and then a piece of brown Physio Tape on top of that to give it padding so I don't feel it. That usually seems to do the trick.

What alterations do you do to your shoe?

I never do anything to my shoes.

Do you Pan-Cake your shoes for performance? What product do you use?

I always use calamine lotion to get rid of the satin look. I love it—it matches the color of my tights much better and makes my foot look like an extension of my leg.

Do you darn your shoes?

No, I don't darn my shoes.

How do you clean your pointe shoes?

If I have black marks on my shoes from the stage, calamine lotion tends to fix that.

Do you have any secret tip for pointe students?

Don't try putting too much padding in your shoes to protect your toes, because it often does more harm than good. If your foot is too tight, then it puts a lot of pressure on your toes, and they are more likely to bruise than if you have less padding. Sometimes less is best.

Could you describe at least one exercise to help strengthen the feet?

I always do this, to warm up my feet or to strengthen: 8 rises in parallel, keeping the knees straight, and then 8 landing in plié. Repeat in first position and second position. Then close into fifth and do 16 échappés. Finish this sequence by doing 16 relevés on one foot right and left. It's an excellent exercise.

Do you use any accessories?

I used to use gel toe separators, but I found they were squishing my feet too much, so now I use no accessories.

What do you do to make your arch look better?

Nothing.

What is your own advice for beginners?

Make sure your first pair of pointe shoes are fitted for you by a professional. It is vital to have the correct shoes for your feet. Don't break them in too much before you wear them. Your feet will get stronger by working through the shoes.

Rebecca Croan
Bolshoi Ballet School

Rebecca spent a year studying at the Boshoi Ballet Academy in Moscow.

She started dancing fairly late, at age thirteen, and started pointe work one year later. She uses Grishkos, XXXX, size 3 UK. She describes her feet as small, narrow, and with a high arch. In order to improve her arch, she usually exercises rolling through her feet. She suggests a good exercise at the barre: 24 relevés in first and second and 20 relevés in fifth. She always uses the same type of pointe shoes. If she gets a blister before a show, she pops it open and soaks it in Epsom salts and then soaks it in Betadine. Rebecca does not use any type of padding.

Nicola Wills-Jones
Silver Medal Winner
Genée International Ballet Competition, Singapore 2009

Nicola started pointe at age twelve. She currently uses Grishko 2007 Pro, size 5 width X, hard shank for rehearsal and class and medium shank for performance.

She started off wearing Bloch Sonata, and then used Bloch Sylphide in performance. She also tried Bloch Balance whenever she couldn't find Grishko's. "Unless you are born with Svetlana Zacharova's feet," she says "students shouldn't try these shoes. No matter how much they are bent, snapped, microwaved, and worn, they are extremely hard to get on pointe and bad to dance in. Grishkos feel nice and light to dance in.

She describes her foot as "very wide, with an average arch on top, but high instep."

She uses Grishko's toe pads and rotates them with Bloch toe pads.

In order to soften her shoes, she puts them in the microwave for ten seconds, not more, to allow the glue to soften slightly, and wears them in a warm-up class so that they mold to her feet.

A pair of pointe shoes with hard shank can last for up to three weeks, depending on how intensively she uses them, while soft-shank shoes would last only for a week and a half.

She does not generally Pan-Cake them for shows, but if she has to, she uses a light face powder.

Depending on how much time she has, she sews practice shoe ribbons and elastics with a sewing machine. For performance shoes, she uses a good-quality thread, to prevent snapping, and sews around the edge of the ribbon and elastic, "making sure I don't go through the satin on the front or through the drawstring." In order to strengthen her instep, she practices slow tendus or uses Thera-Bands to strengthen her ankles. "If reading, watching TV, or sitting down in rehearsal, I put my feet under a heavy couch or piano, making sure my tarsals are directly under the couch, and not my toes. I also bend them manually with my hands.

Any tricks to make her arch look better? "Not really," she says. "I've tried padding my instep with gauze tape to make them look higher, but it doesn't look realistic, so I've never worn it onstage." She suggests practicing slow tendus thinking about going through the foot and quick frappés "to get the ankles moving."

She soaks her blisters in methylated spirit, unless it is an open blister. If it's open, she puts a couple of Band-Aids on it, plus a "corn pad."

Her advice for beginners is to take it easy at first. "Don't go into the center unless you have done a couple of classes on just barre. Your teacher should make sure that you are strong enough in technique to start in the first place, but it is up to the student to know how hard they work on their instep to make it look nice."

Sarah-Elizabeth Johnson
The Ballet Conservatory
Lewisville, Texas
Company Member
LakeCities Ballet Theatre

Trained at the Ballet Conservatory in Lewisville, Texas, Sarah Elizabeth is now a company member with the LakeCities Ballet.

She received scholarships to attend Kirov Academy of Ballet and the Bolshoi Ballet Academy and was accepted into the Pacific Northwest Ballet School 2008 summer intensives. She also attended the American Ballet Theatre's 2008 summer intensive in New York City, and she competed in Youth America Grand Prix and made it to the New York finals twice.

Sarah Elizabeth started pointe work at the age of twelve. She describes her foot as the Giselle type, and she is now wearing custom-made Freed pointe shoes, medium shank and XX width. She always uses the same type of shoe, which she softens by stepping on the box and bending the shank at the arch level, and she generally uses two pairs of shoes a week. She does not Pan-Cake her shoes for performances, and she does not wear toe pads. When it comes to ribbons and elastics, she crisscrosses her elastics and sews them together with the ribbons. She claims that rolling through her feet is an excellent exercise to strengthen her instep. She also recommends executing 24 relevés at the barre in first and second positions and 20 sus sous in fifth. If she gets a blister before a show, she pops it open and soaks it in Epsom salts and then in Betadine.

Here is her advice for beginners: "Pointe shoes are painful the first few weeks, but you will get stronger, and you will grow calluses. Then you will be pain free!"

Aimee Higgs
Royal Ballet School

Aimee started dancing on pointe at age ten. She uses Bob Martin shoes with high vamps and arch support. Her foot has a high arch and instep but weaker metatarsals. In order to soften her pointe shoes, she walks in them and massages them, and she generally uses up to six pairs per month. She Pan-Cakes them for shows using calamine lotion. She sews her elastics and ribbons by hand, using a strong thread, and she crisscrosses her elastics for extra support. She uses Thera-Bands in order to strengthen her instep. No tricks to make her arch look better, although she admits some dancers use fake arches. If she gets a blister before a show, she dries it out with a hair dryer and covers it with Compeed plasters. Her favorite padding is lamb's wool.

Her advice: "Never dance in brand-new shoes as it is uncomfortable and painful and can injure ankles easily."

Ilka Felsen
Graduate of the Rock School
Duke University, Major in Dance

Ilka was fourteen when she started pointe work. Her foot is the peasant type. Her toes are short and slightly tapered so that her big toe is the same length as her second toe, but her third toe is longer than her fourth, which is longer than the fifth. She wears Grishko 2007, size 5.5, XXX, and supersoft shanks. "I would not say that I have a particularly high instep or arch. My left foot is more flexible than my right. I have a little bit of a bunion on my left foot and not so much of one on my right.

Ilka has her own particular ritual to break in her pointe shoes. "I usually pull apart the inside of the shank from the rest of the shoe," she says. "There is a narrow piece of cardboard in Grishko 2007 shoes that is about two inches by one inch in size that can be pulled out. I take out the nail that holds the shank to the bottom of the shoe with either scissors or a hammer, depending on whichever tool is more convenient, and then pull the cardboard insert out."

She says she also steps on the vamps of her shoes to make them a little narrower, and she puts water on the sides to have them form better to her bunions. She usually wears out a pair of shoes in three weeks if pointe work is light (eight to ten hours each week) or in two weeks if pointe is heavy (fifteen-plus hours each week). Basically, it all depends on how many hours she dances each week.

She Pan-Cakes her shoes only when the choreographer or the ballet mistress requests it. She uses Max Factor in the lightest pink she can find for classical ballet pieces. For contemporary performances, she uses NYC brand foundation in the second lightest shade. She likes to try and match her skin color for contemporary.

She sews her elastics on the outside of the shoe about an inch away from her heel. She uses Prima Soft stretch ribbon and sews the tips of the ribbons about two and a half inches from the middle of her heel. She also lightly burns the edges of the ribbons and elastics so they don't fray.

In order to strengthen her instep, she practices the following exercise: "I place my foot on the floor and try to lift my instep off the floor while keeping my sole and heel on the floor, so that the tips of my toes press into the floor while the longer part of each toe gets flatter and also presses into the floor." She also uses Thera-Bands exercises to improve her feet.

She doesn't use any trick to enhance her arch. "I know there are inserts some dancers wear that pad their arches so they appear higher," she says, "but I have never tried those." She declares herself satisfied with her feet and tries to work more on how she uses each foot and its contact with the floor. She feels that stretching her foot so that it gains more flexibility works good for her. She thinks "ankle rolls" are amazing warm-up exercises. Any kind of Thera-Band exercises (pushing the sole of the foot against the Thera-Band, winging the foot with the Thera-Band pulling in the opposite direction) are also helpful in getting the feet to work stronger and bend more. "I like to just point and flex my feet a lot, and sometimes I sit on my heels and pull each knee up to my chest so that my arch stretches."

Grishko 2007 are her favorite shoes so far, after trying Chacott, Bloch Serenade, Bloch Alpha, Freed Studio II, Freed Studio I and Grishko Pro. She didn't get any blister since she started using Grishkos 2007, but she would when she was using Bloch Serenade. If she gets a blister, she coats it with Second Skin and plenty of tape. She also believes that putting her legs up at a ninety-degree angle and letting the blood rush down her legs has some kind of healing effect.

Her advice to beginners: "Try a lot of types of pointe shoes. Pointe work does not have to be painful." She finds that stretching feet using a Thera-Band makes the ankles stronger, and if the ankles are stronger, a dancer can push over the shoes even more. "I think it's more important to have strong, flexible ankles that can push the arches directly over the toes or farther forward."

Her favorite pads are Ouch Pouch Jr. Large. She also sticks a piece of rubber between her big toe and her second toe to prevent her bunions to get larger.

Tiara Watts
Advanced 2 RAD
Prudence Bowen Atelier
320 Chesterfield Drive
Mudgeeraba, Queensland, Australia 4213

 Tiara wears Bloch Heritage pointe shoes, size 5 XX; and she describes her foot as normal, neither wide nor narrow. She likes to wear Bloch toe pads, the ones that are fabric outside and jelly inside.

 She sews her ribbons and elastics by hand with cotton and a needle, by following the instructions on the packet. She uses ribbons with elastics already built in.

 She ties them on by wrapping the ribbons around the ankle one and a half times to join at the inside of the foot (inside ribbon first), with a double knot and no bow.

 She explains that her ballet teacher teaches them many exercises to break pointe shoes in a special way. Facing the barre, doing rises, relevés, échappés, and so on. She uses an average of two to three pointe shoes a month. She hardly gets blisters, but if she gets one before a performance, she covers it with Betadine and tapes them using surgical fabric tape that she finds at the drugstore. She does not like to use Band-Aids. Tiara does not alter her shoes, she does not Pan-Cake them for performances, and she usually starts breaking them in three to five days before a show.

 She sometimes washes her ribbons with soap, but she does not clean her pointe shoes. If you go to a store to get fitted, she suggests you try all the types of pointe shoes on. She believes sharing all the necessary information with the fitter (how many hours a week you dance, what you find hard in pointe shoes, what school you go) will tremendously help in finding the right shoe. Tiara's suggested exercise to strengthen feet is relevés from one foot to another foot in coupé, or cou-de-pied position, facing the barre. Her advice: "Practice makes perfect!"

Brooke Newman
RAD Solo Seal
2009 Genee Competition
Prudence Bowen Atelier
320 Chesterfield Drive
Mudgeeraba, QLD, 4213 Australia

 Brooke wears Bloch Heritage size 5.5, width XXX, with a V-shaped vamp. She describes her foot as extremely wide. She uses Pro Pads by Bloch to protect her toes from blisters and occasionally also wears lamb's wool. She prefers to sew her ribbons quite forward, on the side of the shoe and at a slight angle. "I tie them by crossing the inside ribbon over first and wrapping it around my ankle. Then I cross the outside ribbon over and wrap it around. Then I tie them in a knot and tuck the remaining ribbon underneath so it's hidden away."

Brooke breaks her shoes in by wearing them straightaway and walking in them to soften the sole and the block. "Occasionally, I will bend them slightly with my hands before wearing them. I mostly will go through about two pairs a month." She explains that the padding she wears protects her from blisters; however, she also uses toe tape and lamb's wool if she gets a blister. "I find that when I am performing, I tend not to notice the pain of a blister, so it isn't so bad," she says. She cuts the satin off the tip of the shoe as she finds that it can become quite slippery and fray very easily. If she needs to hide any marks on the shoe for a performance, she applies Pan-Cake and makeup powder. Here Tiara shares her secret tip for pointe students: "Leaving pointe shoes out in the sun after use or in an airy place is great! It helps to get rid of their odor and dries them out, making them last a whole lot longer. I have discovered that doing many relevés on each leg, at the barre or in the center, is great for strengthening the ankle and good for preventing any injuries."

She always sews elastics at the backs of her pointe shoes; she finds it is good for preventing the backs from slipping off the heels. In order to make her arch look better, she says it's important to get right on the block of the shoe, without pulling back. Tiara's advice to young students? "Really try and build strength in your pointe shoes. Once you have sufficient strength, you will be better able to tackle any solos and repertoire you are learning!"

Katie Chachich
Double Major in Dance and Technical Theatre
University of Maryland, Baltimore County

Katie started pointe exactly a week after she turned eleven. She has danced with Harford Dance Theatre and the Bossov Ballet Theatre.

She currently wears Capezio Glissé extra-strong shank for classes and rehearsals and regular shank as performance shoes, after trying, as she likes to say "just about everything under the sun!"

She started with Capezio Infinita, then moved on to Capezio Contempora and Plié, and then moved on to Sansha, followed by Grishko Elite. Then Prima Soft with the V-vamp, Bloch Synergy, Sonata, and Rehearsals. All of these shoes seemed to give her lots of blisters. She continued her search, trying So Danca CK, then Russian Pointe, and finally Capezio Glissés.

Her feet are very wide with slight bunions, and all her toes are the same length, but very small. She wears a size 5 street shoe. In order to soften her shoes, she puts a little bit of water across the front of the vamp to have it stretch around her bunions without giving her a blister. She also bends the shank manually before she wears them. She uses about a pair every week or week and a half when she is training. Katie prefers soft pink stage makeup rather than calamine lotion to mattify her shoes: she buys it from www.discountdance.com. She thinks calamine makes shoes too pink. She sews the ribbons under her foot, so that "even if it breaks, there are no tails of ribbons and still is supporting my foot." Katie strengthens her feet doing lots of relevés with and without her pointe shoes, and knows other dancers also use Thera-Bands. No tricks to make her arch look better: she just slightly bends the shoe where the arch is. When she used to wear Bloch, she would pull the top tack out of the heel to give more flexibility.

If she develops a blister before a show, Katie uses Ora-Gel or Abesol "both for teeth, but work well on sore toes, blisters, or ingrown nails too." Other solutions she suggests are Second Skin burn pads to give extra cushioning or corn cushions "to help relieve pressure from directly hitting a blister." However, she believes that overpadding blisters is not a good idea. Her advice for beginners is to "really think alignment even in your technique classes. Any bad habits you have will be magnified when you get on pointe, so take special care to notice and correct them. Keeping a written journal of your corrections can be very helpful."

After trying all sorts of padding—including cut socks, duct tape, gel pads, and Ouch Pouches—she came to the conclusion that Ouch Pouches were the best. "They aren't sticky like many gel pads and don't have any sharp edges like the old pink Toe Flows," she says. "They allow you to feel the floor, which is important, especially for beginners." She thinks Ouch Pouches are easier to put on than toe tape, and this is particularly useful in quick changes between modern and pointe. They are also washable and more hygienic.

Katie Partridge

Katie started pointe at age twelve. She currently wears Bloch, size 3.5, medium shank, but she sometimes changes. She also wears Grishko size 5 1/2 medium shank, XXXXX (wide). "I am very happy with these shoes at the moment, as they fit securely and do not squash my enlarged big toe joint. The width of the pointe is not too small or too big and the medium shank breaks in quite easily."

Her foot is wide with a large big toe joint, a very narrow heel, and a medium instep. "My toes are long, so it's not ideal!" She uses lamb's wool as padding. She wraps it in a cut-off to a piece from a pair of tights. "I like this because I can wrap the amount of wool I need where I need it, and there are no seams that could dig in as there are in some toe pads."

Katie wears her new shoes around the house with socks over the top. Once they get warm, she takes them off and bends the heel of the shoe against the floor to the point where it would reach the end of her heel, then works on the demi-pointe area. She generally uses one pair every two or three months. She uses calamine lotion to Pan-Cake her shoes, especially before exams and shows. She does not use elastics, only ribbons. "I now sew one whole length of ribbon underneath the instep and up the sides, so that the ribbons do not come off or tear, and it also gives more support where it is needed."

Here is the exercise she practices to strengthen her instep: "Without shoes, spreading all ten toes along the floor, I try to lift my instep from underneath while relaxing the tendon at the front of my heel." She does not use any trick to make her arch look better. "I think it is important to make sure the shank of the shoe breaks at just the right point, so that it fits snuggly against the instep and creates the best support and line as possible, and the shank has complete contact with the whole foot when on pointe."

As warm-up exercise, she practices prances or jogging through the feet to help warm up the shoes and feet without putting pressure on pointe.

If she gets a blister, she pops it immediately and let it dry out. "If I leave them, they just get bigger!"

Her advice for beginners? "Make sure you get the shoes fitted by an expert. Try on as many brands and sizes as you need to, and do not feel pressured to make a quick decision. Once you have the perfect pair, be sure to break them in the right places according to the shape of your foot, and do not just bend them in the middle."

Personal suggestions: "Practice little and often to build up maximum strength . . . I didn't and wish I had!"

Heidi Landford
Australia
Semi-finalist, Genée Competition Singapore 2009

Heidi wears Bloch Heritage, size 4 1/2, width XXX. Her foot is broad with short, even toes and very high arches. Her favorite type of pad is Bunheads Ouch Pouches. In order to better support her arches, she sews the ribbons farther forward than usual, and she doubles the ribbon over to give it a stronger base before she stitches it on. She uses about three pairs of shoes per month and usually breaks them in by doing basic exercises like échappés and rises. If she gets a blister, she uses Second Skin, which doesn't let her feel the pain through. She likes her shoes to be shiny, so no Pan-Cake for performances, and she darns them using the technique called blanket stitch.

Heidi advises students to "get alignment correct from the very first time you go on pointe, and you will have minimal troubles!" She also thinks that the best thing for strengthening feet is to do normal class in pointe shoes.

Kirsten Wicklund
Dancer, Washington Ballet Studio Company

How old were you when you started pointe?

I believe I started pointe at about age thirteen. Though I did start ballet extremely late compared to most dancers, I'm still glad I didn't begin pointe sooner. There should be no rush to begin pointe, because a basic foundation of strong technique is required in order to work properly so as not to injure ourselves.

What pointe shoes do you wear?

I have worn many types and styles of pointe shoes, ranging from Bloch Aspirations and Alphas to Freed Mapleleaf. I have been wearing Suffolk Solos now for quite some time, and I am fairly pleased with them. I wear a 6.5 XX. I think it is very important for young dancers to experiment with many types of shoes. There are so many details that can vary from shoe to shoe and brand, that it doesn't hurt to try many and find out which is right for the individual, based on fit, feel, and look of the shoe.

What type of foot do you have?

I have a wide foot with fairly square-shaped toes. Generally fits into the Egyptian foot category.

How do you soften your pointe shoes?

I often step on the box of my pointe shoes just to initiate the process of molding them to my feet. I don't do much else, so that I can avoid them dying too fast. In fact, I often put extreme hard and strong glue inside the box of the shoe, and also on the shank in the attempt to prolong their life.

How do you make your pointe shoes less noisy?

I work in them, dancing in a somewhat loud hard shoe at first. It is probably the only way for them to break in perfectly. Doing pointe exercises in them helps break them down, and once my shoes have been broken in properly, they usually don't make much noise anymore. That's when they are ready for the stage, in my opinion!

How many pairs do you use weekly or monthly?

Depending on my schedule, I go through two or three pairs a week. In some rehearsals, they are done by the end of it! I usually find a way to salvage one last wear out of them in these cases by either gluing them where they are too soft or using them in a different rehearsal where super-soft shoes are necessary.

Do you Pan-Cake your shoes for shows? What do you use?

I don't, unless I'm required to. I have used face powder, calamine lotion (which I don't really recommend), or just rubbing crushed rosin all over them. This will tend to dull the shine, causing a less noticeable change in color, for a more subtle effect, while still removing the shiny look the pointe shoe originally has.

How do you sew your elastics and ribbons?

I sew ribbons on an angle on each side. I sew two elastics crisscrossing with one end of each at the very back of the heel, and the other end directly on top of the ribbon sewn. This way that part of the elastic is hidden underneath the ribbons once the shoe is on, so that it isn't all visible and distracting to the audience. I make sure they are all sewn around the top of the shoe (the drawstring) so that the shoe is pulled right to my foot, but I can still utilize the drawstring.

Is there any exercise you practice to strengthen your instep?

Many! Any sort of relevé exercise will benefit you if done repetitively. Quick relevés and roll down slowly through the feet, pressing strong into the floor, is great to strengthen; also doing it on one leg is challenging. Doing work with Thera-Bands is also beneficial. Though you aren't in pointe shoes, you will see the difference from the added resistance!

Do you use any tricks to make your arch look better?

I stretch my feet all the time! Get a friend to help, or use underneath furniture, but remember not to sickle! Working on barre basics on pointe shoes and only thinking about pointing your feet as hard as you can will help a lot too!

Can you suggest a warm-up exercise at the barre or in the center?

A great warm-up exercise for pointe that will also help strengthen your feet is to press up to pointe in first position and roll just off your pointe to a high demi-pointe (almost three-quarter pointe!) and then quickly press back to pointe. Roll off pointe with resistance and push to pointe strong and sharp. Do a few slow and then a series quickly before resisting, involving as many as 64 times, alternating slow and fast before coming down. Repeat it as many times as you can to strengthen your pointe work, and it will heat your entire body fast, especially the toes and ankles.

Do you always use the same brand and type of shoes, or do you change?

I like to find a shoe I'm confident in and can trust, but in all honesty, I still play around and try out different brands, styles, and fits!

Do you use any padding?

I use toe pads that aren't too thick so I can still feel my shoe and the floor, but so I don't get too much rubbing of a new shoe against my foot!

What do you do if you get a blister before a show?

Oh, that's bad news! There is a special type of numbing cream I use that you can buy in drugstores and which you can put on about twenty minutes before you go onstage. It might become a much worse blister afterwards, I'll admit; but for the performance, I guarantee it won't hinder your dancing . . . you won't even feel it!

Any advice you would give to beginners?

Work in your basics first. No one expects you to be able to do everything on pointe right away, so master what you can, and be patient with yourself! Never give up on the process, and don't be afraid of it.

Liana Vasconcelos
Dancer, Youth Ballet Company of Rio de Janeiro, Brazil

Liana trained with Ana Elizabeth Alexandre and Maria Angélica Fiorani. The directors are Mariza Estrella and Dalal Achcar.

What pointe shoes do you use?

I use Brazilian-made pointe shoes from So Dança. "The name is Anne, the number is 4 1/2, and the width is B (medium), and they are very hard.

Are your shoes custom-made?

Yes. I always ask So Dança to make them as hard as possible. Because I think this is important in order to work my feet. I have never met my cobbler, though!

How many pairs of shoes does the company allow each month?

As I'm in a youth company, we are just allowed to have one pair of shoes per month.

What type of foot do you have?

My feet are a little bit compressible with a medium arch.

Do you wear any type of padding?

Yes. I use silicone pads.

How do you sew your ribbons and elastics?

I usually sew them with a machine, but sometimes I do it by hand. I use elastic around my ankle, finishing at the shoe's heel, and I tie the ribbons traditionally, with a knot in the inside part of my ankle.

What do you do to make your shoes last longer?

I usually use glue in the sole, to make it last longer.

Do you wear your shoes interchangeably or always on the same foot?

Always on the same foot.

What technique do you use to break in your shoes? How many pairs do you average use in a month?

I always do some exercises at the barre with the new shoes, before starting to rehearse in them. I usually use four pairs of pointe shoes in a month.

How do you protect your toes from blisters, and what do you do if you get a blister the day before a performance?

The silicone pad protects my toes. If I get a blister before a performance, first I put my toes in warm water with salt, and then I put some medicine to scar the blister. When I dance, I protect the blister with cotton and plaster. I also always cut my nails in a squared form, but not so pointed.

Do you Pan-Cake your shoes for performance? What product do you use?

Sometimes yes, but I just use some powder to take off the shine.

Do you darn your shoes?

No, I don't like to darn them.

How do you clean your pointe shoes?

I use a little sponge with water and neuter soap, and then I let them dry in the sun.

Do you have any secret tip for pointe students?

When I have free time during the rehearsals, I'm always trying to balance on one foot (in arabesque, attitude, or passé). It will make it easier, when I am onstage, to get the balance position faster and easier in a variation or pas de deux.

Could you describe at least one exercise at the barre or in the center to help strengthen the feet?

With both feet in sixth position, cross the right leg onto the left leg, putting your right foot on pointe on the side of your left foot, and you do plié with both of your legs. You will feel that this exercise helps you to stretch your instep.

What type of accessories do you use?

I usually don't use any accessories.

What do you do to make your arch look better?

I use a chinerina, or foot stretcher, which is a piece of wood with a strong elastic strap at the top. With this I force my arch every day.

Give your own advice for beginner students.

Don't give up with your first pains and blisters. You will see that year after year, your pointe work will improve, and your performance onstage will become better and better. The secret is, work hard every day!

Sarah Lamkin
Full-time Student, Prudence Bowen Atelier
320 Chesterfield Drive
Mudgeeraba, Goldcoast, Australia

Sarah currently wears Bloch European Balance, size 6 1/2, 2 X.

Bloch describes this shoe as "the pointe shoe that makes the dancer feel like they should stay on pointe all day."

Sarah admits she wasn't gifted with naturally beautiful ballet feet and recently found that Bloch European Balance were the shoes for her narrow, quite small feet.

Do you wear any type of padding, and if yes, which one?

The type of pointe shoe I wear already has a tiny foam piece at the tip . . . , but I also wear Pro Pads as well.

How do you sew your ribbons and elastics?

I sew one loop of elastic around my ankle, and then I fold the ribbon and place it on the inside of my shoe. Then do a stitch around the edge of the ribbon. I sew the ribbons nearer the middle of the shoe, so when I tie them, my arch will be pulled up. I tie my shoes on by wrapping the inside ribbon around my ankle, then the other ribbon, till they meet on my inner anklebone. I tie a tight knot and tuck it underneath my ribbons so that it is not visible.

What technique do you use to break in your shoes? How many pointe shoes do you average use in a month?

When I first put my pointe shoes on, I like to usually go through my feet in the shoes and then face the barre in second position and point one foot and bend over that shoe. I repeat in fourth position, then on the other side. I usually go through three to four pairs of shoes a month.

How do you protect your toes from blisters?

I use closely knitted strapping tape to cover my toes and calluses, and if I get a blister before performing, I use extra tape and blister covers to sponge up the blister so I cannot feel it onstage.

What alterations do you do to your shoe?

I do minor changes to my shoes, only cut the material off the top of the toecap once it starts to fray.

Do you Pan-Cake your shoes for performance? What product do you use?

I sometimes use calamine lotion on my shoes for a nicer, neater look. It changes the color of the shoe and still keeps it the same shape.

Do you darn your shoes?

No, I don't.

How do you clean your pointe shoes?

If they are very dirty and I need them still, I usually repaint them with calamine, then they look nice and clean.

Do you have any secret tip for pointe students?

At first pointe will feel very hard, but keep plodding on because it becomes a lot more natural ad easier.

Could you describe at least one exercise at the barre or in the center to help strengthen the feet?

Relevés on one foot at the barre is always very strengthening. Try a few in the beginning, and eventually you'll be strong enough to be able to do 32.

What type of accessories do you use?

I occasionally use a toe separator between my last two toes because sometimes they rub.

Myriam Ernest
Senior Trainee
School of the Grand Rapids Ballet Company
Grand Rapids, Michigan

Myriam was just turning twelve when she started pointe. She currently wears Russian Pointe Saphir, hard shank, width 6, vamp 2, length 38, with elastic drawstring. She describes her shoe as prearched, "which makes it very easy to dance in." She affirms she has been going through many brands of pointe shoes and found the Jewels Collection started by Russian Pointe really exceptional.

Myriam's foot is extremely arched and flexible. "This has been a blessing and a curse."

In order to soften her shoes, she uses rubbing alcohol and/or water. "If necessary, I bang my shoes against cement to get the sound out."

She generally uses two pairs of shoes per week. Whenever she is required to Pan-Cake her shoes, she uses Max Factor's foundation. Myriam uses Bunhead's Super Spacers for her bunions and Ouch Pouches as pads. If necessary, she also adds small amounts of lamb's wool.

She uses Bloch Elastorib ribbons to help prevent tendonitis. She prefers it because it's wide and supportive. "After burning the ends to prevent fraying, I sew them using a whipstitch and then a blanket stitch at the top." She also crisscrosses her elastics for extra support.

She frequently uses Thera-Bands to strengthen her feet. She also performs toe crunches with a towel to strengthen her arch and relevés on a stair to improve her control and strength. "I make sure to go faster up on the relevé, then slowly down to increase strength.

No trick to show better arches: Myriam prefers focusing on strengthening rather than stretching her feet.

Before class, she combines basic Pilates and breathing exercises with crunches to warm up. Then she stretches out as many areas of her body as she has time for. She finds a foam roller and a tennis ball useful in massaging tight muscles.

Whenever her feet are swollen or she cannot find Saphir, she wears Russian Pointe Almaz, also from the Jewels Collection.

If she gets a blister before a shoe, she sanitizes it with hydrogen peroxide. Then she applies Second Skin on the blister and secures it with duct tape. "This makes the pain go away, even for the most painful blisters. In addition, I sprinkle baby powder in the shoe to soak up excess moisture."

Her advice for beginners? "Pointe is difficult but fun. Make sure to work efficiently in flat shoes to build the strength and good habits for pointe work. Do strengthening exercises on your own to prevent injury and speed [up] progress."

Josephine Cheung
Jean M. Wong School of Ballet (1997-2010)

Josephine has just been accepted for a three-year full-time course at the Bolshoi Ballet Academy in Moscow, Russia.

What pointe shoes do you use?

I am now wearing Freed Classic Pro 5 1/2 XXX by maker Q, and Gaynor Minden 8.5 Med 4 Box Supple. I am planning to try Grishko Elite.

Are your shoes custom-made?

I request the Freed to be made by maker Q.

What type of foot do you have?

Compressible foot with medium arch.

Do you wear any type of padding?

Yes, I wear Ouch Pouches.

How do you sew your ribbons and elastics? How do you tie them on?

I sew ribbons on like a box and a cross in the middle, and just a line through for elastic. I tie the ribbons with the inside one first wrapped around, then the outside one, and tie a double knot, and of course tuck them in.

What do you do to make your shoes last longer?

I Jet-Glue them before I start wearing them, and let them blow dry every time I wear them.

Do you wear your shoes interchangeably or always on the same foot?

Always on the same foot.

What technique do you use to break in your shoes? How many pairs do you average use in a month?

I just break my shoes with my feet. I work in them. I use two to three pairs of shoes a month.

How do you protect your toes from blisters, and what do you do if you get a blister the day before a performance?

I am very lucky. I never got blisters till now.

What alterations do you do to your shoe?

I scratch the sole to make it less slippery and easier to balance on flat, and I also scratch the platform so it's less slippery.

Do you Pan-Cake your shoes for performance?

No.

Do you darn your shoes? If yes, can you describe the technique used?

No, it takes too long.

How do you clean your pointe shoes?

I rub them with a rubber.

Do you have any secret tip for pointe students?

Don't be afraid, and trust that you can do it.

Could you describe at least one exercise to help strengthen the feet?

Using Thera-Bands and doing slow rises on one leg at the barre.

What type of accessories do you use?

I don't use any.

What do you do to make your arch look better?

Always try to push more every time, and find my perfect shoes.

Which is your advice for beginner students?

Don't give up when hard times come, because one day it'll be over, and the joy will come. The only way to do it is to do it.

—Merce Cunningham

Part XI

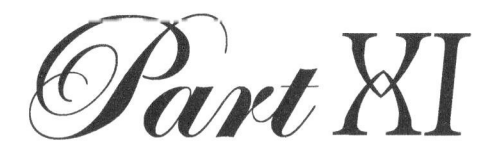

ALL THE SECRETS REVEALED BY THE EXPERTS

Chapter 1

Interviews with Thirteen Ballet Masters

Cem Catbas – Owner of Baltimore Ballet School (Baltimore, USA)
Mara Fusco – Ballet Master/Choreographer – Founder of Il Lyceum di Mara Fusco (Naples, Italy)
Dianne Cheesman – Ballet Teacher/Lecturer, University of Cape Town (South Africa)
Danna Parker – Teacher at Ballet Arizona (Phoenix, Arizona, USA)
Amelia Wander-Vancliffen – Founder of the Vancliffen Arts Foundation (Ontario, Canada)
Luisa Signorelli – Ballet Teacher/Choreographer, Artistic Director of Compagnia Ballet-ex (Rome, Italy)
Kat Wildish – Master Teacher at the Ailey Extension (New York, USA)
Anya Evans – Ballet Teacher at English National Ballet (London)
Ugo Ranieri – Maître de Ballet, Teatro di San Carlo (Naples, Italy)
Jean-Claude Giorgini – Maître de Ballet, Ex-Principal Dancer, Examiner for the French Diploma in Ballet Teaching (Puylaurens, France)
Joanne Morscher – Founder of the Royal School of Ballet (Rocky River, Ohio, USA)
Tanya Pearson – Master Teacher, Founder of the Classical Coaching Academy (St. Leonards, Australia)
Susan Jones - Ballet Master, American Ballet Theatre

Cem Catbas
Owner, Baltimore Ballet School
Cofounder, Baltimore Ballet Company

Cem Catbas's students, who are at least nine to ten years old and who have attended ballet classes at his studio for at least a couple of years, are allowed and encouraged to take pointe classes. They also have to commit to at least three ballet technique classes a week. Cem does not recommend any particular brand of shoe. "Today almost any shoe company makes every possible shape and size," he says. He believes that the shoe that fits is the shoe they have to buy, but he never sends his students to places where they don't have professional fitters.

He thinks dancers should avoid gel pads. "Taping each toe with special toe tape helps a lot, but protecting their toes is their own responsibility."

For beginners, his advice is to get a wider box that "will make it easier to go up and stay up."

He believes that the most important thing is that the shoe fits, but because of their age, the foot will change rapidly, and they will go for different shoes.

According to Catbas, there are two places where the shoe should break: below the toes (for a correct relevé) and underneath the hill. "A beginner should focus on going up on her toes. Breaking the shoe should not be the main concern." He likes for his students to wear ribbons also on their technique shoes. And as an introductory class for pointe, he has the younger ones watch the older girls' pointe class, "to learn different behaviors and preparations as an introductory class."

For the first few months, he avoids exercises in the center but would encourage them to walk in their pointe shoes.

Here is an exercise he uses to strengthen their feet and improve their arch:

"On the floor, sitting in neutral sixth position, knees pulled up, with the hands behind the back, slowly roll up to pointe while distributing the weight gradually forward. The boxes should be perfectly on the floor, and the feet should be the mirror image of each other. Then roll down and repeat it." His personal advice is to do a lot of roll-up exercises to gain strength and learn how to go up on the leg properly. "Hold your upper body constantly and do not drop it when you plié.

Mara Fusco
Ballet Master/Choreographer/Artistic Director
Il Balletto di Napoli and Il Lyceum di Mara Fusco
Naples, Italy

Mara Fusco is an internationally acclaimed ballet teacher. She studied at the Rambert School of Ballet in London and graduated from the Agrippina Vaganova School in St. Petersburg. She is the director and founder of Il Lyceum di Mara Fusco and the artistic director of Il Balletto di Napoli, in Naples, Italy.

It was a pleasure interviewing Mara, whom I had the chance to have as a teacher when I was younger.

What is the age range for going on pointe in your school?

Students start professional classes at nine years old. The class introduces all the principal elements of classical dance beginning with facing the barre (plié, tendu, rond de jambe á terre, frappés, petit adagio, grand battement) and then the same will be studied in the center, approaching the study of all the elementary jumps (temps levé, échappé, assemblé).

Only later, it will be much easier to approach and start pointe work. For this reason, we start pointe work after the first year (elementary class) because we think that children with Latin-structured bodies are able to cope with such a difficult strain from ten or eleven years old, when the body is stronger and when they can surmount the difficulties.

Do you have a special brand of shoes you prefer for your students?

For beginner pupils, it is generally better to use softer shoes, which give them the possibility to go up and down easier, so that they can improve their technique.

For beginners I prefer the Italian shoes Porselli. I don't like the Chinese ones, which are too strong and don't have a nice line. For upper classes, the best shoes are English—Freed or Bloch.

Do you allow your students to use toe pads, and if yes, what type do you think is the best?

In Italy we use something named panno ballerina ("ballerina cloth"), which is a special tissue used generally for cleaning and which has an absorbent characteristic, we think, that is better than the ones which are on the market.

What type of shank, block, and vamp do you prefer for beginners?

If the pupils have big arches, which means for us a very weak type of foot, it's better to use shoes with a vamp providing a strong support, in order to help them.

In other cases, if the pupils have strong arches, which means for us a very strong foot, they can use normal shoes without support.

How do you teach students to break their new pointe shoes in? Do you hold a special introductory pointe class before they start pointe work?

Before teaching how to start pointe work, I generally show my students how to break their new pointe shoes in. When they spring on pointe, I explain that the weight must not be exclusively on the big toe but on the upper part of the foot (ankle), able to execute the movements carefully with completely stretched knees. In the beginning, they spring on pointe from a parallel position, without the feet being turned out.

Do you have special guidelines for students to sew and tie their ribbons? How do you want the elastics to be sewn?

The ribbons must be crossed in the center of the shoe, in such a way that they follow the shape of the foot. The ribbons have to be sewed in the center of the shoe, so that when they are tied, the shoes will adhere to the feet as much as possible. I think it's better to sew the elastic behind the shoe (at the heel), to be sure that the heels will not slip down.

Could you give a sample of a first class on pointe?

The three fundamental exercises of a first class on pointe are all executed facing the barre:

A. Relevés in first, second, and fifth positions. Time 4/4,
   Starting from first position: Demi-plié, spring on pointe with both feet (relevé), lower down the heels in demi-plié, stretch the knees. Repeat 3 times in each position with both right and left foot in front.
B. Assemblé soutenu. Right foot back.
   Fondu on the left leg sliding the right one, to pointe tendue, to second position, then draw up on pointe, closing in fifth position with the right foot in front.

Lower down the heels in demi-plié, stretch the knees.
Repeat the step 4 times going forward (changing legs) and 4 times going backward.
C. Sissonne ordinaire on pointe. Right foot front.
Demi-plié, spring on pointe of left foot and simultaneously lift sur le cou-de-pied devant the right foot. Lower both heels down in demi-plié, stretch the knees.
Repeat 4 times with the working foot devant and 4 times with the working foot derrière.
Repeat on the left side.

What barre exercises do you advise for the first months on pointe? Can you describe?

After three months from the beginning of pointe work, we usually repeat the exercises already described in the center, and we continue to teach new steps facing the barre.

A. Sissonne passée on pointe. Time 4/4.
Right leg front. Starting from a demi-plié in fifth position, spring on pointe with the left leg, simultaneously lifting the right leg in front of the left knee in the relevé devant position. Close fifth and lower down with demi plié. Repeat 4 times then close back.
B. Pas de bourrée (facing the barre). Time 2/4.
Start right foot back. Demi-plié sliding the right foot with toe pointing on the floor to second position. Draw the right leg back to the left leg and simultaneously spring on pointe and, lifting left leg, sur le cou-de-pied devant. Step to left pointe, straightening the knees, and lift the right sur le cou-de-pied devant.
Close in fifth position with both feet in demi-plié.
Repeat all on the left side.

When the pupils are able to perform these exercises correctly, we repeat them in the center.

Is there a particular exercise you teach your dancers in order to improve their arch?

I generally have them do a grand plié in first or in second position on pointe facing the barre, so that the arch is pushing out and then, when they have stretched the knees, encourage them to keep the arch out in the same way as in grand plié.

I usually go very carefully because sometimes there are pupils who can have problems in the Achilles tendon.

What's your personal advice for beginners?

Pointe work is a very important moment for female technique in classical ballet. It's necessary to hold a special introductory pointe class before the start of this work, but what is fundamental is the attention that the teacher must give to musical timing before starting to teach and choose very carefully the type of music for each different step.

At first the exercises must be studied facing the barre with both hands lightly on it. If the exercises are correctly approached, they develop the student gradually, giving her the ability to achieve a balanced control of her movements. At the beginning they must execute each step separately so that the student will feel sure she is not making mistakes. The pupil must be taught to stand correctly, and the placement of the torso over the legs is of great importance. The pelvis must be centered not tipped forward or backward. The abdomen should be slightly drawn in and the diaphragm raised; the shoulders dropped naturally; the head held straight; and the arms, when the student is in the center, held slightly rounded from the shoulder to the fingers.

As the students gain strength, they can try to do all the exercises in the center. In this way, they will feel the difference of balance and will learn to perform all the movements of ballet, from adagio to jumps, and from allegro to pointe work.

Dianne Cheesman
Teacher/Lecturer
University of Cape Town (Africa)

A teacher for over thirty-five years, Dianne was trained in Johannesburg, South Africa, with Majorie Sturman.

How do you assess the ability of a student to start pointe work? What is the age range for going on pointe in your studio?

A dancer should have strong core/posture, secure turnout and weight placement, strong ankles and feet, and have been training for a number of years. The average age is eleven to twelve years, depending on ability, strength of ankles, commitment.

Do you have a special brand of shoes you prefer for your students?

Not any particular brand. Personally, when I danced, I preferred Eva. Many use Gaynor Minden, although I find these not really suitable for beginners. Bloch is good, yet not easily accessible in South Africa. Sansha is another popular brand. Beginners' shoes should be more flexible to enable the dancer to get up and also allow their feet to strengthen.

Do you allow your students to use toe pads, and if yes, what type do you think is the best?

Yes, they can. Not any particular brand, but I do feel that they should be light and not take up too much space in the shoe! Also, they should allow the dancer to feel the floor.

What type of shank, block, and vamp do you want for beginners?

Again this would depend largely on the shape of the dancer's foot.

How do you teach students to break their new pointe shoes in?

Walk in them!

Do you hold a special "introductory" pointe class before they start pointe work?

This has varied over the years. I have had pointe specialists come in and talk to dancers. I have chatted to them before they buy their shoes. I do a lot of demi-pointe exercises leading up to the pointe class and strengthen[ing] exercise classes using Thera-Bands.

Do you prefer soft or hard shanks for beginners?

I prefer soft rather than hard! So they are comfortable and also can feel the toes and work their feet better.

Do you have special guidelines for the students to sew their ribbons? How do you want them to tie their ribbons?

The old fashioned way: at an angle in line with the seam of the shoe. They should tie the inside ribbon first, and then the outside one, and knot them on the inside of the foot, above the ankle.

How do you want the elastics to be sewn? Do you think they should always wear elastics, or only if needed?

Only if needed, sewed at the back, not across the front of [the] ankle. Very high insteps may need an elastic in front of [the] metatarsals.

What is your first pointe class like?

As I said previously, many various classes building up to pointe. Beginners' pointe day:
- Just stepping up onto pointe
- Walking on pointe
- Most exercises only on two feet (I would spend 10-15 minutes only)

What barre exercises do you advise for the first two to three months on pointe? Can you describe two barre and two center exercises?

Just exercises on two feet. Rises, relevés, échappés.
- Facing the barre: Feet parallel, step up onto pointe with right foot, join left foot, lower through feet. Repeat 4 times.
- Fifth position facing barre: 3 relevés, dégagé to second, and repeat with other foot in front.
- Centre: Repeat second barre exercise in the center.
- Three échappés relevés changing feet, one relevé fifth.
- Could you briefly describe two barre and two center exercises for a second-year pointe class?

- Fifth facing barre: Relevé in fifth, lift right foot to retiré devant, lower to fifth on pointe, plié, repeat using back foot, posé de coté foot devant, posé de coté derrière fondu pas de bourrée piqué dessous, relevé fifth.
- Sideways: Échappé fourth/second, changing feet fourth/second/posé en avant 3 times, plié demi detourné, and repeat on other side.

Is there a particular exercise you teach your dancers in order to improve their arch?

We use Thera-Bands, invert feet V (toes in), and raise the instep without lifting the toes off the floor so that you lift the instep. It also helps students rolling ankles.

Which is your personal advice for beginners?

Harden the skin of the toes before commencing with pointe work. Go slow and carefully, and make sure shoes are fitted correctly, and enjoy!

Danna Parker
Artistic Director
Terpsicore Dance Company
PO Box 5202
Scottsdale, Arizona 85261
Teacher at Ballet Arizona (Phoenix)

What pointe shoes do you use?

I use Grishko 2007, size 4.5, width XXX, medium shank.

What type of foot do you have?

I have a wide foot, the Greek type, with a high arch and a longer second toe.

Do you wear any type of padding, and if yes, which one?

I wear lamb's wool pads.

How do you sew your ribbons and elastics? How do you tie them on?

I designate my shoes to a specific foot. I sew my ribbons so one sits at the arch and the outside ribbon sits just a bit higher up on the shoe. Both are slightly angled upward. I tie them with the arch ribbon around first. Then I follow up with the outside ribbon. I tie them in a knot at the inside of the ankle, then tuck the ribbons under.

What do you do to make your shoes last longer?

Usually nothing, but if I'm desperate, I'll get a thick shellac (it works like a hard glue) and put that on the inside of the shoe and around the upper part of the box on the outside.

Do you wear your shoes interchangeably or always on the same foot?

Always on the same foot.

What technique do you use to break in your shoes? How many pointe shoes do you use in average in a month?

I let my shoes break in naturally. The 2007 has a three-quarter shank already, and I like a stiff box, so I don't like to break them in that much! I'll bend the shank a little, but not much. When I was performing more, I would use about two to three pairs a month.

How do you protect your toes from blisters?

I use a gauze tape that sticks to itself, but not my skin. If I have a blister before a performance, I'll usually use a Band-Aid.

What alterations do you do to your shoe?

I will cut the satin off of the toe area.

Do you Pan-Cake your shoes for performance? What product do you use?

Not usually, but if I need to, I use calamine lotion.

Do you darn your shoes?

No, I don't.

How do you clean your pointe shoes?

Usually I don't! Maybe I should start?

Do you have any secret tip for pointe students?

Well, it's not really a secret, but I think it's so important to stay healthy and eat right! Listen to your instructor regarding your shoes and whether or not you need to change them or get new ones. If you're not able to get "up" on your pointe, you need to reevaluate your shoe or strengthen your feet further.

Could you describe at least one exercise at the barre or in the center to help strengthen the feet?

I'm a true believer in slow élevés (rises) at the barre from first position. Not relevés, only élevés. I also really like relevés on one foot with the other in coupé derrière.

What type of accessories do you use?

None. Just my pads and gauze tape.

What do you do to make your arch look better?

Nothing usually.

What is your advice to beginner students?

I feel it's most important to have a proper-fitted shoe. Don't trust that the first shoe you try on is the right one. Make sure you try on several pairs, and be sure you go to someone who is experienced at fitting. Don't trust the salesperson at your local dancewear shop. Chances are they don't know how to properly fit a shoe. Also, it's OK for a pointe shoe to be comfortable! They don't all have to be painful. There is a brand out there that will fit your foot and allow you to pay attention to technique and not pain.

Amelia Wander Vancliffen
Vancliffen Arts Foundation
Malton, Ontario, Canada

How do you assess the ability of a student to start pointe work?

First and foremost is the physical and technical preparation of the child. Today too many teachers are basing themselves on age, years of study, if the child has a pretty foot or not, and on a syllabus that says that at this stage the child should be on pointe. The ability to dance on pointe is the physical capacity of the entire body; therefore, we should look for proper placement and alignment of the entire body, the stability of the foot on the floor, no ankle pronation or sickling and proper distribution of the weight on the entire foot in quarter-, half-, and three-quarter pointe. How the child points the foot, if she breaks at the metatarsal and shortens the toes, or if she lengthens the toes in order that she doesn't buckle in the pointe shoe.

A strong back is necessary. If the child presents a swayback, she will have weak abdominals. The student must be high on her hips in the relevé position, her knees must not be bent, her thighs must be pulled up with the leg elongated and not stiff, and the inner thigh (the two points close to the groin) strong as though they want to meet. There should be no big bulging of the thigh or sinking into the demi-pointe or, in the future, into the pointe. Besides the total physical strength, the preparation given to the child from the earliest lessons is very important. Even the most "ideal ballet body" must be trained, and there are no shortcuts. Unfortunately, it seems common today—those children with very little study on demi-pointe are put on pointe. This, in my humble opinion, is totally wrong.

Much more time must be spent on working with two hands at the barre and work on demi-pointe before attempting pointe. In North America the training is being rushed, and we are destroying the future dancer. The rate of accidents, tendinitis, hip and knee problems has risen because the technical demands are greater. At a younger age, the students are not properly physically or technically prepared for these demands. Every student has the right to be and remain healthy. Everything the dancer does or is not able to do depends on the earliest training. This is why I personally put a great emphasis on what I call the pre-ballet training. In this very early stage, we have the capacity of not only setting the fundamental building blocks of the work that will come once they are at the barre, but we have the possibility of changing and developing what could be lacking in that child's body, like rotation of the hip or flexibility. Even the child with a more rigid foot can be taught how to stretch the foot, with proper exercises aimed to improve the physical aspects.

By doing so and studying a minimum of 3 times a week, I would say by age twelve, a student who has been conscientiously trained is ready for pointe. By age twelve the bones in the foot have reached a point of development that the joints are stronger and able to support the weight of the body. Weight is another factor. Children with a weight problem should not be put on pointe as those children who study once a week. It is impossible for them to receive the proper formation and build the required strength.

Do you have a special brand of shoes you prefer for your students?

There are numerous brands of pointe shoes. This can be very positive, as well as confusing. They all advertise that there is a shoe for every type of foot, and that they outlast the other.

I don't believe there is any one shoe better than another, but it's the student and the teacher—especially in the beginning—that will find a shoe or style that is better suited. I personally feel that when the big moment arrives, the teacher should accompany the student to be properly fitted with a customized shoe and not a commercial one. Every student's foot presents itself differently. Even one foot can be different from the other, and each child has needs. Commercial shoes may not meet those needs.

Today the Gaynor Minden is a very popular shoe used by professionals and students alike. I discourage students from using this shoe (especially in the beginning) because students without proper training or preparation can easily relevé on them. Although these shoes are very well made, we are encouraging defects and putting a strain on the child's body.

Gaynor Minden is better for advanced students or professionals.

Fittings can be tricky. First there should be a preparation, toenails trimmed properly; the child should bring her tights, since heavy socks or nylons can result in an improper fitting. It is important to know the exact street shoe size as every brand fits a bit differently from another. Normally, at the store there is a measuring stick.

Don't be in a rush, and don't take the first pair that you're fitted with. The foot will be changing continuously, so it is also well that every time the child needs a new pair there is someone who is an expert to fit them. Moms should keep a pointe shoe diary and keep track of the type of shoe that their daughters were fitted for and, as changes come about, keep it a record. It is easier in the long run.

First of all, the fitter should see the child's bare foot in order to establish toe length, if the first three toes are equal, or if the big toe is much longer, etc. Normally the beginner shoe should be lightweight, but not too light, and should adhere well to the foot. To establish this, I tell them to do a deep demi-plié on one foot to make sure that the heel doesn't slip down. If they have trouble keeping the heel down on the floor, it means they need another heel cut, or the shoe is too small.

Pointe shoes should not have gaps on the sides with or without drawstrings. In reality a pointe shoe, if it is well fitted, should not need anything but the ribbons. This is why I feel it is necessary to use, especially in the beginning, a customized shoe. Once that is done, the child should go up on them. If they feel pain on the sides or a discomfort on pointe as though their big toe is coming through the shoe, it's time to start again. Pointe shoes should fit like a glove and be comfortable. You should not feel like your foot is in a vise.

Do you allow your students to use toe pads, and if yes, what type do you think is the best?

The only type of padding they should use is lambs' wool, and not much, just as a protection. I personally only used lamb's wool if I had a blister. At times when the shoe became too soft, I used little squares of newspaper. Today there are all sorts of paddings, floorings. I think you need to feel the floor. All these special paddings are more for business reasons than for protection and do not give the dancer the sensitivity in the foot they need to feel secure. Today we think more about pads, special tapes for the feet; and the list goes on and on, when we should be thinking of raising the level of training.

What type of shanks, block, and vamp do you want for beginners?

The type of vamp is determined by the length of the toes, long toes, long vamp; and short toes shorter vamp. Either way the vamp must cover the joint of the big toe. If the vamp is too short, there will be problems because the foot will break at the toes or in the metatarsal. Too high will cause the student to fall back and to strain to rise. I personally tend toward a V-shaped vamp, but then again, it depends on the individual. Shanks should be medium, not too hard and not too soft.

If the shanks are too hard, the student will have problems going up, and too soft she will not feel supported. Same goes for the block. Long toes will need a particular block.

How do you teach students to break in their new shoes?

To break in the box, I have them put some rubbing alcohol (not water) on the upper part and sides of the shoe and just leave them on their feet without walking in them in order not to ruin them, just to take the form of their foot. For the shank, I sometimes use my hands to manipulate the shank, or the day before, have them walk in them and do a bit of relevés on demi-pointe.

I am talking about the day before because I always try to meet with them before and sew the ribbons all together. We speak about how to care for the shoes in order to make them last longer, and then I make the traditional pointe shoe hardener, using rosin and alcohol.

Probably a greater occasion for me than it is for them. It gives you so much watching their faces light up, and keeps the scope of your work fresh in your mind and heart. I think that it is important to pass on our knowledge and experience, in order to form a more knowledgeable public and a new generation of ballet dancers.

Do you prefer soft or hard shanks for beginners?

As I stated previously, I believe a medium shank is better for the beginner. Too hard the child is pulled back, too soft not enough support. A dancer's foot needs to be strong and pliable. The old master teachers would say that "your feet must be like a hand." The child needs to be able to articulate the foot.

Do you have special guidelines for the students to sew their ribbons? How do you want them to tie their ribbons?

I have them fold the heel down and draw a diagonal line with a pencil on each side. They then pin the ribbon on the inside of the shoe far down from heel to side, in order that when they tie the ribbons around the ankle, the heel of the shoe gets support. Then I have them sew with heavy cotton the ribbons. Once they arrive to the border, they sew across. In order to hold the sides better with a finer thread and needle, I have them carefully sew the edge of the border to the ribbon, being careful not to sew the drawstring. Today I often notice that the ribbons are sewn only on the edge of the border. This gives less support, and there is a risk, if the thread breaks, that the ribbon will detach from the shoe. While if the ribbon is sewn deeper in the shoe, the shoe adheres better to the foot; and even if the thread breaks before the entire ribbon detaches, the ballet is over. After they have put the shoe on, using both hands so as to make sure that the shoe isn't twisted when it goes on, I have them kneel on one knee, keeping the foot on the floor flat and pressing a bit forward so that in tying the ribbons they will be comfortable and not too tight stopping the circulation. Take the inside ribbon and then cross the outside ribbon over, passing the back of the ankle, bring them around to the front, return back. I have them tie the knot on the outside of the ankle, by the dimple. Why the outside of the ankle? Making sure that the ribbon is as flat as possible, in this manner, when the student presents the foot or is on pointe, the knot is hidden pretty much from public view.

How do you want the elastics to be sewn? Do you think they should always wear elastics, or only if needed?

If a pointe shoe is properly made and fitted, there should be no need for elastics. Assuming that one feels the need for that extra support, it is common knowledge that there are two methods, one is the elastic sewn on the outside of the heel, creating a loop where to pass the ribbons. This is very tricky because the measurement of the elastic must be very accurate in order that the loop is not too small or too short since that could eventually cause tendinitis of the Achilles tendon.

The most commonly used is the elastic across the foot. This has its pros and cons because a child may have to put extra force as the elastic could hold her back. This is more for the dancer who has an overdeveloped arch or very weak ankles. The same care we take in choosing properly fitted shoes for the child who is beginning to walk must, and should, be applied to the child who dances. Pointe shoe makers are not paying enough attention to the true needs of the child. Only now I'm noticing that some brands are beginning to turn their attention to this matter.

Could you give a sample of a first class on pointe?

The first class on pointe is about 15 minutes, at the end of a one-and-a-half-hour class. Tempo 4/4.
First position, two hands on the barre. Right foot: Roll up to demi-pointe, then full-pointe. Demi-pointe close first position. Repeat with left foot.
Battement tendu à la seconde, press over the foot, moving the weight to the working leg. Return to battement tendu à la seconde, close first position demi-plié, straighten. Repeat with right foot last 8 beats. Repeat all on left side.
Relevés in first, second, and fifth positions—tempo 4/4.
Demi-plié, relevé, demi-plié, straighten.
Relevé is done with a slight spring.
Elevé is rolling through the foot to arrive on pointe and coming down.
I normally maintain just this for at least six to eight lessons.
During this period, I may add bourrée suivi, perhaps échappé.
I prefer to work on a strong relevé on two feet. I make sure there is no jiggling.

What barre exercises do you advise for the first two to three months on pointe? Can you describe two barre and two center exercises?

The norm in my classes is that everything that they do at the barre, they will do in the center once there is a certain amount of proficiency.

Could you briefly describe two barre and two center exercises for second-year pointe class?

Exercise 1 – barre: Tempo 3/4. Relevés in first, second, fifth positions. Two hands at the barre.

Preparation. Demi–plié, relevé, demi-plié sur la pointe, straighten, come down, and repeat 3 times. Battement tendu á la seconde, posé, demi-plié in second position and repeat all.

Exercise 2 - barre: Tempo 2/4 (gavotte), 2 beats for every movement. One hand on the barre.

Fifth position, prepare arm to second. Battement tendu quatrième (fourth position) en avant, demi-plié, arm comes down (preparatory position), relevé in fourth position, arm goes up (in third or fifth position according to method), demi-plié in fourth position, arm opens to second position, battement tendu en avant, closing in demi-plié, fifth position arm comes down, échappé á la seconde, arm goes in second position close fifth, arm closes. Repeat all from the back. Arm to second with the battement tendu derriére.

7 battement tendu á la seconde, arm opens in second position demi-plié, arm comes down, relevé, and arm comes up. Demi-plié, arm comes down, battement tendu á la seconde, arm in second position, close fifth position in demi-plié en avant arm comes down, sus-sous come down, arm comes down.

Four échappés close fifth position.

Center. Example of exercises.

Exercise 1 - Assemblé soutenu, tempo 2/4.

Fifth position en face - soutenu á la seconde, sous-sous fifth position, repeat 3 more times. Back leg does sissonne simple or retiré passé closes front, repeat closing back, repeat closing front, sous-sous fifth position. Repeat all.

The combination is also done en arrière; sissonne simple (retiré passé) begins with the front leg going back.

Exercise 2 - Glissades sur la pointe, tempo 4/4 with and without changing of feet.

Is there a particular exercise you teach your dancers in order to improve their arch?

I really don't think there is any exercise to develop a better arch. If the feet are worked properly from the beginning, they will develop and have the proper form. The more rigid foot needs to work the articulation in the ankle and from when they begin doing circles with their ankles en dehors and en dedans, which are very helpful.

Working on the demi-pointe. Proper execution of battement tendus will give agility to the foot.

What is your personal advice for beginners' pointe?

My advice is for the teachers. Remember, there is no such a thing as "born to dance." Behind every professional dancer of the past, present, or in the future, there was and will always be a dedicated teacher who chooses the higher road, the harder one. The road that might not make you popular or wealthy, but I can assure you, it will bring you a great deal of satisfaction. Teaching is as much of an art as dancing itself. It takes a great deal of patience and lots of passion. Never forget the very first moment that you stepped inside your first studio and placed you hands on that barre. It's going to be those sensations that will carry you.

The responsibility of every teacher is bringing every student to the maximum of their ability, and when a child feels cared for, they will go far beyond your expectations.

Don't rush, take time, and care. The holes that you leave in their education will be there forever no matter what. Work on details—that's the difference at times of realizing a dream or not.

To the students, the art of dance is hard. We ask you to make a commitment before you know what you're getting yourself into. Work hard, stay focused, don't look at others—or better, look but don't compare yourself to anyone. You are unique—there is only one of you, and that's truly a wonderful thing. Focus and listen. The best dancers are listeners. Try not to get discouraged. Dance is like anything else. Some people just need more time to get there, but you will get there. Happy dancing!

Luisa Signorelli
Professional Dancer and Ballet Teacher
Artistic Director
Compagnia Ballet-Ex (Rome, Italy)

How do you assess the ability of a student to start pointe work? What is the age range for going on pointe in your studio?

Pointe work should start around age eleven. The student should already have a good basic placement, at least one or two years of serious ballet and well-developed muscles in order to avoid injuries.

What brand of shoes do you prefer for your students? How do you think a beginner's shoe should fit?

Personally I adore Gaynor Minden, but I think these shoes are better for professional dancers. I do not like very hard shoes, where you feel your foot "compressed" and really very heavy. I like Freed a lot.

Do you allow your students to use toe pads?

The toes have to be protected, but without exaggerating. You should always feel the shoe.

How do you teach students to break their new pointe shoes in?

If the student's feet are not strong yet, it is preferable to soften the shoe, better if using the hands, also working once at the barre to allow the shoes to mold to their feet.

Do you hold a special "introductory" pointe class before they start pointe work? How is that class structured?

It is always preferable to explain how to tie the ribbons in order to avoid having the students coming to class with incorrectly tied ribbons, which is very anesthetic. Everything else is said during classes.

Do you prefer soft or hard shanks for beginners?

It is better to use soft shanks in the beginning. Tendonitis can arise when working in hard shoes.

Do you have special guidelines for the students to sew and tie their ribbons?

Yes, I do, of course. It is very important to know how to tie the ribbons and hide the knot afterwards.

How do you want the elastics to be sewn? Do you think they should always wear elastics, or only if needed?

I believe it is better to have elastics in order to secure the shoe to the foot.

Could you give a sample of a first class on pointe?

Facing the barre and feet parallel, rolling up demi-pointe, then pointe, alternating right and left. They can also perform pliés and relevés in parallel position. Repeat also in first position.

What barre exercises do you advise for the first two to three months on pointe? Can you describe two barre and two center exercises?

In the beginning, I teach a lot of exercises to strengthen the instep, then tendus, bringing weight on the pointe and lunging down, forcing the instep. It is important to practice many relevés in first and second position with two hands at the barre. In the center I insist on échappés and relevés in first and second position.

Could you briefly describe two barre and two center exercises for a second year pointe class?

- 2 échappés, relevé passé, relevé in fifth position with two hands at the barre.
- Pas courus (bourrée) with two hands on the barre.

Center work: it is possible to repeat the same exercises, combining them together. Example:

- 2 échappés, relevé passé, relevé in fifth, 2 échappés, pas couru, glissade
- Piqué first arabesque, failli, piqué first arabesque, failli, balancé, balancé, soutenu en tournant and repeat on other side.

Is there a particular exercise you teach your dancers in order to improve their arch?

I have my students execute many battements tendus trying to articulate the foot using their metatarsals.

Can you give your personal advice for beginners' pointe?

Try to build a solid base and learn without rushing and without overworking because it can be harmful. Warm up feet before putting pointe shoes on. Do not wear shoes that are too tight and . . . take class every day!

Kat Wildish
Master Teacher
The Ailey Extension (New York, USA)

Kat has been teaching for thirty-five years and was trained at the School of American Ballet. She actually teaches as a master instructor at the Ailey Extension in New York. Kat teaches classical ballet, pointe, and partnering. She is certified by the American Ballet Theatre. At present she is a master instructor at the Ailey Extension NYC.

How do you assess the ability of a student to start pointe work?

I generally assess it based on how many years they have been dancing and the strength of their foot work.

What is the age range for going on pointe in your studio?

I don't allow students in my class en pointe until at least twelve years old, when the bones have ossified enough as not to deform.

Do you have a special brand of shoes you prefer for your students?

No.

Any brands you dislike?

Not fond of a performance shoe, on beginners—they need more support while training.

How do you think a beginner's shoe should fit?

Snug, allowing the foot to be supported even when flat, just as a professional's shoe should fit . . . snug.

Do you allow your students to use toe pads, and if yes, what type do you think is the best?

Yes. There are many products available now. I personally like the Happy Toes found at Dance Planet in London. They just cover the tips and tops of the toes and are not bulky. For my students I suggest Bunheads professional Ouch Pouches, also not bulky . . . they seem to work till they find something they personally enjoy. The comfort of ballerinas' toes is a very personal feeling, and I allow the dancers the freedom to adjust that comfort level.

What type of shank, block, and vamp do you want for beginners?

Again I leave this up to the professional fitters that we work with in NYC. Each foot has its own individual needs. It's so important to be fitted properly. I like the high vamp for support, but many beginners are not yet strong enough to get up and over a high vamp and need to begin with a lower vamp. Very nice feet need a stronger shank for support. Medium shank is generally good for most beginners.

How do you teach students to break their new pointe shoes in?

A little water across the demi-pointe position helps them to bend enough to roll through. The exercises at the barre include many rolling through the shoe, to assist in soft landing and give more comfort.

Do you hold a special "introductory" pointe class before they start pointe work? How is that class structured?

Ailey has hosted pointe seminars for teachers, as well as Broadway Dance Center in the past, and I train teachers about pre-pointe procedures. Beginners will be asked to take pointe in soft ballet shoes to learn the combinations and feel more confident when actually putting on the shoes. Also, the men are encouraged to participate in soft ballet shoes to improve their feet in specially designed exercises geared to develop their instep.

Do you prefer soft or hard shanks for beginners?

Neither have I felt a medium shank allows for the majority of students to work at the greatest range. If I see they need more or less support, we adjust accordingly on the next pair purchased.

Do you have special guidelines for the students to sew their ribbons?

I prefer the dancers to sew the ribbons deep down into the shoes next to the shank, to hold the entire shoe against their foot, thereby stabilizing the heel. It seems to prevent injuries.

How do you want the elastics to be sewn?

If elastic is needed, it is placed for the circumstance—i.e., if the heels fall off (generally because of a narrow heel), we need to place the elastic in such a way as not to cause a blister on the heel, yet assists in keeping the shoe snugger.

Do you think they should always wear elastics or only if needed?

Only when needed.

Could you give a sample of a first class on pointe?

We mostly work facing the barre.

1. We begin parallel and gently roll one foot to the demi-pointe, then pointe and roll down, then the other foot, then both.
2. We repeat the same exercise in first position.
3. Tendu: lean into the pointe to force the instep—front, side, back.
4. Demi plié and stretch the knees, demi plié, relevé, and lower down slowly.

What barre exercises do you advise for the first two to three months on pointe?

Relevés going quickly up, then slowly rolling down.

Can you describe two barre and two center exercises?

See above for barre. In the center, we always do just walking en pointe parallel forward 8 counts and back 8 counts. Repeat in a turned-out position, forward and back 8 counts each.

Échappé exercise: Échappé fourth devant, close fifth, soutenu en tournant, repeat the échappé and soutenu, then two échappés to second and retiré hold close back.

Could you briefly describe two barre and two center exercises for a second-year pointe class?

Same as above and add glissades at the barre and center.
Example:

1. Facing the barre: tendu devant, plié in fourth, relevé, lower down, tendu close fifth échappé to fourth. Repeat a'la seconde and derrière, then échappé to fourth, to second, devant and retiré.
2. In the center we add piqué passé after practicing at the barre piqué and maybe turns toward the end of the semester.
3. Piqué arabesque, fall backwards to balancé 3 times, then soutenu en tournant.

Is there a particular exercise you teach your dancers in order to improve their arch?

We overcross the foot in parallel coupé and plié deep to stretch. Also done in overcrossed turned-out coupé, devant, or derrière.

What is your personal advice for beginners' pointe?

Don't rush . . . take it slow and easy for safety. Do not practice badly over and over. It is better to do it good. If it really hurts, take your pointe shoes off. There is no use trying to learn in pain. Develop strength in your upper body to hold you up out of the shoes. Be quiet . . . no one likes a loud ballerina.

Anya Evans
Former Dancer with Royal Ballet
Ballet Teacher, English National Ballet

This interview took place at English National Ballet School in London, England, March 2010.

Anya Evans was born in New York City and began her ballet training at the age of four. When her first teacher recognized her talent, she encouraged Anya to pursue her studies in New York City. At the age of thirteen, Anya studied at the Ballet Russe School under Anatole Vilzak and Madame Schollar, and a year later at the School of American Ballet, studying primarily with Andre Eglevsky, Stanley Williams and Pierre Vladimoroff, and Felia Dubrovska.

At sixteen, Anya was offered a scholarship to study under Dame Alicia Markova, who was then director of the Metropolitan Opera Ballet Company, but declined this in favor of becoming an apprentice with the New York City Ballet, dancing, "Snowflake" and "Spanish" in Balanchine's production of The Nutcracker. The following year, Anya became a member of American Ballet Theatre and spent three years with the company dancing throughout the United States as well as a doing a six-week tour in the Soviet Union.

In 1967, Anya stepped out of the corps de ballet to perform her first major role, the "Pas de trois" in David Blair's production of Swan Lake, opening night at Lincoln Center for the Performing Arts. Following the success of this performance, and with David Blair's encouragement, Anya decided to go to London, where she joined London's Festival Ballet as a soloist. After a year in London, she went to Montreal to dance with Les Grandes Ballets Canadiens. In 1969, Anya realized her childhood dream by becoming a member of the Royal Ballet and was honored to be the first dancer to be admitted to the company without training at the Royal Ballet School. In December 1976, Anya danced the major role of "Giselle" for the first time.

In 1980, Anya left the Royal Ballet to freelance and embark on a teaching career, working at all the major ballet schools in London. In 1991, Anya joined the staff of the English National Ballet School, remaining there until 1997. After returning there in 2006 and 2007 as a guest teacher, Anya will now take up a permanent position once again.

How do you assess the ability of a student to start pointe work? What is the age range for going on pointe in your studio?

Personally, I was on pointe at eight, but I was very motivated. I would say probably at age ten or eleven if they are very seriously trained, certainly not if they attend classes only once a week. You have to really look at the student and make sure that they have the strength before you put them on pointe. I don't think you can make a generalization about the age, it is very questionable.

What type of shank do you prefer for beginners?

I prefer hard shanks, in order to develop their feet.

Is there a particular brand of shoes you advise for beginners?

I think that choosing a brand of pointe shoes is a personal choice.

Do you allow your students to use toe pads?

Personally I wouldn't, but I think all the students do.
I think that now it became so acceptable.

Do you hold a special introductory class when you start pointe work?

It is different in this school, because when they get here, they have already been trained. It is different if I was teaching in my own school. I would start with slow rises, and maybe relevés at the barre to begin with. Certainly not coming in the center until they are really strong in their feet and legs, so mostly I would start at the barre and stay at the barre probably six months.

Are you against elastics on pointe shoes?

No, I am not.

Could you give a sample of a first class on pointe?

Slow rises and lots of relevés. I would surely start on two feet to begin with, and then go to one foot. Once they start in the center, they can execute the same slow exercises.

Is there any exercise you teach your students to improve their arch?

No, not really. Lots of tendus.

In the first year at English National Ballet School, how many pointe classes a week do students attend?

They probably do pointe work every day. If not pointe classes, they have variations, pas de deux, so they're on pointe every day. During the first year, they wear soft pointe shoes for regular classes; second year they wear pointe shoes twice a week for the whole class; and the third year they wear pointe shoes every day.

Could you describe a barre exercise for the first year on pointe?

Demi plié, stretch, rise, lower down twice, and then rise up, down, rise up, down, up, demi plié on pointe, forcing the arch, stretch lower down.

What is your advice to young aspiring dancers?

Work hard. There are lots of dancers out there!

Ugo Ranieri
Principal and Ballet Master
Teatro San Carlo (Naples, Italy)

After a brilliant career as principal dancer, Ugo Ranieri is today maître de ballet of the Teatro San Carlo in Naples, Italy. In his interview, he shared that at the San Carlo, girls on pointe for the first time study a whole year only at the bar. The minimum age requested by the theater to be on pointe is ten to eleven. He likes brands like Freed, Bloch, and Porselli. He believes beginners' shoes have to be comfortable and flexible, with soft shanks, since the girls still do not have enough strength.

Ugo prefers a high vamp in case of strong insteps and is not against the use of toe pads. He advises the soft silicone gel ones. His students soften new shoes by simply using their hands or a little bit of alcohol. When he holds an introductory class, he uses a girl as an example while he explains the various aspects of pointe work. He is not against elastics and likes the ribbons to be sewed in the traditional way, by bending the heel down to find the exact spot. His beginners' classes begin with exercises executed in parallel position and then in first, second, fourth, and fifth. He believes it is very important to control the position of the foot in the shoe going up on pointe and coming down.

Jean-Claude Giorgini
Maître de Ballet
Former Principal Dancer
Examiner, French Diploma in Ballet Teaching
Owner and Director, Giorgini's Dance Center
Lavaur, France.

Jean-Claude Giorgini was simply my ballet teacher, and the best I could ever had. Today, twenty years from these wonderful classes at the Centre de Danse du Sud-Est in Nice, France, Jean-Claude is one of my best friends and a mentor.

Advice for Beginner Dancers on Pointe Taking One Class a Week

I am quite convinced that it is useless to look for the "perfect pointe shoe" when the foot is not strong enough. A well-trained ankle will allow the dancer to go on pointe, not only without effort, but also, and more importantly, in the correct way. Ankles should combine strength and suppleness, these two attributes being the only guarantee for effective and beneficial pointe work. This is why I invented and patented a specific device to work and exercise dancers' feet, allowing to safely "push" the ankle to achieve a better arch and give strength to the joint, especially for dorsal and plantar inflection. Many dancers still force their feet under furniture or other objects in order to improve their arch, and this proves to be very dangerous. This practice will often result in distortion of the bones of the foot, involving significant traumatisms.

Pointe work requires patience, hard work, and time. Furthermore, it should never be attempted before the dancer gains sufficient strength in the ankle, in order to avoid accidents that might provoke permanent damage. If I had to provide an appropriate age to start pointe work—we are discussing dancers who have been seriously studying ballet for several years—I would say the right age would be ten to twelve. There are, of course, particular exceptions of extremely gifted dancers, but these instances should be examined separately. Concerning the choice of pointe shoe type, I prefer to rely on the specialists who offer a wide range of brands. The best shoe will ultimately be the one that fits your foot. In the case of beginners, I often travel to fit them personally for their first shoe. Parents sometimes tend to buy shoes that are too big, and this will cause instability in the ankle, provoking possible accidents.

The rule is trying on as many types of shoes as possible, and always using the toe pads generally worn. Toe pads can alter the fit of the shoe by at least half a size. Padding inside the shoe is good, if not too bulky, in order not to affect the proprioception. I advise the very thin ones made of silicone. I personally always break-in my beginners' pointe shoes and teach them how to do it. The rule is to try not to break the shoe too much and too quickly. The best thing is to let it mold to the dancer's foot. I begin by softening the outer sole by rolling it onto the barre for a few seconds. The second step is to soften the block, paying attention not to break too much the reinforcement that will support the dancer when on pointe. This procedure has to be gently executed with the hands, repeating it several times until the student feels comfortable. At my studio, pointe work always begins with long explanations about how to sew elastics and how to tie the ribbons. When ribbons are tied properly they contribute to make the dancer feel comfortable during the hard work that will follow. The first feeling of the feet in the pointe shoe in contact with the floor is always special.

The first classes will focus on finding the right balance on pointe, and I correct each single foot for eventual mistakes. I work essentially on relevés in order to get the different feeling from relevés executed in soft shoes. It is a slow procedure which requires a lot of dedication from the students. No movement can be executed correctly unless it has been fully understood. I generally start working on pointe after a barre with more relevés on demi-pointe, in order to properly warm up the specific muscles of the heel. I continue with mild exercises in the center, and I dedicate the last fifteen minutes to pointe work. This, of course, is meant for the beginners' level. Talking about shanks, it all depends on the shape of the dancer's arch. Students with strong arches will need harder shanks, but never too hard. A teacher can find the answer only by seeing the student on pointe. For the first two or three months, I have my students work facing the barre, and especially in sixth position. Dancers should learn to feel the inside of the ankles (malleoli), with the axe running through their second metatarsal. Relevés should be executed in first and second position, with plié first and then with straight legs. After a few classes, I add a demi-plié on pointe, to give the students the feeling of their cou–de-pied on pointe.

A few lessons later, I start working in the center with échappés and relevés from two feet to two feet. This is basically what students attending ballet classes twice a week should achieve in a semester. Following the first introductory pointe work, I start with retirés at the barre and in the center. If the result is not satisfactory, I am always ready to stop and go back to the basics.

Joanne Morscher
Royal School of Ballet, Inc.
20771 Beach Cliff Blvd.
Rocky River, Ohio 44116
email: rsb@morscher.com
website: www.morscher.com/dance.com

Mrs. Morscher founded RSB in 1998 and led the program and the school to its many successes. In 2004, she established the Royal Youth Ballet Company (RYBC) as an outgrowth of RSB. Mrs. Morscher, a former principal dancer with North Coast Ballet Theatre, held the position of RYBC artistic director from 2004 to 2008. Originally from Buffalo, New York, she received her initial ballet training from Bernadine DeMike, Janet Springer, and Ginger Burke. She continued her formal training with Troy McCarty, Lynn Brennan Tabor, Dee Hillier, Marguerite Duncan, and Nancy Arcury.

Mrs. Morscher has participated in Continuing Education Seminars such as the Ohio Dance 25th Anniversary Dance Education Day, Nutmeg Conservatory School of the Arts, Youth America Grand Prix Teacher's Course, Vail International Teaching Seminar, Finis Jhung Teacher Workshop sponsored by Ohio Dance Theatre, the Ohio Dance 2005 Festival classes, and was a visiting director at the Eastern Regional Dance America Festival in Harrisburg, Pennsylvania, in 2005.

Students of Mrs. Morscher's have been accepted to prestigious summer programs, university dance programs, and are offered professional contracts around the country. Additionally, her students and choreography have participated and won at the prestigious Youth America Grand Prix (YAGP) Dance Competition.

Mrs. Morscher closed RSB in 2008 to stay at home and raise her son, Hans.

Which do you think is the suitable age to start pointe work?

The age range at our studio was ten to twelve years. I reviewed each student very carefully, looking at the development and strength of the back, feet, and, most importantly, placement. Also, a student was required to study three to four days a week for two years prior to being allowed to train on pointe, as well as continued graded study in ballet training as she became older. I found this last factor (days/hours studied) to be the one that really helped with the training process regardless of the talent of the student.

Is there a specific brand of shoes you recommend to your students?

No, I never had a specific brand that I preferred. I always felt there was a pointe shoe out there for each student. I used all the makers, even ones I was not particularly fond of (Gaynor Minden/Repetto), if I found them to be beneficial for my students. As a teacher, it is your job to help your students find the best shoe for their feet, allowing for the fact that it may take several tries.

Do you allow your students to use padding in their shoes?

Yes, I allowed my students to use a padding of their choice (you really cannot prevent it these days), however, I would not allow them to have their pointe shoes fitted with padding. I find this practice of allowing students to pad the shoes when trying them for an initial fitting leads to, in many cases, a bad fit. I recommended to my students to use a bit of lamb's wool and Saran wrap to make their own pad, which allowed for a very sleek, comfortable padding without the bulk. Also, after a time the Saran wrap would fluff up to twice its size and was quite comfortable in the shoe.

What shanks do you advise for the beginner student?

Again, these specifics of fitting pointe shoes really depend on each individual dancer. Some beginners need very hard shanks, others do not. Some need 3/4 shanks, others need full shanks. For our students, the arch fit was a mandatory requirement. The shoe should fit and mold to each dancer's arch. I would sometimes cut the shanks for dancers as I feel this is the most important aspect of a pointe shoe fit. It is the teacher's responsibility to determine the first fit of her dancers. I always personally took all of my dancers for their pointe shoe fittings.

How do you teach students to break their pointe shoes in?

Through beginning pointe exercises, working the demi, and 3/4. I will also help soften boxes and shanks manually, if I felt it was necessary for proper development. In some cases, we even cut shanks to fit arches if we decided that the shoe was the proper fit everywhere else.

Yes, I did hold a special pointe shoe class for all students and their parents to explain the ins and outs of pointe shoes, their maintenance, how to sew, and my expectations. It was held at the studio after technique class and after everyone was fitted. Students were required to bring their shoes, elastics, ribbons, and sewing supplies. It was a very productive and informative class. The parents and students enjoyed this lecture very much. Once everyone had sewed their pointe shoes and were approved by me, we began the actual pointe class. Sometimes it was a long process, but worth the time and energy.

What types of shanks do you prefer for beginners?

In my opinion, the choice of shank solely depends on the strength of dancer you are fitting.

Do you have special guidelines for sewing the ribbons?

Yes, we had everyone fold the back heel into the pointe shoe, and then sewed the ribbons. Of course, everyone had a different place to sew as all feet/ankle structures are different. I would have all the students pin their ribbons and elastics for approval before sewing. With regard to tying their ribbons, I taught them two ways. Either wrapping one at a time or both simultaneously. I found that some students were better able to tie their shoes if given options. Of course I expected the ends to be tucked in at the indentation of the anklebone, all the while explaining the importance and safety reasons for tying their ribbons properly.

How do you want the elastics to be sewn?

We had a staff member that preferred that we sew all the elastics in cross over the arches with the back elastic deep into the shoe. I agreed with this, but again it does not always work for everyone, and we frequently would have different solutions such as Vamp Elastic for overly developed arches or a loop at the heel for narrow heels. Yes, I do think elastics are very important in helping to support and develop the arch.

A note in response to two previous questions. Every teacher has a different way to accomplish these tasks. I frequently found that students return from the various summer programs with their ribbons and elastics re-sewn. I always advised my students that they should do what is required from each program and each teacher. If they returned from the summer program and wanted to leave their ribbons and elastics a certain way, I generally was agreeable, especially if improvement was apparent.

Could you give a sample of a first class on pointe?

Sample Class:
15-20 minutes after a technique class and conducted facing the barre
- A. Begin in sixth position rolling to the demi, then to the full-pointe, pressing over the shoe, but not up on the pointe. Repeat 8 times on the right and then on the left.
- B. First position, tendu to second pressing over the shoe returning the weight to the supporting leg and closing back to first. Repeat 8 times each side.
- C. First position, gently press in élevé (rise) to the 3/4 only, lowering without plié, 8 times.
- D. First position, have the dancers plié and press with a slight spring to first position on pointe. Repeat 8 times.
- E. Repeat exercise D. And have the dancers plié over the top of the shoe to assess placement.

F. To end I would have them come to the center to do a port de bras study/révérence to practice standing in their pointe shoes. I always found that the last exercise is the hardest because to just stand in pointe shoes can be difficult.

Tanya Pearson
Ballet Master
The Classical Coaching Academy
St. Leonards, NSW 2065, Australia

Russian-born Tanya Pearson is the founder of the Classical Coaching Academy, established in 1993 in St. Leonards, near Sydney. Tanya is one of Australia's most renowned teachers and has produced several coaching DVDs.

Tanya, how do you assess the ability of a student to start pointe work?

Students should reach a maturity level to understand correct posture and placement before attempting pointe work, and preferably have at least three or four years of training in basic ballet technique. The age may vary, however, but not before ten years of age.

Do you have a special brand of shoes you prefer for your students? How do you think a beginner's shoe should fit?

I do not like to recommend a brand of shoe. However, I do recommend that they go to a store where they are carefully fitted for their first pair of pointe shoes. Then before sewing on the ribbons, the students should check with their ballet teachers that the shoe is the correct fit.

Do you allow your students to use toe pads?

It is optional for students to use toe pads. I have no particular preference. However, the thin toecap with a little lamb's wool is comfortable.

What type of shank, block, and vamp do you prefer for beginners?

Preferably not too high a vamp for beginners so they can learn to rise and come down through the demi- and three-quarter pointe, that is, of course, unless the student has a very arched foot. Also not too hard a shank as a young beginner does not do very much or very hard pointe work."

How do you teach your students to break their pointe shoes in?

"Firstly the teacher should bend the shoe at the metatarsal and then show the student or parent how to do it, however this should be done under supervision. The other way is to stand in parallel at the barre and rise up and lower to demi-pointe several times, then repeat in 1st position and then rise and plié en pointe and stretch several times until the shoe begins to feel more pliable.

How is your introductory pointe class structured?

We usually start the student by learning a simple pointe exercise in demi-pointe or flat shoes—when the student knows what to do, we can then explain how to do it correctly once they put their pointe shoes on. I often will use a slightly more advanced student to show the wrong way and then the correct way. I also emphasize how important it is to use correct posture and corsetry muscles to teach the student to come down with resistance, and to go up by using center and not pushing off the barre. The full weight of the body should not sit into the shoes, and it is vital to emphasize to students commencing pointe work the importance of pulling up and out of their shoes and ankles.

Do you prefer hard or soft shanks for beginners?

I prefer a softer shank for beginners as they do not have very much strength in the ankles and metatarsals. It is too difficult to go through demi- or quarter-pointe with hard shoes. Also, they do not yet do anything difficult, so a softer shoe will not wear out, unless a student has a very high arch, as mentioned in question 4.

Do you have special guidelines for sewing and tying the ribbons? How do you want the girls to tie their shoes?

Yes, I show the students where to sew their ribbons. It is preferable to sew them on a slight diagonal from the back of the heel (turn over the heel of the shoe) and also ensure that the ribbon is doubled and stitched in a square so it is less likely to tear. I do show the students how to tie their ribbons correctly.

Are you for or against elastics?

Yes, I prefer elastic sewn, particularly for a performance shoe, not so much for a beginner. I also show the student how to wet the back of the heel before putting on the pointe shoe to allow for a little more security. If the student does not need the elastic, I allow them to make their choice.

Could you give a sample of a first class on pointe?

One of the exercises I find beneficial for both younger and older students is [as follows]:
Facing the barre and stand in parallel position.
Rise on full pointe. Lower to ¼ pointe and rise again to full pointe.
Repeat 3 times and lower into demi-plié.
Repeat the above exercise in first position and second position.

What barre exercises do you advise for the first two to three months on pointe? Can you describe two barre and two center exercises?

A. Relevé in first position and bend knees slightly on pointe then stretch and lower. Repeat 3 times, then repeat all in second position.
B. Échappé to second, lower with resistance in second, then relevé in second and close to fifth. Repeat 3 times.

In the center, have another student preferably behind the beginner and ask them to support the younger student at the waist gently, reminding them to use the correct posture over the toes, and to not sit back or strain with the ribs to go up. Ask them to relevé in fifth, taking the arms slowly up to first position. Repeat 3 times. Then échappé to second taking arms to second. At this point, I ask the younger students to feel that they are hugging me and that I am very fat so they feel the support of their backs as well as arms in second position. Repeat this exercise 3 or 4 times.

Exercise 2: Still with the support of someone behind them, posé forward in fifth croisé, arms in first, and relevé in fifth position. Then posé to the side into fifth position croisé, open arms into demi-seconde, then relevé. Repeat all to the other side and repeat again without the support of the older student.

Could you briefly describe two barre and two center exercises for a second-year pointe class?

For second year's pointe, keep working on the previously stated rising exercises, and add the following:

A. Facing barre: Posé on one foot de coté, emphasizing to lift the supporting hip, then fondu and pas de bourrée piqué under. Repeat this to the other side, then repeat all with one hand on the barre: Posé en avant and arm in first, fondu and pas de bourrée en tournant to the other side and repeat.
B. Facing barre: Relevé in fifth, then relevé devant; again, emphasize to lift supporting hip, plié, then relevé derrière, fondu and courus. Repeat the same side, but replace courus with pas de bourrée under.
C. Still facing the barre, relevé fifth, then relevé into arabesque, fondu and pas de bourrée piqué under and repeat to the other side. Repeat all again (show how not to drop the back in arabesque when in fondu).
D. In the center: Relevé in fifth, relevé devant, échappé to second and then relevé derrière. Then repeat all to other side and repeat everything.
E. Exercise two in the center: Stand croisé right foot front, preparatory position. Courus for 4 counts, emphasizing that the back foot makes you travel, arms through first up to fourth, then turn to right for two counts and pas de bourrée piqué under. Posé de coté upstage devant, then derrière using front then back arm to third position, then another

pas de bourrée piqué and courus back croisé with arms in demi seconde and lower down to preparatory position. Repeat all to other side.

The teacher, of course, can make up other exercises.

Is there a particular exercise you teach your students to improve their arches?

Yes, facing the barre with pointe shoes on, dégagé devant, fondu onto the pointed toes, maintaining turnout and stretch. Repeat 3 times, then repeat derrière with the other foot facing away from the barre, then repeat to second facing the barre and repeat all with the other leg.

What is your advice for girls beginning pointe?

My personal advice for beginners' pointe is not to rely on their shoes—strengthen the posture instead of relying on the posture supporting the dancer en pointe. Also, go quickly up, but always resist when coming down by using strong corsetry muscles and alighting through demi- and quarter-pointe.

Susan Jones
Ballet Master
American Ballet Theatre

How do you assess the ability of a student to start pointe work? What is the age range for going on pointe at ABT?

I generally look for the following things:
- Ability to relevé on one leg with stretched knees on demi-pointe.
- Ability to jump on one leg while supporting body placement and a foot that stretches/pointes with proper alignment and strength.

I would say the age range is about nine, but it depends somewhat on the assets and development of the student.

Do you have a special brand of shoes you prefer for your students? How do you think a beginner's shoe should fit? What is the most used brand of pointe shoes at ABT?

As I haven't been actively teaching pointe to children, this is difficult for me to answer. Shoes should be fit by someone with experience—not too big, not too small.

Do you allow your students to use toe pads?

Toe pads are fine. I'm not familiar with brands.

How do you teach students to break their new pointe shoes in?

I would have them step on the box a bit and wear them at home just to walk in. It gets them used to the shoes. Standing on demi-pointe helps break in the shank. If they bend the shank in the wrong place, it could damage the shank, and they won't have the proper support. That action takes some time to learn about.

Do you hold a special "introductory" pointe class before they start pointe work?

I would introduce pointe work at the barre with two hands in the barre. Nothing on one foot, only on two."

Do you prefer soft or hard shanks for beginners?

It depends somewhat on the structure of the foot, but they do need good support from the shank at first.

Do you have special guidelines for the students to sew their ribbons? How do you want them to tie their ribbons? How do you want the elastics to be sewn?

Fold the center of the back of the shoe in and mark the crease on the side that the fold creates. The ribbons should be sewn on that angle, more or less. Elastics should be worn as needed and sewn from the back of the shoe (on the outside so as not to rub a heel blister).

Could you give a sample of a first class on pointe?

Demi-plié in first (two hands on the barre), rise slowly on pointe, release down to demi-pointe, and back up to pointe. Push over gently still on pointe and back up to first and down to flat, rolling through the demi-pointe.

What barre exercises do you advise for the first two to three months on pointe? Can you describe two barre and two center exercises?

Rising in first and second on pointe, as described above. Doing échappés to second and eventually to fourth from fifth. Doing piqués to fifth to the front, side, and back. Jumping in pointe shoes is important to accustom the foot to working within the shoe as well as grand pliés. Eventually doing piqués onto one foot.

Also doing passé relevés from fifth. Eventually, piqués soutenus turns and later piqués passés, later with a turn.

How do you deal with hyperextended students?

I try to get their heels together in first as much as possible, so they develop some strength in their quads, keeping their kneecaps pulled up. It strengthens their pointe work in general.

What do you advise to beginners' pointe?

Take the time to achieve proper alignment and sufficient strength before attempting "tricks"!

Chapter 2

Interviews with Thirty-One Famous Ballerinas

Cecilia Kerche – Prima Ballerina of Teatro Municipal Rio de Janeiro, Founder of Cecilia Kerche Pointe Shoes
Liliya Aronova – Soloist at Metropolitan Ballet Company (Arlington, Texas)
Celeste Rainier – Corps de Ballet, International Ballet Theatre (Kirkland, Washington)
Charline Dujardin – Soloist at Ballet des Landestheater Detmold (Detmold, Germany)
Anna-Marie Holmes – Ballet Master/Choreographer, Former Artistic Director of Boston Ballet
Molly Smolen – Principal Dancer, San Francisco Ballet
Andrea Maciel de Faria – Company Member, Orlando Ballet
Violeta Angelova – Principal Dancer
Kuei Yao Chu – Artist at English National Ballet (London)
Lucia Lacarra – Principal Dancer, Opera of Munich (Bayerisches Staatsballett – Munich, Germany)
Carolina Maria Aguero – Principal Dancer, Hamburg Ballet (Hamburg, Germany)
Sasha Mukhamedov – Artist at Dutch National Ballet (Amsterdam, the Netherlands)
Jordan-Elizabeth Long – Coryphée, Het National Ballet (Amsterdam, The Netherlands)
Ashley Bouder – Principal Dancer, New York City Ballet
Mila Izotovich – Charleston Ballet Theatre (Charleston, South Carolina)
Daria Klimentova – Prima Ballerina, English National Ballet (London)
Adiarys Almeida Santana – Principal Dancer, Corella Ballet (Madrid, Spain)
Carla Korbes – Principal Dancer, Pacific Northwest Ballet (Seattle, Washington)
Ashlee Dupre – Ballerina
Katia Garza – Company Member– Orlando Ballet
Laura Bösenberg – Principal Dancer, Cape Town City Ballet (Cape Town, South Africa)
Tracy Jones – Artist, Corella Ballet (Madrid, Spain)
Michele Wiles – Principal Dancer, American Ballet Theatre
Katie Williams – Corps de Ballet, American Ballet Theatre
April Giangeruso – Company Member, American Ballet Theatre II
Vanessa Woods – Professional Ballerina
Deanna McBrearty – Ballet Teacher/Fitness Trainer, Former Dancer, New York City Ballet
Megan Wood – Former Dancer, Ballet Opéra du Rhin (Strasbourg, Mulhouse, Colmar)
Celisa Diuana – Artist at the Royal Ballet (London)
Ksenia Ovsyanick – Artist, English National Ballet
Jennifer Florquin – Dancer with the Leipzig Ballet Company (Leipzig, Germany)

Cecilia Kerche
Principal Dancer
Municipal Theatre of Rio de Janeiro
Creator, Pointe Shoes Cecilia Kerche

Cecilia Kerche, world-famous ballerina and creator of the pointe shoes who bear her name, agreed to share with us her "little secrets."

Cecilia wears pointe shoes Cecilia Kerche Bayadère, width B, size 4, normal vamp, and three-quarter shank.

She has a Greek foot, very flexible, and she does not wear any type of padding. She likes to sew her ribbons before the middle seam and the elastics near the back seam. She softens her shoes just by practicing a few exercises, and she can use up to four pairs of pointe shoes a month, depending on what ballet she is rehearsing for and on how many pointe classes she takes. She protects her toes by wrapping them with tape, and if she gets a blister, she cuts the dead skin and tapes her toes. Her shoes are custom-made according to her requirements, so she does not need to modify them. She sometimes clean them using nail polish remover.

As far as special exercises to strengthen her feet, she performs many combinations of battements tendus with flex and rise on demi-pointe.

She uses Jelly Toes as the only accessory. Her advice to young students: "Lots of classes with good teachers, and go for it!"

Liliya Aronova
Soloist, Metropolitan Classical Ballet Company
Arlington, Texas

Liliya started going on pointe pretty late, at age fifteen. "I had to work a lot, in order to catch up," she says. She currently wears Capezio Glissé Pro, size 7.5 M, with either a soft or hard shank, depending on the choreography. Her foot is similar to the Egyptian type, but with the first and second toes of the same length. She describes her bunion area as extremely wide, and her heel really narrow, which makes it really hard to find the proper fit. She softens her pointe shoes by "three-quartering" the shank and putting a nail right before the spot where the shoe breaks. She also performs a few relevés at the barre, paying attention to roll through the whole foot, passing seven-eighth-, three-quarter-, demi- and quarter-pointe. She also likes rising up to first position, then lowering down to three-quarter-pointe and back again to full-pointe. "It strengthens the toes and gets the shoe nice and worked in," she adds.

If she performs a grand pas with fouettés at the end, she might go through up to two pairs of shoes per week. If she dances Balanchine's repertoire, where she can use softer shoes due to the quick footwork required, a pair can last up to one week or more, especially alternating them every day.

She uses elastic around the ankle, and she folds the heel of the shoe in order to sew the ribbons at the place where the folding ends. She sometimes also crisscrosses her elastics and sews the ribbons "in attachment to the elastics that are close to the toes." She adds, "This way, it creates the effect of a ribbon with an elastic, stretching when I plié, and the ribbons cover the elastics so it doesn't look too messy."

In order to strengthen her instep, she sits on the floor with stretched legs, bends forward and grabs her toes, then puts her head as close to her knees as possible and stretches for two minutes. She also stretches using Thera-Bands, keeping the small toes stretched and not knuckled as she points and flexes. She also uses a towel, which she puts on the floor, and then tries to grab with her toes and then release, keeping the toes as straight as possible. In order to make her arch look bigger, she uses a fake arch built out of a sock. "But only in performances," she says. "During rehearsals I never put anything, so I can see my line and try to correct it and work on it as much as I can."

One of her favorite warm-up exercise consists of slow rises in sixth position, alternating the feet and trying to align herself, feeling the Achilles tendon soft and not tight. "After that," she adds, "slow tendus in first, trying to turn out from the hips, and roll through the whole foot as I open and close."

To fight a blister she uses Second Skin. "It alleviates the pain and fastens the regrowth of the new skin." Liliya uses a paper towel as toe pad.

Her advice to beginners' dancers? "Don't give up! It may be very difficult and uncomfortable in the beginning, but work can do wonders!"

Celeste Rainier
Corps de Ballet
International Ballet Theatre
Kirkland, Washington

Céleste joined the International Ballet Theatre in 2006. She appeared in numerous productions with the company, such as Dracula, The Nutcracker, Stars, Giselle, Don Quixote, and Coppélia. Celeste also trained with the American Ballet Theatre in New York City and currently is a member of the Professional Division with the International School of Classical Ballet.

Céleste started pointe work when she was eleven. She used to wear Russian Pointe, width 2 with a medium shank but switched to Grishko. Her foot is in between Egyptian and peasant, her second toe being slightly longer than her big toe, but all the other toes of the same length.

In order to break in her pointe shoes, she smashes the box with the heel of her foot a couple of times, then puts her shoes in the microwave to soften the glue for about ten seconds. When the glue is softened and more pliable, she bends the shank a couple of times, "but not too much, otherwise the shoes die quickly."

Céleste uses gel toe pads, "so I don't really get blisters. If I do get one, then I usually take a gel circle and put it over it [the blister] and then tape it down. I never feel it. I used to use Ouch Pouches by Bunheads, and sometimes I get a tissue and fold it once over my toes if the shoes are new."

She goes through one pair of shoes every two or three weeks, rotating her shoes to make them last longer. "I tie my ribbons so that the knot ends up on the side." If the shoes get dirty before a performance, she uses some light foundation to touch it up. "I generally do not Pan-Cake my shoes unless asked," she says. "But I usually don't clean my shoes. They don't last enough!"

She sews her elastics either in the back or in a cross using one piece, always making sure the thread cannot be seen. She uses Thera-Bands a lot to strengthen her feet, sometimes putting one Thera-Band on top of the other for added strength. Before class she stretches her feet first, and then puts on her booties to keep them warm. She rolls through her feet at the barre and then stretches the Achilles and hamstrings. "Doing relevés on one foot at the barre always helps me warm up my feet," she claims. "I also stretch my neck, my arms in all directions, and my back."

As alternative to Russian Pointe, she sometimes wears Grishkos. Her advice is to find the right pair of shoes according to the type of foot. "When I started pointe, I couldn't find a good pointe shoe," she recalls, "so I wasn't working through my feet as well . . . and of course that held back my process in training. Make sure your pointe shoes fit so your foot can get over the box!" Her advice to beginner students? "Learn how to tie your ribbons correctly so they don't get loose!"

Charline Dujardin
Soloist
Ballett des Landestheater Detmold
Detmold, Germany

How old were you when you started pointe?

I started pointe at the age of nine. Pretty early actually, because all the girls in my ballet group were older, and my teacher decided that I could start with them. She thought that I had enough strength to manage.

What pointe shoes do you use?

I use actually three different brands. My favorite ones are Eva from Karl Heinz Martin (size 4, V-shaped EF). The second ones are Capezio's Partner (size 6 1/2), and I also use Sansha's Ovation (6M).

How would you describe your feet?

My feet are quite wide, and I have a high instep.

How do you soften your pointe shoes?

When I first get them, I will bend them carefully with my hands. But if they are really too strong, I put my shoe in between the space of where the door hangs to the wall, and then close the door a bit. With this technique, you can bend the sole of the shoe, and also the bit at the nose of the shoe where the sole ends and goes into the pointe. By doing this, you can make sure that the shoe bends like your foot does. After this, I will put the shoes on the night before I want to use them and walk around in them at home (I'll put socks above them to protect them against dirt), and then the next day I'll do a barre in them (putting just a bit of water on the line where they bend on to demi-pointe), and then let them dry out. Lastly I apply shellac. At this point, my shoes are about ready to work in the center, rehearse, or perform.

How many pairs do you generally use weekly or monthly?

In performances I will use normally two pairs of shoes. Depending on which show, it can be less or more. In training I'll use about a pair every one or two weeks, also depending [on] what we rehearse, but I always make sure that I alternate my shoes so they can dry out very well and the life of the shoe is extended.

Do you Pan-Cake shoes for shows? What do you use?

For training I don't, because there's no point in Pan-Caking them, but sometimes we need them flesh colored for shows, so I use makeup Pan-Cake from Kryolan. I apply it on the shoes with a wet sponge. If they need to be colored, the people at the costume department of the theater will dye them for me.

How do you sew your elastics and ribbons?

Everybody has a different way of doing this. Some dancers like the ribbons sewn in the front, without elastics. Some absolutely need elastics. During shows I sometimes use only elastics. Again, depending on the show, you adjust your shoes. For training I will use crossed elastics over my arch, with the ribbons sewn at the middle of my foot.

Is there any exercise you practice to strengthen your instep?

Standing in sixth position on pointe in front of the barre, holding the barre with two hands, slowly plié till you sit on your heels, then come back up again and lower through demi-pointe on flat, and start again. Practice lot of relevés—it is an excellent exercise. Use elastic bands to stretch and bend your feet.

Do you use any tricks to make your arch look better?

No, you just have to work your feet all the time, also when you do class without pointe shoes, or even at home when you watch TV. There are a million of exercises you can do to train your metatarsals! You have to use what you've got! I saw people with really ugly feet become people with nice feet! It is possible, through practice!

Can you suggest a warm-up exercise at the barre or in the center?

Relevés, a lot of relevés, and also the exercise that I explained in question 8.

Do you always use the same brand and type of shoes, or do you change?

No, I change, depending on the show. Sometimes I need harder shoes, and sometimes I need softer ones.

What do you do when you get a blister before a show?

Disinfect it, put some types of plaster on it, strap it up with some adhesive tape, and that will normally do it. With the adrenaline of the show, I mostly don't feel the pain onstage.

Any advice you would give to beginners?

Look with somebody, preferably a dancer, for a pair of pointe shoes that really fit your foot. You need to contact someone who knows what is good for you. A wrong pointe shoe can ruin your technique and your way of dancing. Also, pointe shoes will hurt—that's a fact—but treat your blisters well, and continue. If you have blisters in a show, you need to continue. A blister for me is not an excuse for stopping the class, or to take off the shoes. Just take them off, disinfect the blister, and put a plaster on it, eventually with some extra tape so it doesn't come off. Put the shoe back on, and then you can continue. Also, do a million of relevés to strengthen your feet, at the barre, in the center, from two legs, from one leg! That's very important to get that strength for your whole pointe work.

Do you use any padding, and if yes, what type?

No, normally not! I did when I was younger. I used Ouch Pouches, but I think I can't really feel how my foot is in contact with the shoe and the floor, so I prefer without padding. If my feet are full of blisters, I wrap around my toes a sort of dishcloth, the really cheap one with tiny little holes in them. You find them in every supermarket.

The Magic of Pointe Shoes

Anna-Marie Holmes
Ballet Master, International Choreographer
Former Artistic Director
Boston Ballet

Anna-Marie started pointe work at twelve. Her feet were very arched, and her teachers did not want her on pointe before. She started using Capezio pointe shoes at first for more support, then Freed. Her feet are also very wide and with the first two toes of the same length.

Hundreds of relevés and tendus were for her the best way to break her shoes in.

In order to mattify her shoes before performances, she used Max Factor Cake Make-Up. She would sew her elastics at the back so that they would go right around her ankle and the ribbons on an angle to the shoe, careful not to sew through the drawstring.

She suggests to warm up thoroughly [the] legs and ankle muscles with a full ballet class first, and then performing relevés on two and then on one foot.

Her remedy against blisters? "I used to close my eyes, pour alcohol on it, and yell! Put a Band-Aid, and then put lamb's wool around it and dance. Now I see dancers using New Skin to protect their blisters."

Anna-Marie's advice to young dancers: "Don't think of pointe shoes as shoes, but use them as a device to get one up on pointe. Make sure your shoes are not too big as then they will rub and hurt. Also not too small. You need professional advice on it, so do not buy big pointe shoes thinking your foot will grow in them."

Anna-Marie always used lamb's wool as padding. "It absorbs the moisture and softens the pressure on the foot." Her personal suggestion is to make sure you are right up on your pointe shoe and not pulling back off it. She also advises performing hundreds of relevés at the barre before going into the center.

Molly Smolen
Principal Dancer
San Francisco Ballet

Molly wears Freed size 4 1/2, XXX. She has flat but very flexible feet, and she does not wear toe pads. She wears elastics at the heel and ribbons about an inch away. She double-knots her ribbons and always tucks them in on the inside of the ankle. She softens her shoes by smashing the box before sewing the ribbons, and the number of pointe shoes she uses depends on the repertoire she dances. She Pan-Cakes her shoes only if required. She uses rosin to "cut the shine" for Act II of Giselle, and Pan-Cake to match flesh tones of odd-colored tights with Kryolan base make-up." She uses surgical spirit on a cottonpad to clean the satin. "Never use any sort of padding," suggests Molly. "Never wrap your toes. If you start doing it, you'll never be able to stop, and you won't be able to build the necessary calluses.

Her advice to young dancers: "Don't be in a hurry to get started. Your feet will never be the same again!"

Andrea Maciel de Faria
Company Member
Orlando Ballet
Gold Medal, Danza Nino 97
Buenos Aires, Argentina

What pointes shoes do you wear?

I wear Bloch Alpha, size 3 1/2, width XXX. My shoes are not custom-made.

How many pairs of shoes are you allowed each month by Orlando Ballet?

We are allowed about one pair of shoes every working week, so maybe three or four a month, which is really not enough.

How would you describe your foot?

I have the Egyptian type of foot and tapered toes, with high arches.

Do you wear any toe pads?

I wear just a regular silicone toe pad.

How do you prepare your shoes?

I sew my elastics in a way so they hug my ankle, one inch away on both sides from where the heel of the shoe is sewn. I sew my ribbons an inch away from the elastic. I always cut the shank of the shoes according to the curve of my foot.

Very often I have used superglue or Jet Glue on the shank and box of the shoes, to have them last longer. I wear my shoes always on the same foot, and I never break them in. I just do some relevés and start dancing.

I use about two, or sometimes three, pairs of shoes a week, even though in my company we don't get as many. So probably eight pairs of pointe shoes a month.

How do you protect your toes from blisters?

Most of the times just using the toe pad is enough to protect my foot, but when needed I use masking tape around my toes to protect them. If I get a blister on the day of a performance, I pop the blister with a disinfected needle and use Orajel (medicine for teeth pain) on the blister to numb it. The only alternation I do to my shoes is cutting the shank.

Do you Pan-Cake your shoes for performances?

I usually don't Pan-Cake my shoes. I just use some rosin on the shoe satin to eliminate the shine.

Do you darn your pointe shoes?

No, I don't darn my shoes.

Do you clean your shoes?

Usually, whenever the shoe is dirty, it means that it is dead too. So I don't clean it. It goes to the garbage, although I heard that some people use alcohol and a clean cloth.

How do you strengthen your feet?

Always keep your feet strong by exercising with a Thera-Band.
Also practice lots of relevés.
Your advice: "Work hard and keep your feet strong."

Violeta Angelova
Principal Dancer

Violeta Angelova was born and raised in Bulgaria, and her mother was a ballet teacher. She graduated with honors from the National School of Dance Art in Bulgaria and the Vienna State Opera Ballet School in Austria. She was invited to the Royal Festival of Arts in Jordan for a number of international ballet events. She has performed with the Vienna State Opera Ballet, the Ballet Internationale, and is a guest principal for the Eglevsky, New Jersey, and Metropolitan Ballets.

Violeta's repertoire includes solo roles from over fifty ballets, among them Aurora, Kitri, Myrtha, as well as lead roles in Balanchine's Agon and Valse Fantasie. Violeta joined the Suzanne Farrell Ballet in 2006.

What kind of pointe shoes do you wear?

I use all kinds of shoes. I dance in Freeds, Blochs, Grishkos, and Gaynors at the same time. Occasionally in other brands too. The variations of boxes, shanks, and strengths are too many to count.

Are your shoes custom-made?

My Freeds are custom-made. I ask for the hardest possible shoe, and still most die on me in one rehearsal. Without superglue I'd be in big trouble.

I only met the cobbler of my first pointe shoes. They were white satin. My mom took an outline of my foot, and we went to order them from a well-known dance shoe maker in Sofia, who I think used to be one of the National Ballet's shoe makers. He was an old man and adored by his customers.

I was maybe five or six, but remember all this very well. We waited two weeks for the shoes to be made, and when I got them, I was very happy. I have to ask my mom again, but I think I had been nagging her for a pair of my own for a while.

How many pairs of pointe shoes are you allowed by your company?

I've been in many companies, and the assigned shoe amount differs. One thing is common, though—the amount is never large enough for me.

How would you describe your foot?

I have a combination of Giselle/compressible feet. I have long toes. The first and second are the same length, and the rest taper proportionately. I have high arches, and I also underpronate.

Kuei Yao Chu
Artist, English National Ballet

Kuei started pointe when she was eleven. She wears Bloch Serenade B, but she would like to try Freed. She describes her foot as short with even toes, with a wide metatarsus and a medium arch. Her break-in technique is very simple: she just breaks her shoe around the arch and presses the block to make it softer. Whenever she wants her shoes to sound less noisy, she hits the pointe shoe on the wall or uses a hammer. Depending on how often she rehearses, she uses one to two pairs of pointe shoes a week. She does not Pan-Cake her shoes, and she sews the ribbons on the edge of the material and her elastics behind the anklebone. She believes in practicing tendus very carefully and with precision to strengthen her instep. "Pointe work comes from every day's barre work!" she says.

In order to make her arch look better, she cuts her insole, and she also has a fake arch that she seldom uses. Here are the warm-up exercises she suggests: "Circle the ankles. Flex and stretch the ankles. Small jogging to warm up the feet and body—32 échappés and passés."

If she gets a blister before a show, she just puts a thick plaster on it. Her advice to beginners? "Spend some time and money to find the right pair of pointe shoe."

Her personal suggestion: "After a long day of rehearsals and performances, my toes will get quite sore, tired, and aching. I will then use Body Shop's peppermint foot spray that relieves stress. The peppermint in it will lighten my feet and cool my swelling toes."

The Magic of Pointe Shoes

Lucia Lacarra
Principal Dancer
Opera of Munich (Bayerisches Staatsballett)
Munich, Germany

Lucia wears Freed pointe shoes, maker Clove, XX Fortiflex. Her foot is a "square-cut foot," with a very pronounced arch and strong cou-de-pied. She protects her toes using a French natural kind of cotton called coton cardé, and she wraps it with pieces of old tights.

She sews ribbons and elastics in a very traditional way.

She always hardens her shoes with glue before even using them. Then before wearing them the first time for class, she hammers them under the toes to feel the demi-pointe. She was not able to tell how many pairs of shoes she uses per month, since it depends on the ballets she is working on at the moment.

She generally doesn't get blisters, and she doesn't need to protect her toes. "After so many years on pointe, my toes are used to it," she says. "But if I get a rare blister, I put on some Compeed. Lucia does not alter or modify her shoe. She normally never Pan-Cakes her shoes for performance, unless it's the choreographer's wish, or if she needs to color them to match some color tights.

She darns just a double half-circle of the shoe, leaving the bottom untouched. She never cleaned a pair of shoes in her life, since she breaks them much faster than they get dirty. Her secret tip for pointe students? Lucia says that there are no secret tips. "Every foot is different. The only thing that really helps is wearing pointe shoes every single day in class, starting from the beginning of the barre.

Lucia stresses that all exercises at the barre are optimal to help strengthen the foot, but the most important thing, in her opinion, is to always go through the demi-pointe when rising up and lowering down, in order to achieve strength and control.

No accessories for Lucia—"Sorry, just my toes"—and she does not resort to tricks in order to make her arch look better. She was blessed by Mother Nature with a beautiful natural arch!

Here is her advice to beginners: "Work hard on your feet now that you're young, because they will get strong, and that will help you for your whole career. And remember . . . it's very painful at the beginning, but you'll get used to it. Trust me!"

Carolina Maria Aguero
Principal Dancer
Hamburg Ballet
Hamburg, Germany

Carolina is originally from Córdoba, Argentina. She studied in her hometown and was blessed with wonderful teachers like Irupe Pereira Parodi, Jorge Tomin, Olga Ferri, Enrique Lommi, Teresa del Cerro, and Liliana Belfiore.

Carolina wears special-order Capezio pointe shoes, Style 190, size 4 3/4 C, vamp 3 inches with shank number 6, which is the hardest. Her foot is flexible, and she does not use any type of padding, just Second Skin, and she does not alter the shoes in any way. She sews two elastics in her pointe shoes: One over the arch from one side to the other, and the second one from the bottom left side of my heel, stretching over to the right side. From the stitching of the pointe shoes, I sew the ribbon on both sides, and then I naturally tie them around my ankle." She generally uses two to five pairs of shoes per week, depending on the productions. She Pan-Cakes her pointe shoes only if required and cleans them with alcohol. Instead of darning the tips, she just wets the vamp with water.

Here are Carolina's secret tips: "Use comfortable pointe shoes, not too small in order to avoid problems like bunions or bruised toenails. Go on pointe using strength from the ankles and toes, not jumping, and do not let your feet dominate you!"

She suggests doing relevés, with or without plié, in first and second positions, first with both hands at the barre and really using the strength of your toes and ankles, not jumping! Also trying from one foot to one foot, alternating legs.

In order to make the arch look better, she cuts her shoes in the right place; she three-quarters them from the inside and also from the outside.

To Carolina, to be a dancer means "sacrifice, love, and hard work.

"To be able to do all these things without thinking means that you really love this profession. In the end, it's a very good feeling, a pleasure. An artist gives everything onstage—soul, feelings—and shows technique. It's a beautiful feeling when you can project all these things to an audience."

Sasha Mukhamedov
Elève, Dutch National Ballet
(Joined December 2008 as an Aspirante)
Amsterdam, the Netherlands

Sasha is the daughter of Irek Mukhamedov, former principal with the Bolshoi Ballet, and former ballerina Masha Mukhamedov.

How old were you when you started pointe?

Well, I first went on pointe when I was about three years old and used to run around the house in them! But I properly started when I was eight.

What pointe shoes do you use?

I wear two different pairs. For class on pointe and for some solos, I wear Gaynor Minden medium 4 box with the hardest back. And for other solos, I wear Grishko 2007 Pro XXX.

What type of foot do you have?

I'm not really sure how to answer this question, but I have a good pointe and quite a wide foot.

How do you soften your pointe shoes?

I use a hammer.

How do you make your pointe shoes less noisy?

The pointe shoes I wear are made not to make a lot of noise, but if I had to, I would hit them lightly with a hammer under the pointe.

How many pairs do you generally use weekly or monthly?

With Grishko a pair generally lasts about a week, but if we are doing lots of solos, then it is a bit less than a pair a week.

Do you Pan-Cake shoes for shows?

No, I think shoes look nicer as they are.

How do you sew your elastics and ribbons?

Well, I sew the ribbons where it is comfortable and the elastics in a cross close to the heel where my arch is. I also sew my ribbons in correspondence to the arch.

Is there any exercise you practice to strengthen your instep?

I just stretch my feet as hard as possible and bend my toes in every exercise. The best exercise is to just stretch your feet and go through every muscle in every exercise.

Do you use any tricks to make your arch look better?

Stand on full demi-pointe, as high as you can, so that it hurts.

Can you suggest a warm-up exercise at the barre or in the center?

Just lots of échappés and relevés.

Do you always use the same brand and type of shoes, or do you change?

I change because I find Gaynor Minden more comfortable for jumps, because they are softer.

What do you do when you get a blister before a show?

I try not to get any blisters by always making sure everything is covered properly. I have had a few bad ones, and I just try to let them breathe as much as I can. When I have to put my shoes on, I use on a big gel plaster.

Any advice you would give to beginners?

The advice I would give is just do little by little, not once a week but every day, so that your feet can get used to being on pointe. Even if it's only a couple of échappés, you will start to find it more comfortable.

Do you use any padding, and if yes, what type?

Yes, I use Ouch Pouches.

Jordan-Elizabeth Long
Coryphée
Het Nationale Ballet Amsterdam
(The Netherlands)

Elizabeth wears custom-made shoes from Freed of London, Makers Maltese Cross and V, size 4 XX. Her feet are small, with a wide metatarsal and narrow heel, and she uses Ouch Pouches toe pads. She sews her ribbons by folding the edge of them over the elastic. Then she sews both of them together just behind the seam of the shoe. She sews the other end of the elastic next to her heel on the back of the shoe. When she ties her shoe, she always takes the inside ribbon first so that she can pull up the material on the arch.

She first flattens the box by stepping on it before she puts the shoe on. Then she performs a couple of relevés so that the shoe forms to her foot. After this, she takes them off and puts Jet Glue inside the tip of the box and cuts the satin off the tip. Depending on what she is dancing, she uses six to eight pairs of shoes per month. If she gets a blister, she usually tapes it, and this works. When she was younger, she used to sew down the sides of her shoes. Now she has them special-ordered, and they come the way she wants. Elizabeth only Pan-Cakes her shoes if it is specifically asked for. She usually uses any type of liquid foundation, but always tries her shoes out before the show, to make sure the Pan-Cake does not cause her to slip. She darns her shoes occasionally. She does it by sewing a loop stitch around the tip of the shoe and then going back around and sewing that stitch down. She generally doesn't get to the point of cleaning her pointe shoes because they "die" before she needs to clean them.

Do you have any secret tip for pointe students?

When you are beginning pointe, having properly fitted shoes is very important. If you live in a more rural area, it might mean traveling to a ballet shop in a larger city, but it is worth it. For students who have been doing pointe for a while, I find that it can be very beneficial to take a regular class on pointe as often as possible, so that one can get used to working each part of their foot before it is time to go onstage.

Could you describe at least one exercise at the barre or in the center to help strengthen feet?

Doing slow relevés on pointe, on both one and two feet, can really improve control and ability to roll through three-quarter and demi-pointe. It is very important to think about using each part of the foot.

What type of accessories do you use?

I do not use anything other than toe pads.

What do you do to make your arch look better?

I stretch my feet as often as possible. I try to remember to use each part of my foot, especially when rolling onto and off of pointe and when jumping.

What is your advice to beginners?

I would recommend to beginner students to find the most highly qualified teacher that they can, and then to listen. Be patient. Don't try to go on to advanced steps when you are not ready. Learning how to do everything properly from the beginning is much easier than having to go back and relearn when you are older.

Ashley Bouder
Principal Dancer
New York City Ballet

What pointe shoes do you use?

I currently am switching from Freed to Suffolk. In Freed, I wear 5 XX hp (heel pin). I three-quarter my shoes and have a combined shank (double). I get extra glue in my vamps, and I also put my own glue called Hot Stuff in the tips before I ever put them on. The sides of my pointe shoes are cut very low to allow more of my ankle to show when I point my foot.

Are your shoes custom-made? What are your requirements of the shoemaker? Have you ever met your cobbler?

My shoes are custom-made. I have never met any of my Freed makers over the years, but now that I am switching to the Suffolk brand, I have been working directly with Mark Suffolk. He is the owner and company founder and also makes shoes. He flew to NY and came to my dressing room at my theater with some trial pairs he had created from my spec cards from Freed. We tried everything on, discussed what I liked, what was comfortable, and what he thought might work better. It was amazingly helpful to hear directly from the maker and have an actual discussion about making my pointe shoes the best they can be.

How many pairs of shoes are you allowed each month?

There is no pointe shoe limit in NYCB, but if we are performing that month, I will typically wear between one and three pairs a day. I always wear a brand-new pair for each performance and start my day with either the pair from the night before or a brand-new pair. So in a performing month, I'll go through twenty-five to fifty pairs of shoes.

What type of foot do you have?

I have a square foot with short toes. I don't have bunions, but I do have a bunionette on the outside. I have a fairly high arch that allows light to show through when standing flat.

Do you wear any type of padding, and if yes, which one?

I do wear padding. I always wear a bit of lamb's wool between my fourth and fifth toes because I tend to get corns in there. And I cannot put my pointe shoes on without my Ouch Pouches, made by Bunheads. I wear the Ouch Pouch Jr., large size. A friend of mine is the founder of that company and used to be soloist with NYCB, so she really knows what a dancer needs. I would not dance without her products.

How do you sew your ribbons and elastics? How do you tie them on?

Yes, I sew my own pointe shoes. It takes me about five minutes per pair. I crisscross my elastics and attach them with the ribbons directly at my three-quarter cut in my shank. The other end is sewn at the back heel. I use the Bunheads tendonitis ribbons with elastic sewn where it goes over my Achilles tendon. I wrap the outside ribbon first, and then the inside over that and tie my knot on the inside of my ankle and tuck it under the crossed ribbons from the bottom right behind my anklebone.

What do you do to make your shoes last longer?

I always use very hard glue called Hot Stuff before I put my shoes on, but I also add glue as needed.

Do you wear your shoes interchangeably or always on the same foot?

I always wear my shoes on the same foot.

What technique do you use to break in your shoes? How many pointe shoes do you use on average in a month?

Before I wear my shoes, I apply glue in the tips, step on the shank, and mash it a bit with my hands and bang the edges so that I won't slip and I don't make too much noise running and landing from jumps.

How do you protect your toes from blisters, and what do you do if you get a blister the day before a performance?

The kind of toe pads I wear really prevent me from getting blisters, but they do happen. I usually either tape some Second Skin on it or a get a blister cover made by Band-Aid brand at the pharmacy. Those really help take away the pain.

What alterations do you do to your shoe?

I have my sides cut very low. They are one inch from the shank. I put extra glue up the sides of the vamp. My shank is combined, so doubled, and cut at the three-quarter mark. I also have a heel pin, which means I have a little extra height at the heel.

Do you Pan-Cake your shoes for performance?

I never Pan-Cake my shoes. It is not allowed at NYCB.

Do you darn your shoes?

I don't darn my shoes. I find it is a lot of extra work. I'd rather just put on a new pair of shoes and go.

How do you clean your pointe shoes?

I don't clean my pointe shoes. I don't really wear them long enough to be concerned with them being dirty.

Do you have any secret tip for pointe students?

Glue your shoes as soon as you feel them dying! Dancing on dead pointe shoes can cause injuries. You start using your foot in a weird way to compensate, and you can strain the top of your foot very easily.

Could you describe at least one exercise at the barre or in the center to help strengthen the feet?

I think one of the best exercises is attaching a Thera-Band to a pole or the end of the barre, inserting your leg in it, so that it pulls on your ankle and doing relevés facing every direction. This builds great strength and muscle awareness for every step you could do.

What type of accessories do you use?

I just use lamb's wool and Ouch Pouches.

What do you do to make your arch look better?

I never use anything to make my arch look better or different. I just have my shoes cut down so more of my arch shows.

What is your advice to beginner students?

From my teaching experience, I would say, please, please put your weight on the big toe! No sickle!

Mila Izotovich
Charleston Ballet Theatre
Charleston, South Carolina

Mila dances with the Charleston Ballet Theatre, danced with Metropolitan Classical Ballet, and spent two seasons as a guest principal artist for ballet companies in the United States.

What brand of pointe shoes do you wear?

I currently wear Mirella's. I started out in Repetto's when I was twelve years old. I have worn Chacott Veronese, Sansha, Bloch, Grishko, and Russian Pointe (Celeste and Entrada).

How would you describe your foot?

I have a low-profile foot with small sloping toes.

Do you wear any type of padding?

When I wore Blochs and Grishkos, I did not wear padding. However, the current fit of my Mirellas requires something to fill the spaces. Blisters are formed from friction. Thus, if your foot doesn't completely fill the shoe, or if the shoe is not the correct shape for your foot, you will have spaces, sliding, and blisters. I have preformed lamb's wool pads. I trim them down to cover just my toes and not my knuckles or the ball of my foot. I have worn paper towels, but I don't like how it rolls up and creates ridges.

How do you sew your ribbons?

I sew my ribbons generally along the seam in the pointe shoe. The idea is for the ribbon to elongate the look of my foot on pointe. If it is sewn too high, it cuts my ankle in half and decreases the appearance of curve and arch. Depending on the cut and shape of my pointe shoe, I have either criss-crossed elastic or a single one. If the shoe fits snugly and stays on my heel, I sew a single elastic from the corner of my heel to go under the anklebones and decrease wrinkling and bulging when en pointe.

If the style of pointe shoe I am wearing slips off my foot, I will sew crossed elastic, both of which are hidden or camouflaged by the ribbons. I sew the back of the elastic to keep the shoe on my heel and the front end of my elastic to help my ribbons pull the shoe closer to my foot when en pointe. Elastics should never be sewn so that they are visible past the ribbon (unless you have such arched feet that you need to keep your metatarsals in the shoe!) as it creates bulk and ugly lines.

I tie the inside ribbon one and a half times around my ankle, the outside ribbon twice around, and then tie them behind the outer anklebone. This hides the knot from the audience when I am in a turned-out position.

How do you soften your shoes?

If my shoes are hard (Grishko, Bloch, Sansha), I work the shoe to bend it and really work the demi-pointe flexibility. I never broke in Veronese or Mirella or Russian Pointes. My usage of shoes depends on the répertoire I am dancing, and how many rehearsals I have en pointe. A pair of shoes can generally last three performances in principal roles (like Sugar Plum pas de deux or three full-length Swan Lake). I need harder shoes for Sugar Plum as there are many pirouettes, piqués, and jumps on pointe. Swan Lake however, requires a softer shoe in spite of all the pas de deux work, because there is a lot of rolling onto and off of pointe. Sugar Plum is bright and sharp whereas Swan Lake is soft and like taffy.

What do you do to prevent blisters?

If I think I am getting blisters, I will either readjust my padding or tape my toes. Any kind of tape is good as long as it doesn't stick to the shoe and increases the friction! In case of blisters, raw egg white has been an extraordinary aid in healing broken skin. Once the blister area is clean, make an omelet and smear some egg white on before you throw away the shells. The egg white will dry in less than a minute. If I get a small blister the day before a performance, I'll tape it really tight the next day. If I get a big puffy blister, I'll clean it; pop it with a sterilized sharp object, just like a balloon; empty it; and tape it really tight.

How do you alter your shoes?

I don't like to buy shoes which need alteration because that means they do not fit correctly. I do spray clear acrylic spray paint in the boxes of my shoes (as opposed to Jet Glue or superglue) to increase the lifespan. Contrary to other methods, like glue or floor polish, the Kryolan does not make the shoe clack or bang once applied and can be applied multiple times. I usually wear my shoes once or twice to get the box as I like it, then spray a decent coat and let dry overnight. This prolongs the life of the shoe really significantly!

Do you Pan-Cake your shoes?

The appearance of my shoes is at the discretion of whichever director I am dancing for. NYCB likes shiny pointe shoes as does Bolshoi Ballet. However, I have heard directors say that only amateurs have shiny pointe shoes. If I need to Pan-Cake my shoes, I use whatever foundation I have on hand. Either a wet/dry foundation, or liquid, applied with a sponge.

Do you darn your shoes?

I darned my Grishkos and Russian Pointes as they have exceptionally narrow tips and the satin tended to tear in that area. I now trim my Mirella's when they begin to tear, and then I apply superglue to the edges so as not to get wrinkles!

Do you clean your shoes?

I don't clean my pointe shoes. If they are dirty, I Pan-Cake them. I do wash my lamb's wool pads.

What exercise do you suggest in order to strengthen feet?

Slow relevés without plié. No pliés. If you are trying to strengthen your feet, don't use your legs.

What type of accessories do you use?

I am now using makeup sponges cut in half as a toe spacer for an injury. I don't like objects in my shoes. They remind me of stones or pebbles while hiking!

How to you stretch your feet?

The arch of the foot comes from the top of the foot and is supported underneath. I stretch my feet by rolling a yoga mat into itself, placing my toe knuckles on at least midpoint of the roll and sitting on my heels. It is very important to remember to stretch the ankle and not the toes! Toes don't make an arch, the ankle does. The less fabric my pointe shoe has, the higher my arch looks because there is nothing hiding it. Stretch the tops of your ankles!

What is your advice?

Listen to your teachers. Find as many good teachers as you can. Expose yourself to as many wise and experienced teachers as possible!

Daria Klimentova
Prima Ballerina
English National Ballet

Daria wears Grishko ProFlex, size 3, super hard, 3 crosses. These shoes are especially made for her foot, and she describes them as "perfect." Her foot is narrow with short toes and a nice arch. She doesn't use any padding and any elastic. She sews the ribbons on the side of the shoe using a sewing machine.

Daria breaks her shoes in naturally, by putting them on and using them in class. She uses about five pairs a month. In order to protect her toes, she puts masking tape around them every time she uses pointe shoes, but she says she does not get blisters. She does not need to alter her shoes since Grishko does it for her: super hard, lower sides. She does Pan-Cake her shoes for performance using pink paint by Kryolan. She does not darn her shoes. In order to clean her shoes, she puts more wet paint or she throws them away.

She says she doesn't really have a secret tip for pointe students, but she believes you damage your feet less with Grishko shoes.

Here is an exercise she suggests to help strengthen the feet: "Sitting on the floor, flexing and pointing feet using Thera-Bands in order to get stronger calves."

Daria does not use any accessory, but she says that Grishko bends the heel on the shoe; she doesn't do anything herself.

Her advice for beginners' students: "Tape each toe. Don't wear shoes that are too soft but not too hard. Do a lot of exercises, step by step."

Adiarys Almeida Santana
Principal Dancer since 2008
Corella Ballet Castilla y Leon, Spain
(Artistic Director: Angel Corella)
Previously of Ballet Nacional de Cuba and Cincinnati Ballet

What pointe shoes do you use?

I use Bloch Serenade, special order. Maker Professional. Size/fit 2 1/2 C, platform – flat, vamp shape – STK, color fabric - European pink, drawstring – cord, insole – STK, Bloch formula - POP 6 cm.

Are your feet very arched?

I have a medium arch.

Do you wear any type of padding in your shoes?

Yes! I wear Bunheads Ouch Pouches Jr. Small.

How do you sew your ribbons and elastics? How do you tie them on?

The type of ribbon I use is Prima Soft Extension Stretch Ribbon, and my elastics are Freed Bulk 3/4 Wide Elastics. I sew the elastic and ribbon together in the middle of my arch, the ribbon on top of the elastic. Then I cross the elastics and sew it in the back by my heel. In order to tie them, I cross the ribbon that is on the outside of my foot and tie it around my ankle twice. Then I slide it through from down to up in the inside of my ankle to hold it. I do the same with the other ribbon and tie it to the first ribbon. I tie the knot on the top in the inside of my ankle, and I hide it into the ribbon. I used to sew it for security, but these ribbons I'm using now will never come undone.

What technique do you use to break in your shoes? How many pointe shoes do you average use in a month?

I usually use my pointe shoes in class first, and then I glue them to have them stay the way I like. I generally don't wear very new shoes for performances, but if I'm doing many shows, I sometimes have no choice. How many pointe shoes I use in a month depends on how much I'm dancing and what I'm dancing. If I'm doing contemporary ballets, where you don't really need hard shoes, I could say I use about three or four pairs a month. If I'm dancing something classic, I use more, maybe about five or six pairs a month, also counting that I wear them for class. I also use Daniel's pointe shoe glue, which helps a lot to make shoes last longer.

How do you protect your toes from blisters, and what do you do if you get a blister the day before a performance?

I usually don't put anything. Sometimes I tape my big toe. I usually don't get blisters anymore, but I remember I used to get a lot of them in school, I guess, because my feet were more sensitive. If I get one before a show, it is always going to be very painful, but you can always do something to make it a little better. Usually the best thing is Second Skin and also some product with a little numbing agent in it. I think all dancers are used to different pain. It's part of our profession, so we have to learn how to take care and balance it out and be professional enough that the audience won't know something is wrong.

What alterations do you do to your shoe?

I cut them three quarters inside. Then I slice the insole a little bit so it's not so sharp, and that way it won't make blisters in my arch. I take the sock liner and put it back in the original place and sew it inside the shoes. That way it won't roll up and make me feel uncomfortable while I'm dancing. I also sew the ribbons in the front for better balance and support. Also that way, they don't slip as much. I tie the drawstring into a knot and cut it. Then I sew it and hide it inside, putting a little piece of elastic on top. This elastic protects my toes from coming out of the shoes and hurting myself.

Do you Pan-Cake your shoes for performance? What product do you use?

I like them shiny. But when I dance bare legs, then I Pan-Cake them with Kryolan Aquacolor Makeup.

What technique do you use to darn your shoes?

I darn them in the front, for better balance and support. I cut a little piece of the satin in a circle. Then I start darning just on the satin all around the base of the shoe. After this, I repeat the darning taking the satin and the material below, so that way it won't come undone.

How do you clean your pointe shoes?

I use nail polish remover and a little piece of cotton.

Do you have any secret tip for pointe students?

Not really . . . just the crazy things I do to my shoes . . . but I think as a student, it's better not to do anything to them, at least the first few years. It's important to get the strength in your toes, ankles, demi-pointe, and arches. If they wear their pointe shoes the way they come, they will know if they are going on pointe correctly and if the position of the foot inside the shoes is correct.

Could you describe at least one exercise at the barre or in the center to help strengthening feet?

I think it's important to focus on using your demi-pointe, especially at the barre in every battement tendu, every rond de jambe par terre, etc.

I also recommend to take a pair of used pointe shoes, take the insole completely out, and smash them in the front with a hammer to make them softer, then use them at the barre as demi-pointe shoes, not as pointe shoes. This will make you work your arches better and will give you strength on pointe.

What type of accessories do you use?

None.

What do you do to make your arch look better?

Nothing. I just work on my pointe shoes and my foot works in class.

What is your advice for beginner students?

Ballet is a very hard career. You have to love it in order to do it. There are many things you have to go through—bad things, good things, it's all part of the experience, the discipline, it's all about learning. The lovely thing about it is that you can dance and act at the same time, and you get to express yourself, and that's what you bring onstage. I believe we all dance the way we are. We bring onstage our personalities, our feelings, our emotions, our passion for ballet—everything you have you give it out there. We are always learning. It doesn't matter if you are a student or a professional—you can always learn something new or improve on many things, and you can always dance better. Please enjoy it every second and work harder every day. "Don't leave for tomorrow what you can do today." But of course, very important, take care of your body.

Carla Korbes
Principal Dancer
Pacific Northwest Ballet
Seattle, Washington

Carla wears Innovation by Bob Martin. Bob Martin used to work for Freed and now runs his own company. Her shoe size is 4.5 XX with a heel pin. Carla's foot is pretty square, with short toes and flexible arches. She likes Innovations because they last longer, since her feet tend to break shoes very quickly. She always wears Ouch Pouches in her shoes—the large ones. She also needs a toe spacer between her big toe and second toe to make her feet feel more aligned.

She describes herself as very fast in sewing her shoes. Due to the large amount of shoes she generally needs, she figured out a way of using thicker thread and bigger stitches so that she can sew a pair of shoes in less than ten minutes.

She always glues the tips of her shoes with Hot Stuff before she wears them, in order to make them last longer. Once they are dry, she steps on the shanks with her heels to get them wider and softer. If the shoes are still too hard, she sprays some water on the fabric to soften the box. Since her shoes come already three-quartered, her shank is usually "ready to go."

If she is working on something like Swan Lake, she wears a pair of shoes a day. Otherwise she can wear a pair for three to four days.

She rarely gets blisters because she wears Ouch Pouches in her shoes. "The only toes that I tape are my little toes because I have calluses on them and sometimes they can be torn off if I don't tape them. If I do get a blister and I have to perform, I buy corn pads, cut the hole a little bit bigger than the blister, and then put it around the blister. That way there is less pressure on the blister itself.

Since Carla's shoes are custom-made, she doesn't need to make any alteration. "Every inch is measured to fit my foot. I like lower boxes so it doesn't cut into my insteps. And I like my heels to feel like they hug my foot, so not too short. And I order my shoes with a three-quarter shank."

She does not Pan-Cake her shoes for shows. If she needs flesh-colored shoes, her costume shop at Pacific Northwest ballet dyes them for her with spray paint.

She does not darn her shoes, and she does not clean her shoes. "By the time my shoes get dirty, they are also too soft for me to wear. So in that case, I need a new pair."

Her secret tip for pointe students: "When going on pointe, always remember to be completely over your arches. That way, when you go on pointe, your feet will look better and will also be stronger."

She suggests practicing simple relevés at the barre in order to strengthen the feet for pointe work. "You should do them with plié and also with straight legs. If I am coming back from vacation or I feel I don't have enough control and articulation on my feet, I usually do a lot of relevés to reconnect the muscles on my feet, as well as around my ankles, thighs, and gluts."

In order to make her arch look better, she suggests finding a shoe that hugs the foot. "A shoe that is too big hides the lines of your foot. And a shoe that is too small prevents dancers from articulating their feet and having their feet look at their best. Also, stretching the arches of your feet is always recommended so you can keep your flexibility."

She advises beginner students starting on pointe to "be smart and listen to your body. Pointe shoes can hurt in the beginning, and you just need to get used to them. But if you are hurting too much, take a break before the pain turns into an injury. Respect and love your body!"

Ashlee Dupre
Ballerina

Ashlee is currently working as a ballet chorus girl in The Phantom of the Opera in Vegas. She has also worked with Twyla Tharp in Moving Out, with NYTB as a soloist, and with Colorado Ballet as a corps de ballet. She originally trained at Kirov.

Ashlee wears Grishko 2007 (X-SS), and she describes her foot as narrow with a high arch. She wears Bunheads Ouch Pouch Jr.

How do you sew your elastics?

I sew my elastics by the heel and the ribbons at the top of my arch. I tie the ribbons starting with the outside one and then the inside, I double-knot by the inside bone and tuck them under.

When my shoes "die," I do not throw them out. I put them away, and in a couple of weeks or months, I use them again, maybe not for as long, but I still get to use them because they have hardened a little.

I wear my shoes on the same foot since my feet are different.

I usually step on the box and bend the arch, but not too much. I put them on and pour water over the top of the shoe so the pointe shoe molds to my feet, do some exercises in them, and take them off to dry. I repeat the next time I put them on. After the third use, they are perfect, and then possibly dead afterwards.

I don't usually get blisters, but when I do, I just handle the pain because nothing really takes it away.

I cut the top satin on the pointe shoes so it's less possible to slip. I do not Pan-Cake my shoes, unless my employer asks for them to be Pan-Caked. Otherwise, they usually recommend a product.

I do not do any darning. My tip for students is . . . find a pointe shoe you like. It might take a while, but in the end, you will be so much happier and healthier.

Exercise: Barre, relevés in first without hanging on the barre. Center. Piqués without turning, to learn where your center is and [to be sure] that you are really getting on to your shoe.

I don't use any accessories. I would not advise using fake arches (unless it looks natural). Put a towel on the floor with bare feet. Curl the towel using only your toes. Do not come off the barre until you feel ready. Be confident in yourself; otherwise you will be afraid to do a lot. Pointe is hard work, but once you get the hang of it, can feel really good.

Katia Garza
Company Member
Orlando Ballet

What pointe shoes do you use?

I wear Gaynor Minden 3-212-22.

What type of foot do you have?

Wide, short toes in diagonal with medium-high arch.

Do you wear any type of padding?

I just wear masking tape on my toes.

How do you sew your ribbons and elastics? How do you tie them on?

I sew the elastic in a cross from the heel to the arch, and the ribbons from the arch, trying to pull up the fabric of the pointe shoe as much as I can. I always try to have it almost like a sock.

What do you do to make your shoes last longer?

Gaynors last long, but I use moleskin, that I can buy at Walgreens or Walmart, and I cut it in squares and put it on the pointe shoe platform with tape. Then I put some makeup on it, so it looks the same color as the fabric.

Do you wear your shoes interchangeably or always on the same foot?

Always on the same foot.

The Magic of Pointe Shoes

What technique do you use to break in your shoes? How many pointe shoes do you use at an average in a month?

I use a hair dryer to break them in. Maybe I use two pairs in a month if I dance a lot.

How do you protect your toes from blisters, and what do you do if you get a blister the day before a performance?

I protect my toes with tape, and sometimes with Second Skin. Before a show, I usually put my feet in ice and leave them dry outside of the sheets of the bed.

What alterations do you do to your shoe?

None. Just the hair dryer in performances, so they look better.

Do you Pan-Cake your shoes for performance? What product do you use?

Powder is faster. And sometimes the Chacott Pan-Cake for body.

Do you darn your shoes?

No, I don't darn them.

How do you clean your pointe shoes?

If I need to, I clean them with a toothbrush little by little. So they don't get wet.

Do you have any secret tip for pointe students?

Pointe shoes have to feel comfortable even if it is painful in the beginning. They should feel good on your feet, at least when you are walking without dancing.

Could you describe at least one exercise at the barre or in the center to help strengthen the feet?

Very slow relevés with two fingers on the barre without plié. Just up and down, and with one foot in cou-de-pied; 16 pliés relevé and in passé. The same can be done in arabesque.

What type of accessories do you use?

Moleskin.

What do you do to make your arch look better?

Well-sewn elastics will make the ballet shoes look good. Breaking them [in] in the correct place is also very important. When I used Capezio, what helped me to make my shoes look better were the jelly pads because the jelly gets in the parts that my toes do not reach and make me stand better like if I had longer toes.

What is your advice for beginner students?

In the beginning, it is painful, but the skin will get used to it eventually. Do extra exercises to get stronger. This will give you freedom onstage and better jumps. It is important to strengthen every part of the body, not just the toes . . . the back, the stomach, and the legs.

Laura Bösenberg
Principal Dancer (since 2009)
Cape Town City Ballet
Cape Town, South Africa

Laura, what brand are your pointe shoes?

My pointe shoes are Gaynor Mindens size 8.5M 3-211-22 (right foot) and 9N-211-33 (left foot). Due to a toe injury a while back, I had to lengthen my left shoe. My toes are long, and I use the large Ouch Pouches for comfort and protection.

How do you like your ribbons sewn?

I like to sew my ribbons just before the side seams of my shoe attaching the elastics behind, then crisscross the elastic so that they meet at the back of the shoe.

Which is your break-in "ritual"?

To break in the shoe, I only need to sometimes blow-dry the backs for an extra curve in the back.

Do you Pan-Cake shoes for performances?

Yes, I do Pan-Cake my shoes for performances. I use Kryolan.
I just wipe my shoes with Pan-Cake to clean them.

Would you describe an exercise to strengthen feet?

Slow rises in parallel and first position at the barre, rising through the foot are always good, and relevés in first and second position.

Do you use any accessories?

I like to use toe separators to correct the alignment of my big toe.

Could you give advice to young students?

My advice would be to always enjoy what you do, do it for yourself and . . . practice makes perfect!

The Magic of Pointe Shoes

Tracy Jones
Artist
Corella Ballet, Spain
Madrid Spain

What pointe shoes do you use?

I use Bob Martin Innovation pointe shoes, size 5.5, X, extra insole.

Are your shoes custom-made? What are your requirements for the shoemaker?

Yes they are custom-made. I have been wearing them since I was fifteen, and I have met my shoemaker. My requirements are high vamp and a very hard shank, but cut at a specific point to where my arch bends.

How many pairs of shoes are you allowed each month in your company?

It depends on the repertoire and rehearsal/show timetable of each month.

Do you wear any type of padding, and if yes, which one?

I wear Ouch Pouches.

How do you sew your ribbons and elastics?

I sew them in crisscross, and I use special elastic ribbons that I order from the USA that let my tendons always move easily.

What do you do to make your shoes last longer?

I use shellac and Jet Glue around the areas that normally go soft first. I also darn the tops, as I feel that makes the shoe last longer and gives you a little extra support.

Do you wear your shoes interchangeably or always on the same foot?

Always on the same foot.

What technique do you use to break in your shoes?

I cut them about three quarters of the way up. I then bang them out on concrete so as to take out the sound and soften the demi-pointe. I wear them in class a few times before using them in a show.

How many pointe shoes do you use at an average in a month?

About eight pairs.

How do you protect your toes from blisters?

I use silicone gel toe pads called Ouch Pouches. If a blister does come up, though, I usually use Second Skin on it and tape.

What alterations do you do to your shoe?

I cut the shank.

Do you Pan-Cake your shoes for performance?

No, our director likes them shiny.

Do you darn your shoes? Can you describe the technique used?

I do darn my shoes, but only in a ring around the tip of the shoe. It gives me extra support and helps me to balance.

How do you clean your pointe shoes?

I use surgical spirit.

Do you have any secret tip for pointe students?

Make sure that you break your shoe in to fit your foot exactly. You will find it a lot easier to dance in.

Could you describe at least one exercise at the barre or in the center to help strengthen the feet?

I advise performing lots of relevés at the barre, especially executed on one leg and really going through the foot. You can also use a Thera-Band to help strengthen the toes.

What type of accessories do you use?

Just Ouch Pouches.

What do you do to make your arch look better?

I just make sure that the shoe is broken in so that it highlights my foot.

The Magic of Pointe Shoes

Michele Wiles
Principal Dancer
American Ballet Theatre

What pointe shoes do you use?

I use Bloch Synergy pointe shoes. I wear a size 5, width Y. High vamp and hard shank.

What type of foot do you have?

I have strong feet and a high arch.

Do you wear any type of padding?

I use one Handi Wipe and cut it up into two pieces. It protects my toes from blisters and keeps the sweat from melting my shoes.

How do you sew your ribbons and elastics? How do you tie them on?

I tie my pointe shoes, starting with the inside ribbon; wrap it once; then tie the outside ribbon once, tie both ribbons in a knot, and tuck them in. I also sew the ribbons to my tights for a performance, so I don't have to worry about them falling out. Another necessary ritual for my pointe shoes before performance is to add rosin to my heels (a squeaking noise lets me know I've put enough on) and feet, so I don't feel like I am slipping around.

What do you do to make your shoes last longer?

To make my shoes last longer, I leave them out at night to dry. During our performance weeks, the shoes last longer because I am in shape and I don't depend on the shoe as much.

Do you wear your shoes interchangeably or always on the same foot?

I cannot interchange my shoes because my feet are completely different from each other.

What do you do if you get a blister the day before a performance?

I wear Handi Wipes and the occasional tape to protect my toes from blisters. I usually get blisters from rehearsing. So I take an Advil or take a couple of days off because there is no sense in dealing with the ridiculous pain.

What alterations do you do to your shoe?

I cut the left shank down because my arch is lower on that side. Bloch has cut the sides down, given me a heel pin because I'm in between sizes, and made the box more flat."

How do you soften your shoes?

I use water to soften the box. Usually, taking center in your pointe shoes during class will break them in.

Do you have any secret tip for pointe students?

The key to strength on pointe is the relevé. You must remember you can't just go up. You have to push down into the floor to relevé.
Give your own advice for beginner students.
My advice is, these things take time. Be patient and . . . relevé!

Katie Williams
Dancer, Corps de Ballet (Second Year)
American Ballet Theatre

What pointe shoes do you use?

I currently wear the Bloch Sonata Mark II in a size 4C. This is a stock shoe with a full shank of medium hardness.

What type of foot do you have?

I have a Greek-type foot, with the second toe longer than the big toe, and a low arch.

Do you wear any type of padding?

I use the Ouch Pouch Pro Pads, which offer a thin layer of padding without gel on the bottom so you can still feel the floor.

How do you sew your ribbons and elastics? How do you tie them on?

I sew my ribbons from the crease in the shoe and use the Bloch kind with Achilles elastic sewn in to the ribbon. I use single wide elastic around the back of the heel, rather than two crossing elastics.

What do you do to make your shoes last longer?

My shoes are generally pretty durable, but to make them last longer, I will alternate between pairs to let them breathe, even waiting as long as a week, and then reusing a pair. After a while, the shoes will re-harden somewhat, so their life can be prolonged if you don't constantly use the same pair.

Do you wear your shoes interchangeably or always on the same foot?

I always wear my shoes on the same foot, because the arch of my left foot breaks slightly lower than my right, and so I cut the shank accordingly.

What technique do you use to break in your shoes, and how many do you use at an average in a month?

To break in my shoes, I cut the shank about three quarters of the way and remove the nail, then step on the box to widen it for my foot. In a month, I probably go through between eight and fifteen pairs of shoes, depending [on] if we are performing, which requires new shoes much more often, or just rehearsing.

How do you protect your toes from blisters, and what do you do if you get a blister the day before a performance?

I actually haven't had a blister in many years, because my Ouch Pouches really help to cushion my foot. However, I have used numbing gel and band-aids in the past to help with blisters.

What alterations do you do to your shoe?

My shoe is stock, so the only thing that I alter is the shank, by cutting it.

Do you Pan-Cake your shoes for performance? What product do you use?

For our classical productions, I don't need to Pan-Cake my shoes. But if we do a bare-legged ballet requiring nude shoes, I will use a liquid foundation from the drugstore and a sponge to Pan-Cake my shoes.

Do you darn your shoes?

No.

How do you clean your pointe shoes?

I go through my shoes so quickly that I don't have to clean them. They just go in the trash instead!

Do you have any secret tip for pointe students?

Try to experiment as much as possible with pointe shoes, because everyone's foot is different. A shoe that looks great on a friend may not fit your foot the same way, and a badly fitting pair of shoes can really affect your dancing and the health of your feet!

Could you describe at least one exercise at the barre or in the center to help strengthen the feet?

Relevés are the number one exercise for strengthening feet. At the barre, start in first position and do slow roll-ups with and without plié to gain strength and mold the shoe to your foot. It's also smart to do relevés on one foot, in coupé, passé, attitude, etc., because these will help you in the center when it comes time to turn.

What type of accessories do you use?

I put a makeup wedge in between my first and second toes to help align them in the shoe and protect my bunion. This also helps to even out my toes since I often have pain in my longer second toes.

What do you do to make your arch to look better?

I think rather than relying on a fake arch, it is best to find the right shoe to maximize the shape of your foot. The place where your arch is highest should match the place where the shoe breaks.

What is your advice to young students?

Be very patient when first starting out on pointe, and make sure to get the basics before attempting difficult steps or tricks. Having a good foundation will ultimately help you much more in the long run than being able to do 32 fouettés on pointe but with bad technique. Take it slow and focus on building strength first, and eventually the fouettés will be much easier!

April Giangeruso
Company Member
American Ballet Theatre II

What pointe shoes do you use?

I use Capezio Elan size 10.

What type of foot do you have?

Greek foot, high arch.

Do you wear any type of padding?

Ouch Pouch Jr. medium.

How do you sew your ribbons and elastics? How do you tie them on?

I crisscross thin elastic with ribbons, and I tie them around the ankle.

What do you do to make your shoes last longer?

I don't do anything special to make shoes last longer. I use one or two pairs a week.

Do you wear your shoes interchangeably or always on the same foot?

Always on the same foot.

What technique do you use to break in your shoes? How many pointe shoes do you average use in a month?

I just bend them slightly before I put them on, do a few relevés, and am ready to dance. I use about six pairs a month. I have always preferred the feeling of new shoes for most ballets, though there is the occasion where I prefer more broken-in shoes. If the stage is slippery or if the choreography is very fast or very slow, I need more broken-in shoes.

How do you protect your toes from blisters?

I have never had a problem getting blisters. My pointe shoes are very comfortable now. I have worn the same shoe for a long time and could basically wear them all day without taking them off. If by chance I would get a blister, I use Second Skin to cover it, and it works like magic.

What alterations do you do to your shoe?

I don't do anything to my shoes except have Capezio put in their quiet piece to lessen the noise.

What product do you use to Pan-Cake your shoes?

I use a little baby powder on the top and sides to lessen the shine. I am careful not to get it on the sole or tip because it could cause them to be slippery. I think that very shiny shoes are sometimes distracting.

Do you darn your shoes?

No, I don't.

How do you clean your pointe shoes?

I do not clean my pointe shoes.

Do you have any secret tip for pointe students?

It is important to get used [to] having pointe shoes on for long periods of time, so wear your shoes around the house: when you are cooking, eating, reading, watching TV, doing homework. It builds up your calluses and resistance to pain. It has really helped me to do that on long vacations because otherwise your skin gets soft, and then you come back and get blisters or sore toes. When you don't have to think about your feet hurting, you can just focus on the dancing.

Could you describe at least one exercise at the barre or in the center to help strengthen the feet?

I do a lot of relevés and Thera-Band exercises to strengthen my feet. I also love to do "toe pushups" at barre in my pointe shoes because it really strengthens your toes. Toe pushups are when you go to pointe and lower to demi-pointe and then push back up.

What type of accessories do you use?

I use toe spacers between my big and second toes and corn cushions between my fourth and fifth toes.

What do you do to make your arch look better?

Nothing.

What do you advise beginner students?

Do lots of Thera-Band exercises and relevés and listen to your teachers. They know what is best and do not practice without them present. Don't get discouraged if at first your feet hurt or you have difficulty. Once your strength improves, things will get easier.

Vanessa Woods
Professional Ballerina

Vanessa Woods is originally from Cinnaminson, New Jersey. She received her training from the Princeton Ballet School, Miami City Ballet, and at Purchase College (State University of New York). Upon completing her training in Miami, she moved to Denver to perform with the second company of the Colorado Ballet for two years. Following, she then performed with the Suzanne Farrell Ballet, Connecticut Ballet, Opera New Jersey, New Chamber Ballet, and the Pennsylvania Ballet. In August 2009, Vanessa moved to New York City to continue her freelance dance career.

What pointe shoes do you use?

Funny enough, I'm in the midst of changing pointe shoes again. Even after dancing on pointe for over thirteen years, I still am not convinced I found the perfect pair for me yet. I've been wearing Freed Studio Professionals, and now I'm trying Capezio Sylphide special order.

What type of foot do you have?

Tapered, with compressible toes and middle arch.

Do you wear any type of padding, and if yes, which one?

Very old Ouch Pouches.

How do you sew your ribbons and elastics? How do you tie them on?

I sew the elastics on the inside on the very back of the shoe and the ribbons right at the side inseam, leaving enough ribbon on each side to go around my ankle at least twice. I have the ribbon length down to a science, so that when I cut ribbons off old pairs, the new ones always tie in the same place on my ankle.

What do you do to make your shoes last longer?

Jet Glue! I couldn't live without it. I call it "liquid gold" and always joke that the best present for Christmas . . . would be a stocking full of Jet Glue. I also rotate my shoes and put them on my windowsill to dry every night.

Do you wear your shoes interchangeably or always on the same foot?

Always on the same foot. If not, they have a tendency to look sickled.

What technique do you use to break in your shoes? How many pointe shoes do you use at an average in a month?

I don't do too much to my shoes prior to wearing them. Depending on how hard the pair of shoes is, I might bend the arch and step on the box to make it flatter. I also sometimes wet my foot just around the demi-pointe of the box to soften it if I'm wearing it for barre. The amount of shoes I go through in a month always varies depending on what I'm performing. On average, my shoes tend to last a week, two if I am using a lot of glue and rotating several times for rehearsals and class.

How do you protect your toes from blisters, and what do you do if you get a blister the day before a performance?

I don't do anything to protect myself from blisters anymore. My feet are very used to pointe, so blisters are not an issue. If it happens before performance time, New Skin burn patches are a lifesaver.

What alterations do you do to your shoe?

I have a three-quarter shank, or skived shank, lowered sides and vamp and, depending on the shoe, a reinforced shank.

Do you Pan-Cake your shoes for performance? What product do you use?

I Pan-Cake my shoes only if we're doing a ballet that requires us to. If the company doesn't provide the exact color they want us to Pan-Cake with, I use rosin.

Do you darn your shoes?

No, I don't. Way too much time and effort!

How do you clean your pointe shoes?

Very simply, I don't.

Do you have any secret tip for pointe students?

The more you wear your pointe shoes, the less your feet will hurt. It seems the opposite, but just get through the pain in the beginning, and you'll eventually get to a state where you can go hours without them hurting.

Could you describe at least one exercise at the barre or in the center to help strengthen the feet?

Slow relevés at the barre in first and in coupé back, rolling through each and every part of the toe and foot, keeping your shoulders down and using your feet and legs and not your upper body.

What type of accessories do you use?

I don't use any accessories, except regular old masking tape if I need to.

What do you do to make your arch look better?

I work my feet every day to keep them strong and use a Thera-Band to strengthen my foot, toes, and arch so it continues to look better class by class.

What is your advice for beginner students?

Don't compare yourself to other girls in your class. Everyone learns at a different pace, as well as they develop and grow. I remember always feeling like the last to pick up new steps when I was in school, and I always compared myself to my best friend, who got the better parts, but you just have to work your hardest and block the competition out. If you stay positive and focused, you can remain motivated and passionate to work at your own personal best . . . and at the end of the day, what more could you ask for?

Deanna McBrearty
Ballet Teacher/Fitness Trainer
New York City Ballet
Former Dancer (1992-2004, NYCB)

What pointe shoes do you use?

I use special-order Capezio Odette, size 7 1/2 E, square vamp, and medium-strength shank.

Are your shoes custom-made? What are your requirements for the shoemaker?

Yes, they are custom-made. I specify to have the toe surface slant back slightly to assure the balance is over the toes and not straight up and down, because that is how my arch is shaped.

When you were in a ballet company, how many pairs of shoes were you allowed each month?

In NYCB we were allowed as many as we would go through. NYCB's pointe shoe specialist, Angel, keeps track of how many each dancer uses per month and orders accordingly to keep stock.

What type of foot do you have?

High arch.

Do you wear any type of padding?

Masking tape around individual toes, a bunion spacer between the big toe and the second toe, and one paper towel wrapped around all toes.

How do you sew your ribbons and elastics? How do you tie them on?

I sew them in eight minutes flat! I use heavy yarn/thread and make three loops around each end of elastic at the back of [the] heel of the shoe. Then I sew the elastic and ribbon on top of each other right behind the seam of the middle of the shoe to form and "X" shape to the elastics. I use ribbon with elastic presewn into it so that when I loop the ribbons around my ankles, the elastic part lies across the Achilles and allows for more flexibility and lessens the chances of tendonitis. The ribbons loop twice around the ankle, get tied on inside of the ankle, get cut to that length and the short ends, then get tucked in.

What do you do to make your shoes last longer?

I apply superglue to the inside of the tip of the toe vamp prior to wearing.

Do you wear your shoes interchangeably or always on the same foot?

I wear them on the same foot. I pronate so much on pointe due to my bunions that it makes it too unstable to switch because they get broken in on a slight slant towards the big toe.

What technique do you use to break in your shoes? How many pointe shoes do you use at an average in a month?

I use my fingers to place a bit of water across the demi-pointe to make them more pliable to roll through from demi onto pointe.

I bend the shank both ways, back and forth, to loosen the arch prior to wearing. When I do that, I make sure to hold the inside top of the shank down with my thumb so the staple doesn't pop out.

I probably went through approximately sixteen to twenty per month depending on the roles I had. If I had a lot of turning solos or parts that required long balancing, then I went through more shoes because I would wear a new pair each time. If I tried to wear soft shoes for roles like that, my balance wasn't as good. If I had a lot of jumping roles, then wearing shoes over again wasn't an issue. You want to wear a more broken-in shoe as it wouldn't be as loud for landings and it would be more pliable for pointing in the air.

How do you protect your toes from blisters?

Dancers have a high threshold for pain, so blisters don't keep you from dancing, and you don't even feel the pain while dancing because the adrenaline kicks in. You do, however, feel it afterwards, so it's best to protect the feet in advance. I used to wrap each toe with masking tape to cut down on friction on the skin. As well, I would wear a gel cap on my little toes to avoid the extra pressure the shoe would put on my pinky nails.

What alterations do you do to your shoe?

I take the paper insert out and line the shank with masking tape instead. The tape gave me a better grip for my foot and lasted longer than the paper, which would curl up under my arch.

What product do you use to Pan-Cake your shoes?

Regular face base for a role such as Arabian in Nutcracker, otherwise I didn't alter the color of the shoe.

Do you darn your shoes?

No.

How do you clean your pointe shoes?

I don't.

Do you have any secret tip for pointe students?

Pointe shoes last longer if you let them air out in between uses and if you superglue the inside tip.

Could you describe at least one exercise at the barre or in the center to help strengthen the feet?

Staying on relevé and slowly lowering from relevé on pointe to demi off pointe and back to relevé (never bending the knees and never lowering the heels down all the way to flat, just to demi-pointe).

What type of accessories do you use?

Gel toecaps for little toes, gel bunion spacers, masking tape, and superglue.

What do you do to make your arch look better?

All natural!

What is your own advice for beginner students?

The feet get stronger with practice. Just remember to start out slowly with exercises at the barre before trying anything in the center. You want a strong foundation built (which means strong ankles, toes, and toughened skin) prior to trying moves without support. You don't want to form any bad habits like jumping up onto pointe before you've learned the technique of rolling onto pointe, which comes from foot, ankle, and seat strength.

Megan Wood
Former Dancer
Ballet Opéra du Rhin
(Strasbourg, Mulhouse, Colmar)

What type of pointe shoes do you wear?

I mostly wear Freed's Classic SBT shoe, because they mold to my feet very well and are like a second skin. I am a size 3 1/2 XX, and I have an extra hard wing, so my foot is supported. And also, they last a bit longer.

Are your pointe shoes custom-made?

Fortunately, the pointe shoes I like to wear are standard shoes. I don't have to get them custom-made, which is lucky because I can get them straightaway without having to wait. I do prefer a couple of makers' style as they have a wider platform so it is better for balancing.

How many pairs of pointe shoes do you generally use in a month?

Normally I start off with six pairs, and then I take it from there, as it all depends on what kind of repertoire you are doing and how demanding the pointe work is.

How would you describe your foot?

I think I have a peasant foot, because my toes are quite similar in length starting from the second toe, and the ball of my foot is wider than the heel. However, I do have very slender feet with a very high arch, which in theory is perfect for a ballet dancer, but they do come with their problems. I feel very fortunate to have my feet.

Do you use padding?

I tried a lot of different paddings from lamb's wool to spongy inserts, but the best one I have found is called Happy Toes, (although I like to call them Happy Feet), and they really do keep my feet happy.

How do you sew your ribbons?

Firstly I choose which shoe I will wear on the right foot and left. Then I take a full length of ribbon (around 2 meters) and put it evenly under the arch of my foot in the pointe shoe. Once placed—where it will support my arch when en pointe—I will start to sew it either side. I have the ribbon under my arch in order to make sewing easier, but also for more support when working on pointe. Then I cut the ends of the ribbons so as they don't fray into inverted arrows. After this, I get four pieces of elastic and sew each of them at the back of the pointe shoe about two inches apart. Then I cross them over, and I sew the other ends just behind the ribbon. I need to crisscross my elastic to support my high arch in the shoe, otherwise my foot will slip out as the arch sits away from the shank. This could also cause injury. When I tie my ribbons, I start with the inside one wrapping it all the way around the ankle, then the same with the outside and tie them together just behind my anklebone in the small groove.

Do you re-harden your shoes?

Once my shoes are starting to get soft, I use wood hardener and a rotation of different pairs of shoes.

Do you always wear your shoes in the same foot?

I prefer to wear them on the same foot because of the way my foot works. Once the shoes mold to that individual foot, it is uncomfortable to change them around, and it throws me off balance.

What do you do to protect your feet from blisters?

To make the skin harder, I will use surgical spirit; however, if a blister does appear, I try to use waterproof plasters and wash it again with surgical spirit to try to stop infection and dry it out. Blisters can be very painful, so if I have a performance, luckily, the adrenaline takes over, and you can forget the pain, with the use of plasters.

What type of alterations do you perform on your shoes?

I don't make any alterations to my shoe as they are made just how I like them, and they support my foot extremely well.

Do you Pan-Cake your shoes?

I don't often Pan-Cake my shoes. I normally leave them shiny, but if we are required to, I will use calamine lotion if I wear pink tights. If I need to match my skin tone, I will use a Pan-Cake/foundation a shade darker than my skin so it matches when the stage lights hit the shoes.

Do you darn your shoes?

I don't darn my shoes anymore because it is time consuming, and also I go through my shoes too quickly. I darned when I was younger and used a spiral chain stitch starting from the middle of the platform to the edge. Sometimes if the satin is coming away from the platform, I cut it off to prevent fraying and slipping.

Do you clean your pointe shoes?

Normally I keep a clean pair for performance, but if I need to, I will either use calamine or use a strong product which the company has.

Can you suggest a valid exercise for strengthening feet?

The most important exercise for strengthening your feet in class is tendu. You should go through your foot on the way out and then exactly the same when coming back into your closed position. Doing this will build up your metatarsal muscles but will also help with precision and placement in all your work.

Do you use any accessories?

I tend not to use any accessories other than the Happy Toes padding as I feel it is important not to stuff your foot too much inside the pointe shoe. It could cause more damage because your feet cannot breathe, and you cannot feel the floor efficiently enough.

What would you advise beginner students?

Make sure you really look after your feet by having a proper pointe shoe fitting with someone who knows what they are doing, and who takes time and effort into getting you the perfect starter shoe. As your feet grow in strength and you get more advanced, you may have to change and try lots of different pointe shoes to find the perfect ones for you. This takes time, so be patient, and you will find the right pair.

It is vital that you continuously strengthen your feet with tendus, metatarsal raises and dyna band work so you don't injure yourself and you feel secure en pointe. Make sure you also have a strong core stability so you hold yourself properly en pointe, not sitting into your pointe shoes but pulling up out of them. If you sit into your shoes, you will hurt your toes because all of your weight is going through them, but also you could hurt your back if your stomach muscles are not supporting it during ballet. If your body and feet are strong, you will find pointe work easier, and you will advance more quickly, feeling secure and confident. Keep pushing through, and you will get there.

Celisa Diuana
Artist
The Royal Ballet, London

What are your current pointe shoes?

I use Freed's pointe shoes, single X, Anchor maker.

I see your shoes are custom-made. What type of specifications do you give your maker?

I want them flexible, so I ask them to take the pin off the heel. I haven't met my cobbler in person, but I know he's one of the oldest pointe shoe makers and very experienced.

How many pairs of pointe shoes do you use in a month?

I usually ask for four pairs a month, but sometimes I don't need that many. It all depends on the work I'm doing, the amount of dancing, and the type of choreography.

How would you describe your foot?

I have a Greek square foot with medium arch.

Do you use any type of toe pads?

I wear lamb's wool toe pads.

What do you do to re-harden your shoes?

I use shellac (it's a type of glue). I use a bit inside my shoes when they are brand new, and then let them dry in en pointe position, straight up with the block facing down.

Do you always wear them on the same foot?

Once they are worn the first time, I like to keep wearing them always on the same foot.

How do you break your shoes in?

I don't use any technique to break my shoes for one reason: they are never that hard!
Breaking them in with my feet helps them [in] molding with my foot shape. I usually go through four pairs a month, but again it depends how much work I have (considering rehearsals and shows) and what type of dancing I do. For example, if I'm doing Swan Lake shows and rehearsals, I need more shoes as the pointe work technique is more demanding.

How do you protect your feet from blisters?

I usually don't protect them, as they are naturally protected by the hard skin that I've developed over the years. But yes, I protect them if I have a blister on the day of a performance. I'd put an antiseptic cream or a numbing cream, and then a plaster on it.

What alterations do you do on your shoes?

I cut off the satin on the platform and shave (with a Stanley knife) the outside of the sole, so it's flatter.

Do you Pan-Cake your shoes for performances?

I do Pan-Cake them if it's required in the ballet. It depends on the style of the ballet or choice of the choreographer. I use a Pan-Cake used by professional makeup artists.

How do you clean your pointe shoes?

I clean them with surgical spirit.

How do you take care of your pointe shoes?

After wearing them for rehearsal, they are usually wet, so I hang them up, always with the block facing down, so it dries in the right position. If you are not careful, they can change shape while they dry, [which] can affect [their] balance ... and make them unstable. Sometimes I like to put a pointe shoe "shaper" in them after I wear them.

Can you share an exercise to strengthen the instep?

One really basic exercise is the metatarsal strengthening. Take the barre with both hands, then go up to full-pointe. From there lower to a high demi-pointe very slowly and then up again. Do that repetition about 10 times every day. It's an excellent first exercise on pointe to warm up, and also to keep the strength of your feet. In the center, relevés are really good. You can do them in first position and second.

Also, échappés from first to second position then back to first, 10 times, same from fifth position, really crossing the top of your thighs.

What do you do to make your feet look better?

I don't do anything to make my feet look better.

What advice can you give to beginners?

Start pointe work when your bones are strong enough to do it. I advise to start when you are twelve or thirteen years old—that is when I started. So you don't damage your feet bones and your bones are much stronger. Wait until your body is really ready for it. It's very important to be wise at the start point, so you can get things right from the very beginning. Dance with your heart. Make it appear as light as you can!

Ksenia Ovsyanick
Artist, English National Ballet

Ksenia is originally from Belarus. She started as a student at the English National Ballet School, then joined the ENB Company, where she actually dances.

What pointe shoes do you use?

I wear Grishko Fouetté, size 5 XXX, hard shank, ProFlex.

Are your shoes custom-made?

No, they aren't, but negotiating on it at the moment.

How many pairs of shoes are you allowed each month?

We are allowed ten pairs of shoes each month.

What type of foot do you have?

I have a Greek foot with medium arch.

Do you wear any type of padding?

No.

How do you sew and tie your ribbons and elastics?

I sew two invisible elastics so that they cross on top of the arch and the ribbons in between of them.

What do you do to make your shoes last longer?

With Grishko shoes, I find that they last quite long, so I never actually do anything.

Do you wear your shoes always on the same foot?

Always the same foot. My shoes tend to take the shape of my foot after a while.

What technique do you use to break in your shoes? How many pointe shoes do you use at an average in a month?

I averagely use four to six pairs a month, sometimes more depending on the intensity of the performances. I use my hands to soften the back of the shoe. I also step with my heel and all my weight on the vamp of the shoe to make it flatter and a bit wider. Sometimes, when I put my shoes on, I put some water on the bunion area to conform the shoes to the shape of my foot. It works perfectly with Grishko shoes, but I can't promise the same effect with other makers.

How do you protect your toes from blisters?

I've been quite lucky with blisters, as I always make sure that there is no space between the shoe and my foot. But if I do get a blister, I'd use some antiseptic cream and put plaster on it and, unfortunately, would have to deal with the pain.

What alterations do you do on your shoe?

I used to sew the backs of my shoe near the heel area, so that there is no extra material, but I find it not necessary anymore.

Do you pancake your shoes for performance? What product do you use?

"We usually have to pancake them for the performances. We're provided with Kryoline Pancake, but I usually just use rosin, putting it on my shoes with a tissue."

Do you darn your shoes?

Yes, I darn it around the edge of the shoe platform. Not sure how to describe it, but I go around about three times.

How do you clean your pointe shoes?

Just put some more Pan-Cake or rosin on the dirty patches.

Do you have any secret tip for pointe students?

If the shoes don't fit you perfectly, just experiment with sewing or cutting all the necessary parts.

Could you describe at least one exercise at the barre or in the center to help strengthen the feet?

All types of relevés on one leg or both are good for strengthening, but also doing all kinds of rolling through the foot and pushing over the arch (holding the barre) help to develop a beautiful arch. Balancing on one leg for a long time (aiming for a minute) is a great exercise too.

What type of accessories do you use?

I use toe spacers between my first and second toes, as I have quite big bunions.

What do you do to make your arch look better?

I tried to use fake arches, but it made my footwork weaker, so at the moment no tricks.

What is your advice for beginner students?

Personally I feel a bit scared if I don't feel the floor when I stand on pointe. It makes me dance worse, or even makes me fall. So make sure that you wear shoes that you feel confident in.

Jennifer Florquin
Dancer
Leipzig Ballet Company
Leipzig, Germany

Jennifer danced with Leipzig Ballet, Germany, and received her main education at the Jacqueline Kennedy Onassis School of American Ballet Theatre in New York and the English National Ballet School in London.

She also trained with the San Diego Academy of Ballet, Conservatoire National de Région de Montpellier, and San Francisco Ballet School.

What pointe shoes do you use?

I wear Capezio Glissés MS 10 medium with hard shank and long vamp.

Are your shoes custom-made?

No, they are not.

When you were in a ballet company, how many pairs of shoes were you allowed each month?

We were meant to try and not go over twelve pairs a month. Naturally, this amount is surpassed depending on the dancer's foot, rehearsals, and amount of performances.

What type of foot do you have?

I have the Giselle type of foot with a high arch.

Do you wear any type of padding?

Yes, I wear lamb's wool.

How do you sew your ribbons and elastics? How do you tie them on?

I crisscross thick Bloch elastics. I sew my Freed soft, not shiny ribbons with the front part of my elastics in a slight diagonal away from the ankle.

What do you do to make your shoes last longer?

First, I start by using Jet Glue on the tip of the shoe. Then I put some on the shank just about under the heel and when needed right at demi-pointe. When I am done with class, rehearsal, or performance, I put my shoes to dry upside down and let gravity get the moisture out of the box. Most importantly, I alternate my shoes a lot, to allow them to dry. Often, I will find a pair that is usable weeks or even months later!

Do you wear your shoes interchangeably or always on the same foot?

I would never alternate shoes on my feet. I find that to be dangerous, because all of a sudden your feet are asked to use slightly different muscles. Pointe shoes should be like gloves and mold to your feet.

What technique do you use to break in your shoes?

I really don't do much at all. I slightly bend the shoe under my arch. I put a little bit of water with a piece of cloth at the top of the vamp. There is nothing like a good pointe barre to break in your shoes properly.

How do you protect your toes from blisters?

I am rarely bothered by blisters. If I do get one, I disinfect it, and simply put a Band-Aid and roll it up with toe tape.

What alterations do you do on your shoe?

I don't do alterations to my shoes.

Do you Pan-Cake your shoes for performance? What product do you use?

Yes, but that would depend on the ballet. I use calamine lotion to Pan-Cake my shoes.

Do you darn your shoes?

No, I don't.

How do you clean your pointe shoes?

My shoes don't last that long, so I don't find that I have to clean them. Like I said, it is important that you aerate them in a dry place. Also, calamine is great for hiding dirty spots.

Do you have any secret tip for pointe students?

Even if pointe barre can be long and sometimes painful and you would just like to get to do center exercises such as pirouettes, it is nevertheless so important in your training whether you are a student or a professional.

Could you describe at least one exercise at the barre or in the center to help strengthen the feet?

I think it is important to have a balance of different exercises: rolling through the feet exercises, rising with almost a slight jump on pointe exercises, and consecutive relevés.

What type of accessories do you use?

I don't use any accessories.

What do you do to make your arch look better?

During all of my dance training, and still now as a professional, I always think of how my feet look in every angle! Your feet are just as expressive as your hands in dance. Especially in ballet, your pointe finishes the line of your leg just like the period in a phrase. Your feet should not only point, but also tell a story.

What is your advice for beginner students?

Be sure to have teachers that teach dance technique in a healthy way and that clearly understand how anatomy works with dance. When injured, heal it completely, or you may regret it!

Really getting exposure to dance is important—from seeing a performance, to going to a summer course, to competitions and auditions. This is how you will meet other dancers, teachers, and possibly directors who might want to work with you.

Most importantly, it is your determination that will get you far. Not one teacher or dance school can make you become a professional dancer, but it has to come from you. It is a really hard career, and that is why you have to constantly remind yourself why you are dancing. That is because you love it and that you have that drive in you to keep going and not give up.

Chapter 3

Sample Pointe Exercises

Here I will provide some examples of beginners pointe classes.

Beginners Class

First Trimester

Barre

Start with parallel feet (sixth position) facing the barre. Arms bras bas.

1-2: Hold
3-4: Place hands on barre

1 Right foot to demi-pointe
2 Full-pointe
3 Demi-pointe
4 Lower down
4-8 Repeat with the same foot

1 Cross right foot across left with fully pointed foot
2 Bend supporting leg, pushing right instep to bend shoe.
3-4 Stretch devant off the ground parallel and close parallel.
5-8 Repeat with left foot.
8-16 Repeat the whole exercise.

Facing the barre, feet in first position:

1-2 Tendu to second position closing first.
3-4 Repeat closing with demi-plié.
5-8 Tendu to second and lunge pushing on the instep then close first position.
1-8 Repeat to left.
1-32 Repeat all.

Second Trimester

Facing the barre –, feet in first position:

1 Demi-plié in first position.

2   Rise on pointe, retaining the plié.
3   Stretch the knees.
4   Lower down the heels.
    Repeat 3 times then reverse the exercise.

1   1 rise in first position.
2   Demi-plié on pointe.
3   Lower down the heels in demi-plié.
4   Stretch the knees.

Repeat the whole exercise in second position.

Famous Dancers' Statements About Shoes

If no pointe existed, I would not be a choreographer!

—George Balanchine

A la question "Qu'est-ce-que pour vous la Danse? à laquelle je n'ai jamais su répondre, quatre lignes me sont venues à l'esprit. Quand les mots manquent, Quand le geste ne suffit plus, du fond du corps, à fleur des sens, l'art prend son envol ... le vécu devient DANSE."

—Jean- Claude Giorgini

" If something is wrong with my shoes, what I'm dancing can be destroyed." Sorine, D. and Sorine, S. (1979) Dancer Shoes. New York: Alfred A. Knopf, Inc.

—Carla Fracci

"If I happen to have on a really special pair of shoes for a performance, it can make all the difference in the world." Sorine, D. and Sorine, S. (1979) Dancer Shoes. New York: Alfred A. Knopf, Inc.

—Victoria Tennant

"I take care of them; otherwise they will neve take care of me." Sorine, D. and Sorine, S. (1979) Dancer Shoes. New York: Alfred A. Knopf, Inc.

—Mikhail Baryshnikov

"Because some shoes have lumpy, distorted tips, heels that are too long, or shanks that aren't equal in lengths, I have to treat each shoe individually." Sorine, D. and Sorine, S. (1979) Dancer Shoes. New York: Alfred A. Knopf, Inc.

—Gelsey Kirkland

Glossary

Achilles tendon: The largest tendon in the body, connecting the calf muscles to the heel bone.
Aplomb: Self-confidence
Arabesque: Position of the body where the dancer stands on one leg, while the other leg is extended behind the body, with both knees straight.
Articulation: Place where bones meet to form a joint.
Cartilage: Specialized form of connective tissue with varying amounts of intercellular matrix that is nonvascular and found in various parts of the body.
Corps de ballet: Group of dancers who are not soloists
Échappé: Opening of both feet from a closed to an open position
Étoile: French word for "principal dancer"
Fracture: Broken bone
Genu valgum: Knock-knee
Genu varum: Bow leg
Hammertoes: Deformity of the second, third, or fourth toe.
Hyperextension: The extension of joints, muscles, or tendons beyond the normal limit.
Ligament: Band of strong fibers connecting bones
Maître de ballet: Ballet master
Metatarsal area: The area just before the toes, also known as "ball of the foot."
Metatarsalgia: Painful condition affecting the ball of the foot or metatarsal area
Plantar fasciitis: Irritation and swelling of the thick tissue on the bottom of the foot
Podiatrist: Doctor specializing in the diagnosis and treatment of problems and diseases related to the foot
Principal: Highest rank a dancer can reach within a ballet company
Pronation: The act of rolling to the inner side of the foot when standing
Relevé: Rising on the demi-pointe or pointe with a slight springing action
Scoliosis: Lateral curvature of the spine
Shin splints: Painful condition in the shin
Sprain: Injury to ligaments due to their stretching beyond normal capacity
Stress fracture: Small crack in a bone
Supination: Excessive outward rolling motion of foot or ankle
Tendinitis: Irritation, inflammation, and selling of a tendon.
Tendon: Band of fibrous connective tissue that forms the end of a muscle and inserts into a bone controlling the direction of muscle pull

Bibliography

Books

Arnheim, Daniel D. Dance Injuries Their Prevention and Care. Princeton, NJ: Princeton Book Company, 1991.
Arnot, Michelle. Foot Notes. New York: Doubleday/Dolphin, 1980.
Barringer, Janice and Sarah Schlesinger. The Pointe Book: Shoes, Training and Technique. Hightstown, NJ: Princeton Book Company, 2004.
Dandré, Victor. Anna Pavlova in Art and Life. London: Benjamin Bloom, 1932.
Guest, Ivor. The Romantic Ballet in Paris. London: Isaac Pitman, 1966.
Hall, Coryne. Imperial Dancer. Gloucestershire: Sutton Publishing Ltd., Phoenix Mill Thrupp,Stroud, 2005.
Hyden, Walford. Pavlova the Genius of Dance. Boston: Little, Brown and Company, 1931.
Howell, Lisa. The Perfect Pointe. 2006.
Jeannin, Christine. Chaussons de Pointes. Paris: Editions DesIris, 2007.
Juon, Esther. Pointe Shoe Secrets. Switzerland: Ebnother Druck AG, 1995.
Levinson, André. Marie Taglioni. London: Dance Books Ltd., 1930.
Lawson, Joan. Teaching Young Dancers. London: A & C Black, 1984.
Lawson, Joan. The Teaching of Classical Ballet. London: A & C Black, 1983.
Mara, Thalia. On Your Toes. New York: Dance Horizons, 1972.
Mara, Thalia and Barringer, Janice. On Pointe: Basic Pointe Work – Beginner - Low Intermediate and a Look at the USA International Ballet Competition. Hightstown, NJ: Princeton Book Company Publishers, 2005.
Page, Ruth. Class Notes on Dance Classes Around the World: 1915-1980. Princeton, NJ: Princeton Book Company, 1984.
Priddin, Deirdre. The Art of the Dance in French Literature from Theophile Gautier to Paul Valery. London: Adam and Charles Black, 1952.
Reinhardt, Angela. Ponte Shoes: Tips and Tricks. Alton, Hampshire, England: Dance Books Ltd., 2008.
Roberts, Elizabeth H. On Your Feet. Rodale Press, Book Division, 1975, 1980.
Ryman, Rhonda. Dictionary of Classical Ballet Terminology. London: Royal Academy of Dance, 1995.
Sorine, Daniel and Stephanie Sorine. Dancershoes. New York: Alfred Knopf, 1979.
Sparger, Celia. Anatomy and Ballet. London: A & C Black Ltd., 1970
Spilken, Terry L. The Dancer's Foot Book. Princeton, NJ: Princeton Book Company, 1990.
Terry, Walter. On Pointe. New York: Dodd Mead, 1962.
The Royal Academy of Dance. The Foundations of Classical Ballet Technique. London: Royal Academy of Dance, 1997.

Vaillat, Leandre. La Taglioni ou La Vie d'une Danseuse. Editions Albin Michel, Paris, 1942.

Vincent, L. M. The Dancer's Book of Health. Princeton, NJ: Princeton Book Company, 1988.

———. Competing with the Sylph: Dancers and the Pursuits of the Ideal Body. New York: Berkeley, 1979.

Articles

Attfield, Michele. "Evolution of the Pointe." Dancing Times (July 2003): 25, 27.

Bentley, Tony. "The Heart and Sole of a Ballerina's Art: Her Toe Shoes." Smithsonian 15 (June 1984).

Glasstone, Richard. "Some thoughts on Pointe Work." Dancing Times (1997).

Guest, Ivor. "Pioneers of the Pointes." Dancing Times: 5-7.

Horosko, Marian. "If the Shoe Fits. Part I: Guide to Pointe Shoes." Dance Magazine (April 1986): 80-81.

McCormack, Moira. "Straight to the Pointe." Dance Gazette. No. 3 (2001): 44-45.

Nuckey, Jean. "Pointe Work at Pre-Elementary and Elementary Level." Dance Gazette. No. 3 (1997): 32-33.

Russel, Jacob Hale. "Unhappy Feet: Ballerinas' New Lament." The Wall Street Journal (December 1966).

Taylor, Angela. "The Making of a Pointe Shoe: Part II." Dancing Times (August 1991): 1043-1044.

Tobias, Tobi. "Toe Shoes: The Satin Thorns Under Every Ballerina's Feet." New York Times (21 September 1975): III, 26:1.

Trucco, Terry. "Pointe of No Return. Dance Magazine (December 1993): 60-65.

Electronic Sources

Buxton, D. M.,
http://www.foot.com

Ballet News

Videography
Patricia Barker "On Pointe Shoes".

Resources
Pointe Shoe Experts

Michele Attfield – Freed of London Ltd., London
Mary Carpenter – Professional pointe shoe fitter, New York
Zoe Cleland – Fitter, Capezio Pointe Shoe Factory, New York
Michael Clifford – Pointe shoe master at Birmingham Royal Ballet, Birmingham, England
Julie Heggie – Pointe shoe mistress at English National Ballet, London
Jane Latimer – Pointe shoe mistress at London's Royal Ballet
Judy Weiss – Grishko Fitter, New York
Marlena Juniman – President of Prima-Soft Pointe Shoes
Pointe Shoe Makers
Bob Martin – Innovations Pointe Shoes
Ushi Nagar – Pointe shoe maker
Gary Brooks – Factory manager at Freed of London
Dawn Terlizzzi – Manager, Special Makeup Wholesale Division, Capezio Pointe Shoe Factory
Michael Thoraval - Founder of Capulet Pointe Shoes
Luca Bogarelli – Founder of Coppelia Pointe Shoes, Italy
Vanna Porselli – President of Porselli Pointe Shoes, Italy
Eliza Minden – Founder of Gaynor Minden Pointe Shoes
Jean Teplitsky – Teplov Pointe Shoes
Doctors, Podiatrists, Osteopaths, and Physiotherapists
Dr. Frank M. Sinkoe – Podiatrist for Atlanta Ballet
Dr. Margaret Papoutsis – Osteopath – The Margaret Papoutsis Practice, London
Dr. Simon Costain – Podiatrist, founder of The Gait and Posture Clinic, London
Ginette Van Hamel – Sports physiotherapist, consultant physiotherapist at National Ballet of Canada

Index

A

Académie de Danse Princesse Grace,217,223
Accademia Nazionale de Danza, Roma,58,59
accessories, pointe shoe
accessories, 4, 96,105,113,191,198,232,243, 293,308,320,326,332
Achilles tendinitis,57,62,187,205
Achilles tendon,62,81,83,95,171,187,202, 203,206,210,254,263,285,337
age to begin pointe work,202,205,210,260, 265,271,273,275,277,280
Aguero, Carolina Maria,283,293
alcohol, to soften shoes,67,78,89,90,96,100, 189,245,262,272
Almeida, Adyaris,127,283,303
alterations in shoes,72,89,157,158,325
American Ballet Theatre,School, 330
analgesic,194,195
Angelova, Violeta,283,291
Alekzander, Aria,156
ankles,33,35,37,38,48,50,65,77,81,82,92, 167,173,185,190,205,233-235,241,255,263, 264,273,274,278,292,294,302,305,306, 321,323
anklebone,81,83,170,179,244,276,292,298, 301,324
ankle joint,49,92
arabesque,10,
arches of foot,15,
Ardizzone, Remy,49
Arnheim, Daniel,57
Arnot, Michelle,42,187
articulation,55,117,168,169,171,264,307
Ash, Aesha,99
Asylmouratova, Altynai,221,222
Atlanta Ballet,28,126,130,202,340
Attfield, Michele,13,14,15,17,19,
Avdotia, Istomina,1

B

back seam of pointe shoe,27,33,77,82,95,284
Balanchine, George,3,4,47,50,64,70,72,130, 220,221,284,291,336
Balle, Niels,219
Ballet du Nord,28
Ballets Russes de Monte Carlo,220
Barker, Patricia,62,127,336,339
Baronova, Irina,98,105
Beauchamps, Pierre,216
Bedells, Phyllis,216
Beevers, Carol,36,62
beginner classes, samples,334
Béjart, Maurice,148
Belyea, Suzanne,192
Bentley, Toni,15,89
Beretta, Caterina,221
Besobrasova, Marika,217
bespoke shoes,18,21,
Bias, Fanny,6,
binding room, 19,22,
Birmingham Royal Ballet,129,131,215,340
Blasis, Carlo,221
Blessington, Lady,1
blisters, vi,67,68,72,84,85,188-190,194,198,

201, 226-228,229,231,233,236-238,246, 247,286,288,289,293,296,299-301,303, 304,306, 313,315,317-319,322,325,329, 332
Bloch, Jacob,105
Blocks (pointe shoe blocks),3,20,21,27, 30-35, 50,65,72,73,74-78,82,87,88,90, 92 ,96, 97-100,106,124,125,128,132,135, 136, 147,157, 166,180,190,196,199,210, 212, 224,229,237,260, 262,273,292,320, 327
Bogarelli, Luca,148,340
Bolle, Roberto,116
bones of foot,41,56,58,59,260,301,328
Boone, Kristi,156
Bouder, Ashley,128,283,297
Bournonville, August,218,219
Bosenberg, Laura,127,283,310
Boston Ballet,74,85,127,128,145,150,155,156, 283,289
bowlegs,43
box. See toe boxes
Braver, Richard T.,58
breaking in of new shoes,75,86,88,169,170
Brill, Ruth,2,73
Broadway, Dance Center,268
Bromberg, Emily,150
Brooks, Gary,17-18-19-20-21,23
Brothers, Crystal,82,97
Brynd, Bryony,80
Brugnoli Amalia,1,6,
Bunheads Dance Accessories,67,76,84,169, 174,191,198,200,224,227,228,239,268,286, 298,299,304,307

bunionettes,298
bunions,vi,57,70,117,124,188,190,191,198, 200,202,204,211,234,235,237,246,294,298, 322
Burke, Ginger,274
bursitis,57
Bussel, Darcey,47,72,96
Butler, University,172
Buxton, Dianne M,48

C

Calamine lotion,78,90,226,227,229,231,234, 237,238,245,258,325,332
calcaneous (heel bone),41
calluses,47,60,67,193,199,212,234,244,289, 306,318
canvas,22,30,36,67,97,11,116,119,129
Capezio, Salvatore,10,107
Capezio Ballet Makers,15,174,198
Capulet, Pointe Shoes,14,15,
cardboard,34,64,75,113,115,149,234
Carolina Ballet, 24
Carpenter, Mary,172
cartilage,335,361
Caselli, Mark,202,361
Castellini, Cecilia,1,361
Catbas, Cem,251,269
Cecchetti, Enrico,10,28,215,221,233,239
Chalendard, Anaïs,64
Chazin Bennahum, Judith,1
Cheesman, Dianne,251,255
Cheung, Josephine,224,246
Chivers, Beth,110
Chung, Chris E., 49

Ciapponi, Nicole,227
Cincinnati Ballet Company,172
Cleland, Zoe,167,340
clicker, 23
Clifford, Michael,129,131,340
cobbler,18-19, 20,75,107,111,112,115,122, 144,145, 149,151,158,242
Cojocaru, Alina,127,156
compressible foot,246
Contin-Souza,74
Conti, Stephen, F.,45,183,193
Coppelia, Pointe Shoes,109,148,340
Cormani, Lucia,216
Costain, Simon,210,340
Coulon, Jean Francois,1,6
Cornejo, Erica,156
corn padding,233,306
corns,74,193,198,200,212,298
Cornwall, Verena,223
cost of pointe shoes,65
costumes,22,113,134,
Coulon, Jean-Francois, 5
Covent Garden, 2
Crait, 2
crown,31,168,169,170
custom-made shoes,18,22,75,88,107,121,122 126,165,296

D

dancer's heel,32, 173
Dandré, Victor,3,10
Danilova, Alexandra,220
Danilova, Maria,1
DanzTech, Inc.,200

darning of shoes,10
Del Caro, Maria,1
DeMike, Bernadine,274
demi-plié,52,92,164,187,224,253,254,261, 263,264,269,272,274,279,334,335
De Valois, Ninette,215
De Voisins, Gilbert,7
Didelot, Charles Louis,1
Diuana, Celisa,74,283,326
drawstrings,22,23,27,30,31,33,62,76,78,108, 116,119,121,132,176,201,228,229,233,240, 261,262,289,305
   cotton,108
   elastic,108,117,121,245
   tying,
drying of shoes,19,100,133,144,171
Dvorovenko, Irina,128
Dudin, Hélène,220
Dujardin, Charline,283,286
Dupont, Aurélie,128
Duval, Franck Raoul,119
dyeing of shoes,132,133,135,211,287

E

Eagling, Wayne,223
Ebermann, 2
échappé,58,86,92,175,236,239,252,256,257, 263,269,274,279,292,295,337
Egyptian foot,230
Eks, Mat,13
elastic,vi,31,37,48,63,64,72-74,77,78,80-82, 87,89,95,98,106,108,110,,117,121,165,170, 174,187,198-200, 202,205,206,224,227-230, 233-236,238,240,242,243-247,253,

256,263,266,269,272,273,276,278,281,
284-287,289,292-296,298, 301,303-305,
307,308,310,314,317,319,321, 324,329,331
elastomeric, materials,113
Elmhurst, School of Dance,134
Elssler Fanny,2,7
Espinosa, Edouard,215,216
Evans, Anya,iii,251,270
Exacto knife,96,201

F
Fabulon,90,99
Factor, Max,100,245,289
Fairchild, Megan,81
Fallen arches,192,209
Fang, Zhong-Jing,156
Farrell, Suzanne,80,156,220,291,318
Fatigue,6,51,206
Feet, v,vi,vii,1,5,9,13-15,28,31,35-37,41-43,
    45,47-50,55,57-66,70-76,78,79,82,84,86-92
    105,114,115,117,121,124,126,128, 131,137,
    151-153,158,163-166,169-173,175,179,180,
    183,185,189,191,193,196,200,204,205,207,
    208,211,212,224-226,229,231-244,246,247,
    253,255-257,259,261-266,268,271,274-276,
    284-297,301-304,306,307,309,313,315,318-
    320,322,323,325-328,331,332,334,337
    types of,44
Filpi, Francesca,156
first fitting,61
first pointe class,
fit of shoes,70
flat feet,46,51,192
Flore et Zéphyre,1

Flyte, pointe shoes, 1
Fokine, Mikhail,10,
Fonteyn, Margot,148,216
foot,
    Giselle,228
    Grecian or Greek,316
    Egyptian,230
    peasant,324
Forskitt, Hayley,74
Forsythe, William,13
Fracci, Carla,78,116,336
Freed Frederick, Ltd.,18,110
Freed of London, Ltd.,14,15,17,20-21-22
Fuchs, Arthur,114
fouetté,2,124,284,316,328
Fuoco, Sofia,2
Fusco, Mara,251,252
Fuzi,111,174

G
Gamba, Ltd.,15,18-19,28,30,34,36 ,74,75,86,
    110,111,112,123-125,143,144,146,174
Gamba, Luigi,112
Gardner, Kim,49
Garza, Katia,127,282,308
Gautier, Theophile,2,5
Gaynor,Minden,14,15,28,32,34,64,73,86,89,
    112,113,123,124,127,128,153,155,157,174,
    198-200,229,246,260,261,265,294,308,310,
    340
Genée, Adeline,2,112,216,227
Genée Competition,227,236,239
Georges –Philippe Marie,7
genu valgum,43,337

Giangeruso, April,128,283,316
Giorgini, Jean-Claude,251,272,336
Giselle, ballet,44,65,78,285
Giselle foot,57,228
Glasstone, Richard,51,52
Golders Green Crematorium, 10
Gonchar, Nadia,156
Gorman, Keri,80
Gosselin Geneviève,1
Govrin, Gloria,49
Graham, Martha,148
Grahn, Lucile,2
Gregory, Cynthia,336
Grishko,14,15,36,69,75,87,95,113,123,124,125 127,175,178,224,227,228,232,234, 235,237, 238, 246,257,285,291,294,295,300-303,307, 328,329,340
Guest, Ivor,2,6,8

F

hallux Valgus,190,208,365
Hamilton, William,57
hammertoes,57,191,192,337
hamstrings,203,221,286,304,365
Hancock, Shirley,207,225,
hand-turned shoes, 15,33,115
hardening pointe shoes,98,99,136,229
Harrod, Elizabeth,365
heat therapy,187,188,203,210
heel, 6,14,24,32,33,35,41,42,43,45,47,50,62, 63,70,73,75-77,82,84,87,88,92,95,101,102, 106-108,121,124,125,135,147,153, 154,164 168-174,176-178,183,186-188,196,199,200, 206,211,226,227,229,230,235,237,238,240, 253,254,261-263,269,276,278,281,285,287 289,290,294-299,301-304,306-307, 314,321, 329, 331,336,337
heel bone (calcaneous),41,337
heel grippers,199
Heggie, Julie,iii,129,130,134,340
Heinz, William,187,190
hessian,14,20,27,29,33,34
history of pointe dancing,1,110
Holmes, Anna-Marie,289
Howard, David,172,192
Howard, Merrit,223,227
Howell, Lisa,338
Howse, Justin,58,207
Hudson, Anjuli,73,86
Hugo, Victor,5

I

icing of feet,184,186,207,211
ingrown toenails,62,188,189,238
injuries,vi,4,34,43,45,57,59,63, 70,135,183-185, 194,196,203,209,210,217,237,265,268, 299
insoles,27,72,120,121,186,200
instep,3,35,45,50,58,63,81-83, 92,116,117,133, 164,168,200,232,233,234,235,238,243,256, 257,266,268,269,272,286,292,334
Iozzo, Nadia,74,128
Istomina, Avdotia,1
Ivy House,9,10

J

Jansen Dance Project,iii
Janssen of Pairs, 2,7

Jarvis, Theresa,219
Jensen, Carrie,85
Jeppesen, Lis,218
Johnson, Sarah Elizabeth,223,233
Jones, Susan,251,280
Jones, Tracy,73,283,311
Juniman, Marlena,152,340
Juon, Esther,79,177

K
Kansas City Ballet,28,74,128,348
Kaplan, Joe,61,64,84,90
Karsten, Sophie,6
Kechacha, Rym,73
Kerche, Cecilia,284
Killian, Katrina,220
Kirkland, Gelsey,96,220,336
Kirstein, Lincoln,220
Kistler, Darci,220
Kitchens, Kylee,128
Klimentova, Daria,283,303
Kochetkova, Maria,150
Kondaurova, Ekaterina,128,156
Korbes, Carla,127,306
Kraszczuck, Pedro,109
Kschessinska, Mathilde,3

L
Lacarra, Lucia,127,283,293
Lakecities, Ballet,233
Lamy, Eugène,8
La Scala, Teatro,2,59,116,155,221
Lassenne, Pierre,115
last of shoe,15,18,20,21,22,27,28,106,143, 150,152
La Sylphide,5,7,8
Latimer, Jane,129,137,340
Lawson, Joan,58,63
Legnani, Pierina,2
Léon, Michel,2
Leonova, Marina,221
Les Ballets de Monte Carlo, 24,111,155,217
Les Grands Ballets Canadiens, 24,111,145
Levinson, André,8,
Lifar, Serge,148
ligaments,41-43,46,50,184,191,192, 204,208, 209,337
Littlefield, Dorothie,220
Livry, Emma,7,14
Long, Jordan-Elizabeth,283,296
Lully, Jean-Baptiste,216
lumbricles,45

M
Maciel De Faria, Andrea,283,290
Makarova, Natalia,148
maker symbol,18,21,33
Mara, Thalia,190
Margarosyan, Talar,55
Marlow, Jill,128
Martin, Karl Heinz,114,127,286
Martin, Bob and Pat,306
Martin, Michaela,114
Martins, Peter,336,220
Maryinsky Theatre,3,113,128,155,156,176,222
Masala, Luca,217
Maximova, Ekaterina,13,
McBrearty Deanna,283,321

McCormack, Moira,81,82
Melendez, Anne Marie,74,128
Merlet,115,124,125
Merlet, Roger James,115
metatarsalgia,185,337
metatarsals,47-50,67,99,117,119,120,164,166,
    168,170,173,185,186,191,199,204,212,234,
    256,259,261,267,274,278,288,296,301,325,
    326,328,337
Miami City Ballet School,4,222
Milwaukee Ballet,28,127
Minnesota Dance Theatre,49
moleskin,44,97,190,193,199,201,308,309
Montessu, Pauline,2
Moran, Linda,62
Morscher, Joanne,68,251,274
Mukhamedov, Irek,294
Mukhamedov, Sasha,283,294
Mullin, Michael J,187
Murphy, Gillian,127,156
muscles,1,7,35,37,41,42,45,48,49,51,59,187,
    188,194-196,202-207,209,211,246,265,278,
    280,289,307,325,326,331,337
Muus, Henriette,219

N

Nagar, Ushi,iii,26,28,31,75,87,122,340
nails,188,189,238,243,261,294,322,
National Ballet of Canada,55,85,155,205,340
narrow shoes,45
Neale, Wendy,60
neuromas,57,60
New York City Ballet, 15,50,57,81,89,128,
    129,220-222,283,297,321
Nichols, Kyra,70
Nicolini, Romeo,2,3,9
North Carolina Dance Theatre,128
Nourrit, Adolphe,7
Novella, Thomas,42,50
Noverre, Jean Georges,1
Nuckey, Jean,49,50,59

O

Obrasztsova, Yevghenia,156
Ogden, Heather,85
Olivieri, Frédéric,221
Onward, Kashiyama,111
Orlando Ballet,127,283,290,308
orthotics,187,208,212
Osmolkina, Ekaterina,156
osteopaths,340
Papoutsis, Margaret,iv,42,183,192,209,340
Ostergren, Tempe,74,85,128
Ovsyanick, Ksenia,283,328
Owens, Kyla,iii

P

Pacific Northwest Ballet,24,306
    School,227
padding of shoes,44,67,74,84,85,100,119,136,
    167,168,174,185,189,191,192,204,227,229-
    234,238,244,261,275,289,301,303,314,324,
    326
Palmer, Vanessa,156
pancake makeup on shoes,100,245,289,329
Papoutsis, Margaret,iv,42,183,192,209,340
    270,277-279,285,287,302,307,309,316,335
Parker, Danna,251,257

Paris Opéra,2,7,14,118,128,130,218
  Ballet School,216,217
Part, Veronika,156
Parrondo, Dalay,150
pas de Deux,65,74,78,221,224,229,243,301
paste,18,20,21,27,33,34,86,88,144,145
paste room, 22,23
Pavlova, Anna 2,3,9,10
  and pointe shoes, 3,14
  and shoemakers,3
Pearson, Michele,67,82
Pearson, Tanya,230,251,277
Pennsylvania Ballet, 24,111,145,318
Père Lachaise Cemetery, 8
Petipa, Marius,2
Petit, Roland,118
phalanges,173
physical therapists,205,340
  Hancock, Shirley,207
Pilates, Joseph,173,204,210,246
Pillows for Pointe, Inc.,227
piqué,1,269,279,280,282,301
pirouette,78,102,301,332
plantar fasciitis,51,183,185,186,337
Platel, Elisabeth,216
platform of shoe,3,10,13,18,21,23,27,28,30,
  31,35,65,73,74,75,77,87,89,90,96,99,106,
  107,108,113,115,116,121,124,133,136,
  145,147,150,151,154,169,178,199,229,
  247,308,324,325,327,330
pleats of shoe,21,27,32,33,77,84,96,97,113,
  135,144,199
plié,45,46,52,208,243,252,257,261,263,264,
  148,150,157

demi,52,164,187,224,228,253,254,269,272,
  274,279,334,335
grand,4,92,282
podiatrists,41,42,55,57,58,185,189,196,202,
  203,210,211,212,337
  Braver, Richard T.,58
  Costain, Simon,iv,210,340
  Lowell, Scott Weil,191
  Novella, Thomas,42,50
Poggini, Luana,58
pointe dancing,5
pointe,
  on,58,59,62,63,65,70,71,75,79,84,91,92,105
  113,121,133,134,136,147,150,157,164,166,
  168,169,171,185,187,189,198,202,205,210,
  227,232,234,238, 239,241,244,253,254,256,
  259-261,263,271-275,287,289,293,294,297,
  301,305,307,314,316,318,322-324, 332,
  335,336
Pointe shoes,
  alternating,266,284
  anatomy of,30
  and Romantic ballet,2,6,7
  breaking in,75,86-88,169,170
  cleaning,132,296
  cost of,65,126
  custom-made or
  bespoke,3,18,19,21,22,27,28,33,73,75,77,86,
  89,107,110,121,122,126-129,132,135,148,
  149,157,165,233,284,290,291,296,298,306,
  321,324
  fitting,46,61,69,121,144,261
  handmade,19,64,73,79,105,108, 134,143,
  narrow,5,10,13,45,70,106,107,108,113,117,

121,122,124,125,132,150,154, 164,167,169, 178,190,199,200,227,228,232,234,236,238, 244,269,276,302
  making of,13,15,18,19,20,26-29,34,105,107, 110-112,114,118,144,146,153
  unblocked shoes,2
  unpadded slippers, 2
pointe tendue,254
pointe training,35,57
polymers, 14,64,165
Porselli, co. Ltd.,14,15,97,116,148,253,272, 340
Porselli, Eugenio,116,148
Porselli, Vanna,14,116,148,340
posture,48,217,255,277-280
Preobrajenska, Olga,221
preparation of shoes,261
pre-pointe training,57
Pribisco, Pamela J.,99
Priddin, Deirdre,5
Prima Soft,116,117,123-125,152,153,198,235, 237,304,340
Prina, Annamaria,221
Principal pointe shoes, 117
Prix de Lausanne,230
pronation,49,187,192,211,337

R

Rambert Dance Company, 13
Ranieri, Ugo,251,272
readiness for pointe training,57
rehardening of shoes,98,99,136
Reid Lobatto, Linda,177
relevé,44,48,52,58,59,86,88,92,175,187,203, 205,226,228,229,236-238,245, 246,252,254, 257,259,260,262,264,269,271,273,274,279, 280,284,286, 288,291,295,296,297,300,302, 307,309,312,314,316-318,323,328,330,332, 337
Repetto,36,75,86,112,118,123,124,130,143, 174,300
  Repetto, Rose,118
Riaboushinska, Tatiana,105
ribbons,
  sewing of,76,80,199
  types of,80
Ricci, Benedetto,221
Richmond, Ballet,28,150
rises,49,52,55,58,59,73,86,92,229,231,236, 239,248,256,271,285
Roberts, Elizabeth H.,338
Roche, Nora,52
rock rosin,132,170,178,199
Roqueplan, Camille,1
Rojo, Tamara,111
rolling onto pointe,232,234,263,266,268,269, 276,297,301,323,330,332
romantic ballet,2,8
Royal Academy of Dance,28,35,37,49,52,58, 59,63,163,216
Royal Ballet,24
Royal Ballet School,15
Royal Danish Ballet,24
  school,
Royal Opera House,129,215
Royal Swedish Ballet School,218 258,284,306,320
Royal Winnipeg,28,155,205

Russian Pointe,14,36,105,118,119,123-125, 228,245,285,300,302
Ryman, Rhonda,52

S

San Francisco Ballet,24,28,49,111,128,150, 283,289,330
San Jose, Ballet,145,150,155
Sansha, Inc.,36,74,119,123-125,128,149,174, 225,226,237,255,286,300,301
Scacchi, Massimiliano,59
School of American Ballet,50,59,81,220,221, 270,330
schools,vi,55,149,163,172,179,202,205,218, 221,223,270
Schwartz, Keira,150
Sciturro, Christie,72
Scott, Weil, Lowrell,191
Seay, Deanna,156
sesamoiditis,183
shanks,2,3,14,27,28,64,73-75,89,101,111-113, 122,147-150,152,154,158,168,173,176,261, 262,266,271,274,275,291,306,336
  cardboard shanks,64,75,113,115,149
  cutting,87,101,290,315
  graduated,117,152,153
  hard,64,112,113,123,127,150,228,230 232,233,245,271,275,284,313,328,330
  leather shanks,148
  medium,108,113,114,178,227,232,233,238, 257,262,268,285
  memory,117
  three-quarter,75,88,114,123,151,168,169
  Heinz-Martin,114,127,286

shin splints,51,183,192,208,209,212,337
Shipulina, Ekaterina,156
shoe cleaning,132,296
darning,1,13,14,73,133,294,305
drying,100,133,171
re-hardening,98,99,136
softening,86,88,199,273
sewing ribbons,76,80,199
sewing elastics,73,77,81,82
Shoemakers, 3,10,18-19,26-28,135,144
  Bloch,15,34,36,75,86,88,105,106,123-125, 127,128,164,198,227,228,230,235-239,244, 253,272,290-292,300,301,303,313,314
  Bob Martin,87,107,112,127,128,143,234, 306,311,340
  Capezio, 10,15,28,30,34,36,58,86, 97,107, 108,123-125,127,128,130,144 ,145,167-171, 174,175,237,284,286,294,309,316, 317,319, 321,331,340
  Chacott,15,28,109,123-125,174,198,235,300, 309
  Coppelia,109,148,340
  Freed of London,17,109,128,163,198,296,340
  Fuzi International,111,174
  Gamba,18,19,28,30,34,36,74,75,86,107, 110-112,123-125,143,144,146,174
  Gaynor Minden,14,15,28,32,34,64,73,86,89, 112,113,123,124,127,128,153,155,157,174, 246,260,261,265,294,308,310,340
  Grishko,14,15,36,69,75,87,95,113,123-125, 127,175,178,224,227,228,232,234,235,237, 238,246,257,285,291,294,295,300-303,307, 328,329,340
  Mark Suffolk Pointe Shoe Co.,80,87,120,

121,124,128,174,227,239,297,298
Merlet,115,124,125
Nicolini,2,3,9,10
Prima Soft,116,117,123-125,152,153,198,
235,237,304,340
Principal,118
Porselli,14,15,97,116,148,253,272,340
Repetto,36,75,86,112,118,123,124,130,143,
174,300
Russian Pointe,14,36,105,118,119,123,124,
125,227,228,245,285,300,302
Sansha,36,74,119,123-125,128,149,174,225,
226,237,255,286,300,301
So Dança,109,119,123,242
Teplov,157,340
Triunfo,121-125
Ushi Nagar,26,28,31,75,87,122,340
Schwartz, Keiria,150
Sibley, Antoinette,28,216
sickling of feet,32,48,177
Signorelli, Luisa,251,265
Sinkoe, Frank, Doctor,202,340
shoes,
    bespoke shoes,19,77,132,149
    traditional shoes,34,154
Schorer,Suki,50,51,59
sickling of feet,32,48,177
Sleeping Beauty,78
Smith, Emily,223,229
Smolen, Molly,283,289
Snyder, Heather,55,57
soles,3,4,6,22,23,27,31,36,37,49,72-75,86,87,
89,96,112,120,164
Somova, Alina,156

Soto, Jack,220
Sparger, Celia,41-43,58
Spessiva, Olga,105
sprain,57,184,185,194-196,205,337
sprained ankles,185
Springer, Janet,274
Stannus, Edris,215
Stock, Gailene,215
stress fracture,50,185,337
stretching,6,48,49,187,203,204,209-212,224,
227,246,285,294,307,337
strain,50,51,168,187,194-196,202,260,261,299
Stuart, Muriel,220
Sturman, Majorie,255
Stuttgart Ballet, 24,
surgical spirit,289,311,325,327
Suffolk, Mark,80,87,120,121,124,128,174,
227,239,297,298
supination,49,337
Swan Lake,2,65,78,129,165,270,301,306,327
sylph,2
Sylphide, La,6,8

T
Taglioni, Filippo,4,5,7
Taglioni, Marie, 1,2,5,7,8,14,338
taglionniser, 5,
talcum powder,132
talus (ankle bone),41
tarsal bones,41
tarsus,58
Teatro di San Carlo, Napoli,272
tendonitis,46,57,62,82,187,203,205,207,209,
246,266,298,321

tendons,41,82,171,196,203,224,311,337
Tennant, Victoria,336
Teplitsky, Jean,157,340
   Georges,157
   Diane,157
Teplov, Pointe Shoes,157,340
Terabust, Elisabetta,80
Terlizzi, Dawn,144
Theleur, E. A.,2
thermoplastic, elastomerics,154
Thomas, Melissa,42,50
Thoraval, Michael,146
tibia,43,192,209
Tiger balm,195,201,356
tights,4,25,62,68,80,100,102,135,152,172,188, 190,196,231,238,293,325
toe boxes,154
   construction of,20
   plastic,64
toecaps,136,323
toenails,47,167,185,188,189,261,294,347
toepads,61,67,98,199,200,224,226,227,232,233 236,238,272,273,277,286,289,296,297,299, 312,327
Toumanova, Tamara,105
Trockadero, Ballets,150,155
Tsuchiya, Makoto,109
turnout,52,177,183,190,202,255,280
tutu,v,8,111,151,172,176
Tweedie, Valrene,97,98

U

Ulanova, Galina,148
upper of shoe,20,21,22,144,146,154,157,165, 176
urethane , foam, 14

V

Vaganova, Academy,222
   Agrippina,222,252
vamp of shoe,3,13,22,30,31,34,35,50,62,70, 74,75,82,105,106,108,111,112,115-117,119, 120,123,124,127,137,138,145,149,151-154, 167-169,176,199, 227,228,230,234,236,237, 245,253,261,268,272,277,294,297,299,303, 313,320-322,331
Vasconcelos, Liana,224,242
Vassiliev, Vladimir,13
Vessel Schluter, Anne Marie,219
Villella, Edward,126,222
   Linda,iii,222
Vishneva, Diana,127,176
Vladimiroff, Pierre,220
Vogel, Deborah,49

W

Wallis, Lynn,63,216
Wander Vancliffen, Amelia,251,259
warm-up,51,187,194,205,224,228,231,232, 235,239,241,246,267,285,286,289,292
Watts, Tiara,223,236
Weiss, David, Dr.57
Weiss, Judy,iii,69,175,340
Weiss, Robert,220
Wildish, Kat,251,267
Wiles, Michele,128,283,313
Wilkenfeld, David,105
Williams, Katie,283,314

Williams, Stanley, 220, 270
Willis, Nathaniel, 5, 7,
Wills-Jones, Nicola, 223, 232
wings of pointe shoes, 31, 32, 78, 99, 174
Wong, Yue Shuen, 183
Wood, Megan, 283, 323
Woodbury, Lacy, 149
Woods, Vanessa, 283, 318
Wyon, Matthew, Doctor, 115

Y
Yao Chu, Kuei, 283, 292
Yanowsky, Zenaida, 156
Youth American Grand Prix, 230
Yuan Yuan, Tan, 128

Z
Zakharova, Svetlana, 127